Nuclear Cardiology

Editors

SHARMILA DORBALA
PIOTR SLOMKA

CARDIOLOGY CLINICS

www.cardiology.theclinics.com

Consulting Editors
ROSARIO FREEMAN
JORDAN M. PRUTKIN
DAVID M. SHAVELLE
AUDREY H. WU

February 2016 • Volume 34 • Number 1

ELSEVIER

1600 John F. Kennedy Boulevard • Suite 1800 • Philadelphia, Pennsylvania, 19103-2899

http://www.theclinics.com

CARDIOLOGY CLINICS Volume 34, Number 1
February 2016 ISSN 0733-8651, ISBN-13: 978-0-323-41682-5

Editor: Lauren Boyle
Developmental Editor: Alison Swety

Cardiology Clinics (ISSN 0733-8651) is published quarterly by Elsevier Inc., 360 Park Avenue South, New York, NY 10010-1710. Months of issue are February, May, August, and November. Business and Editorial Offices: 1600 John F. Kennedy Blvd., Ste. 1800, Philadelphia, PA 19103-2899. Customer Service Office: 3251 Riverport Lane, Maryland Heights, MO 63043. Periodicals postage paid at New York, NY and additional mailing offices. Subscription prices are $320.00 per year for US individuals, $581.00 per year for US institutions, $100.00 per year for US students and residents, $390.00 per year for Canadian individuals, $729.00 per year for Canadian institutions, $455.00 per year for international individuals, $729.00 per year for international institutions and $220.00 per year for Canadian and international students/residents. To receive student/resident rate, orders must be accompanied by name of affiliated institution, data of term, and the *signature* of program/residency coordinator on institution letterhead. Orders will be billed at individual rate until proof of status is received. Foreign air speed delivery is included in all *Clinics* subscription prices. All prices are subject to change without notice. **POSTMASTER:** Send address changes to *Cardiology Clinics*, Elsevier Health Sciences Division, Subscription Customer Service, 3251 Riverport Lane, Maryland Heights, MO 63043. **Customer Service: 1-800-654-2452 (U.S. and Canada); 314-447-8871 (outside U.S. and Canada). Fax: 314-447-8029. E-mail: journalscustomerservice-usa@elsevier.com (for print support); journalsonlinesupport-usa@elsevier.com (for online support).**

Reprints. For copies of 100 or more, of articles in this publication, please contact the Commercial Reprints Department, Elsevier Inc., 360 Park Avenue South, New York, NY 10010-1710. Tel.: 212-633-3874; Fax: 212-633-3820; E-mail: reprints@elsevier.com.

Cardiology Clinics is also published in Spanish by McGraw-Hill Interamericana Editores S. A., P.O. Box 5-237, 06500, Mexico D. F., Mexico; in Portuguese by Reichmann and Alfonso Editores Rio de Janeiro, Brazil; and in Greek by Dimitrios P. Lagos, 8 Pondon Street, GR115-28 Ilissia, Greece.

Cardiology Clinics is covered in *MEDLINE/PubMed (Index Medicus), Excerpta Medica, The Cumulative Index to Nursing and Allied Health Literature* (CINAHL).

Contributors

EDITORIAL BOARD

ROSARIO FREEMAN, MD, MS, FACC
Associate Professor of Medicine; Director, Coronary Care Unit; Director, Echocardiography Laboratory, University of Washington Medical Center, Seattle, Washington

JORDAN M. PRUTKIN, MD, MHS, FHRS
Assistant Professor of Medicine, Division of Cardiology/Electrophysiology, University of Washington Medical Center, Seattle, Washington

DAVID M. SHAVELLE, MD, FACC, FSCAI
Associate Professor, Keck School of Medicine; Director, General Cardiovascular Fellowship Program; Director, Cardiac Catheterization Laboratory, Los Angeles County + USC Medical Center; Division of Cardiovascular Medicine, University of Southern California, Los Angeles, California

AUDREY H. WU, MD
Assistant Professor, Internal Medicine, University of Michigan, Ann Arbor, Michigan

EDITORS

SHARMILA DORBALA, MD, MPH, FACC
Director of Nuclear Cardiology, Noninvasive Cardiovascular Imaging Program, Heart and Vascular Institute, Division of Cardiovascular Medicine, Department of Medicine; Division of Nuclear Medicine, Department of Radiology, Brigham and Women's Hospital, Associate Professor of Radiology, Harvard Medical School, Boston, Massachusetts

PIOTR SLOMKA, PhD, FACC
Research Scientist, Artificial Intelligence in Medicine Program, Cedars-Sinai Medical Center; Professor of Medicine, David Geffen School of Medicine, University of California at Los Angeles; Departments of Imaging and Medicine, Cedars-Sinai Medical Center, Los Angeles, California

AUTHORS

HUSSEIN ABU DAYA, MD
Division of Cardiology, Department of Medicine, University of Pittsburgh Medical Center, Pittsburgh, Pennsylvania

PHILIP D. ADAMSON, MBChB
Centre for Cardiovascular Science, University of Edinburgh, Edinburgh, United Kingdom

FOZIA ZAHIR AHMED, MBChB, MRCP
Department of Cardiology, Manchester Heart Centre, Central Manchester University Hospitals NHS Foundation Trust, Manchester, United Kingdom

PARTHIBAN ARUMUGAM, MBBS, MSc, FRCP
Department of Nuclear Medicine, Central Manchester University Hospitals NHS Foundation Trust, Manchester, United Kingdom

ROB S.B. BEANLANDS, MD, FRCPC, FACC
Vered Chair and Chief, Division of Cardiology, Department of Medicine; Chief of Cardiology and Director, National Cardiac PET Centre, Cardiac Imaging Department, University of Ottawa Heart Institute; Professor of Medicine, Department of Cardiology, Ottawa, Ontario, Canada

FRANK M. BENGEL, MD
Department of Nuclear Medicine, Hannover Medical School, Hannover, Germany

DANIEL S. BERMAN, MD
Professor of Imaging, Departments of Imaging and Medicine, Burns and Allen Research Institute, Cedars-Sinai Medical Center; Medical Director, Artificial Intelligence in Medicine Program, Cedars-Sinai Medical Center; Professor of Medicine, David Geffen School of Medicine, University of California at Los Angeles, Los Angeles, California

JOHN P. BOIS, MD
Division of Cardiovascular Diseases, Mayo Clinic, Rochester, Minnesota

PANITHAYA CHAREONTHAITAWEE, MD
Division of Cardiovascular Diseases, Mayo Clinic, Rochester, Minnesota

ROBERT A. deKEMP, PhD, PEng, PPhys
Division of Cardiology, Department of Medicine; Head Imaging Physicist, National Cardiac PET Centre, Cardiac Imaging Department, University of Ottawa Heart Institute, Associate Professor of Medicine (Cardiology), University of Ottawa, Ottawa, Ontario, Canada

WILLIAM LANE DUVALL, MD
Division of Cardiology, Hartford Hospital, Hartford, Connecticut

MARC R. DWECK, PhD
Centre for Cardiovascular Science, University of Edinburgh, Edinburgh, United Kingdom

FERNANDA ERTHAL, MD
Fellow in Cardiac Imaging, Division of Cardiology, Department of Medicine, National Cardiac PET Centre, University of Ottawa Heart Institute, Ottawa, Ontario, Canada

ERNEST V. GARCIA, PhD
Department of Radiology and Imaging Sciences, Emory University Hospital, Emory University School of Medicine, Atlanta, Georgia

GUIDO GERMANO, PhD
Scientific Director, Artificial Intelligence in Medicine Program, Cedars-Sinai Medical Center; Professor of Medicine, David Geffen School of Medicine, University of California at Los Angeles; Department of Medicine, Cedars-Sinai Medical Center, Los Angeles, California

ROBERT J. GROPLER, MD
Mallinckrodt Institute of Radiology, Washington University School of Medicine, St Louis, Missouri

MILENA J. HENZLOVA, MD
Mount Sinai Heart, Mount Hospital, New York, New York

RENÉE HESSIAN, MD, FRCPC
Division of Cardiology, Department of Medicine, National Cardiac PET Centre, University of Ottawa Heart Institute, Ottawa, Ontario, Canada

NASIR HUSSAIN, MD
Division of Cardiology, Hartford Hospital, Hartford, Connecticut

JACKIE JAMES, MBChB, MSc, MD, FRCP
Department of Nuclear Medicine, Central Manchester University Hospitals NHS Foundation Trust, Manchester, United Kingdom

DANIEL JUNEAU, MD, FRCPC
Division of Cardiology, Department of Medicine, Fellow in Cardiac Imaging, National Cardiac PET Centre, University of Ottawa Heart Institute, Ottawa, Ontario, Canada

RAN KLEIN, PhD
Imaging Physicist; Assistant Professor, Division of Nuclear Medicine, Department of Medicine, University of Ottawa, Ottawa, Ontario, Canada

RICHARD LaFOREST, PhD
Mallinckrodt Institute of Radiology, Washington University School of Medicine, St Louis, Missouri

SAURABH MALHOTRA, MD, MPH
Division of Cardiology, University of Buffalo, Buffalo, New York

BRIAN Mc ARDLE, MD
Division of Cardiology, Department of Medicine, National Cardiac PET Centre, University of Ottawa Heart Institute, Ottawa, Ontario, Canada

MATTHEW J. MEMMOTT, MSci, MSc
Department of Nuclear Medicine, Central Manchester University Hospitals NHS Foundation Trust, Manchester, United Kingdom

MANISH MOTWANI, PhD
Advanced Cardiac Imaging Fellow; Departments of Imaging and Medicine, Cedars-Sinai Medical Center, Los Angeles, California

DAVID E. NEWBY, DSc
Centre for Cardiovascular Science, University of Edinburgh, Edinburgh, United Kingdom

HIROSHI OHIRA, MD, PhD
Division of Cardiology, Department of Medicine, National Cardiac PET Centre, University of Ottawa Heart Institute, Ottawa, Ontario, Canada; First Department of Medicine, Hokkaido University Graduate School of Medicine, Kita-Ku, Sapporo, Hokkaido, Japan

MATTHEW W. PARKER, MD
Division of Cardiology, Hartford Hospital, Hartford, Connecticut

MARINA PICCINELLI, PhD
Department of Radiology and Imaging Sciences, Emory University Hospital, Emory University School of Medicine, Atlanta, Georgia

JENNIFER M. RENAUD, MSc
Research Analyst, National Cardiac PET Centre, Cardiac Imaging Department, University of Ottawa Heart Institute, Ottawa, Ontario, Canada

ALAN ROZANSKI, MD
Division of Cardiology, Department of Medicine, Mt Sinai St. Lukes and Roosevelt Hospitals, New York, New York

ALBERT J. SINUSAS, MD
Departments of Internal Medicine and Diagnostic Radiology, Yale University School of Medicine, New Haven, Connecticut

PIOTR SLOMKA, PhD, FACC
Research Scientist, Artificial Intelligence in Medicine Program, Cedars-Sinai Medical Center; Professor of Medicine, David Geffen School of Medicine, University of California at Los Angeles; Departments of Imaging and Medicine, Cedars-Sinai Medical Center, Los Angeles, California

PREM SOMAN, MD, PhD, FRCP (UK), FACC
Associate Professor of Medicine (Cardiology); Associate Professor of Clinical and Translational Science, Division of Cardiology, Department of Medicine, University of Pittsburgh Medical Center, Pittsburgh, Pennsylvania

MITCHEL R. STACY, PhD
Department of Internal Medicine, Yale University School of Medicine, New Haven, Connecticut

JAMES T. THACKERAY, PhD
Department of Nuclear Medicine, Hannover Medical School, Hannover, Germany

MARK I. TRAVIN, MD
Director of Cardiovascular Nuclear Medicine, Montefiore Medical Center; Professor of Clinical Radiology and Clinical Medicine, Albert Einstein College of Medicine, Bronx, New York

PAMELA K. WOODARD, MD
Mallinckrodt Institute of Radiology, Washington University School of Medicine, St Louis, Missouri

Contents

Preface: Frontiers of Nuclear Cardiology **xiii**

Sharmila Dorbala and Piotr Slomka

Advances in Single-Photon Emission Computed Tomography Hardware and Software **1**

Marina Piccinelli and Ernest V. Garcia

Nuclear imaging techniques remain today's most reliable modality for the assessment and quantification of myocardial perfusion. In recent years, the field has experienced tremendous progress both in terms of dedicated cameras for cardiac applications and software techniques for image reconstruction. The most recent advances in single-photon emission computed tomography hardware and software are reviewed, focusing on how these improvements have resulted in an even more powerful diagnostic tool with reduced injected radiation dose and acquisition time.

Technical Aspects of Cardiac PET Imaging and Recent Advances **13**

Guido Germano, Daniel S. Berman, and Piotr Slomka

As the number of myocardial perfusion single emission photon computed tomography studies performed in the United States has steadily declined over the past several years, an opposite trend can be seen for myocardial perfusion PET. This review covers basic technical aspects of cardiac PET imaging and recent advances that maximize the quality and efficiency of cardiac PET. The covered topics include radioisotopes used in cardiac PET and basics of acquisition and reconstruction, including time-of-flight techniques, PET detectors, attenuation correction, and respiratory gating techniques.

Cardiovascular PET/MRI: Challenges and Opportunities **25**

Richard LaForest, Pamela K. Woodard, and Robert J. Gropler

Recently, systems combining PET and MRI have appeared on the market. The 2 main advantages of these systems over PET/computed tomography are the improved soft tissue contrast with MRI obtained without ionizing radiation and the potential for simultaneous acquisition of the PET and magnetic resonance images. However, its clinical acceptance has been slow for several reasons. Moreover, there are significant technical challenges that must be overcome from an image acquisition, processing, display, and laboratory workflow perspective for implementing cardiovascular PET/MRI on a routine clinical basis. The potential is high for PET/MRI to become a critical tool in the management of disease.

Radionuclide Tracers for Myocardial Perfusion Imaging and Blood Flow Quantification **37**

Robert A. deKemp, Jennifer M. Renaud, Ran Klein, and Rob S.B. Beanlands

Myocardial perfusion imaging is performed most commonly using Tc-99m-sestamibi or tetrofosmin SPECT as well as Rb-82-rubidium or N-13-ammonia PET. Diseased-to-normal tissue contrast is determined by the tracer retention fraction, which decreases nonlinearly with flow. Reduced tissue perfusion results in reduced tracer retention, but the severity of perfusion defects is typically

data indicate that long-term risk is highly influenced by both the magnitude of ischemia and various baseline clinical factors. An optimized assessment of stress MPI, which includes long-term risk prediction, might improve the potential future clinical effectiveness of this imaging modality.

Radionuclide Assessment of Left Ventricular Dyssynchrony **101**

Hussein Abu Daya, Saurabh Malhotra, and Prem Soman

Phase analysis of gated myocardial perfusion single-photon emission computed tomography is a widely available and reproducible measure of left ventricular (LV) dyssynchrony, which also provides comprehensive assessment of LV function, global and regional scar burden, and patterns of LV mechanical activation. Preliminary studies indicate potential use in predicting cardiac resynchronization therapy response and elucidation of mechanisms. Because advances in technology may expand capabilities for precise LV lead placement in the future, identification of specific patterns of dyssynchrony may have a critical role in guiding cardiac resynchronization therapy.

Radionuclide Imaging in Congestive Heart Failure: Assessment of Viability, Sarcoidosis, and Amyloidosis **119**

John P. Bois and Panithaya Chareonthaitawee

Radionuclide imaging provides both established and emerging diagnostic and prognostic tools to assist clinicians in the management of patients with ischemic cardiomyopathy, cardiac sarcoidosis, and cardiac amyloidosis. This review highlights the underlying pathophysiology of each entity and associated diagnostic and clinical challenges, and describes the available radionuclide imaging techniques. Specific protocols, advantages and disadvantages, comparison with other noninvasive imaging modalities, and discussion of the evolving role of hybrid imaging are also included.

Clinical Applications of Myocardial Innervation Imaging **133**

Mark I. Travin

Cardiac autonomic innervation plays an important role in regulating function. Adrenergic innervation imaging is possible with the norepinephrine analogue radiotracer iodine 123 *meta*-iodobenzylguanidine (^{123}I-*m*IBG) and positron emitting tracers such as carbon-11 hydroxyephedrine. ^{123}I-*m*IBG uptake is assessed globally via the heart to mediastinum ratio on planar images and regionally with tomographic imaging and has utility in various cardiac diseases. There is promise for guiding expensive invasive therapies such as implantable defibrillators, ventricular assist devices, and transplant. There are reports of utility in primary arrhythmic conditions, ischemic heart disease, and diabetes and after cardiac damaging chemotherapy.

Radionuclide Imaging of Cardiovascular Infection **149**

Fozia Zahir Ahmed, Jackie James, Matthew J. Memmott, and Parthiban Arumugam

Owing to expanding clinical indications, cardiac implantable electronic devices (CIEDs) are being increasingly used. Despite improved surgical techniques and the use of prophylactic antimicrobial therapy, the rate of CIED-related infection is also increasing. Infection is a potentially serious complication, with clinical manifestations ranging from surgical site infection and local symptoms in the region of the

CARDIOLOGY CLINICS

FORTHCOMING ISSUES

May 2016
Cardioembolic Stroke
Ranjan K. Thakur, Andrea Natale, and Ziyad Hijazi, *Editors*

August 2016
Pulmonary Hypertension
Ronald J. Oudiz, *Editor*

November 2016
Sports Cardiology
Aaron Baggish and Andre La Gerche, *Editors*

RECENT ISSUES

November 2015
Adult Congenital Heart Disease
Karen K. Stout, *Editor*

August 2015
Clinical and Electrophysiologic Management of Syncope
Antonio Raviele and Andrea Natale, *Editors*

May 2015
Lipidology
Edward A. Gill, Christie M. Ballantyne, and Kathleen L. Wyne, *Editors*

ISSUE OF RELATED INTEREST

Interventional Cardiology Clinics, July 2015 (Vol. 4, No. 3)
Intravascular Imaging: OCT and IVUS
Matthew J. Price, *Editor*
Available at: http://www.interventional.theclinics.com/

THE CLINICS ARE AVAILABLE ONLINE!
Access your subscription at:
www.theclinics.com

Preface
Frontiers of Nuclear Cardiology

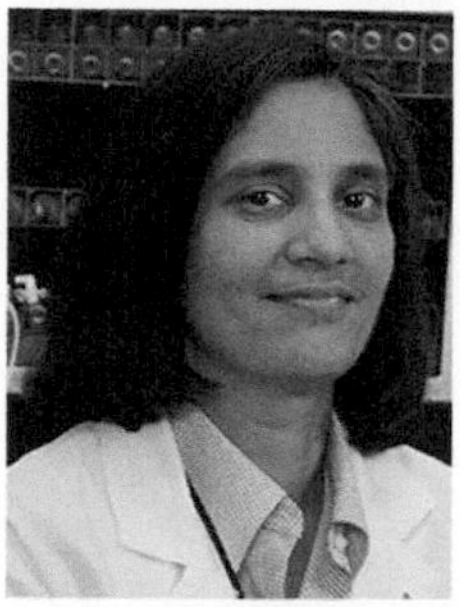

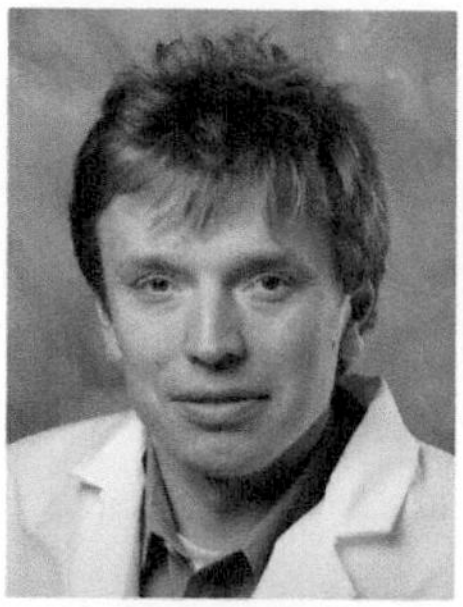

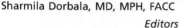

Sharmila Dorbala, MD, MPH, FACC Piotr Slomka, PhD, FACC
Editors

Forty years ago, radionuclide myocardial perfusion imaging, a breakthrough in noninvasive imaging, began as a robust clinical tool for evaluating coronary artery disease (CAD). Today, radionuclide imaging has progressed into a molecular technique that can detect an expanding array of cardiovascular diseases, paving the way for personalized therapies. Of course, these developments couldn't have come to the fore without the rapid technical innovations in the imaging technologies. New devices, including hybrid PET/CT and PET/MR scanners as well as novel image reconstruction software, have brought the best research ideas to clinical practice. The selection of articles in this issue of *Cardiology Clinics* illustrates the multitude of technological and radiotracer advances that are transforming the field of nuclear cardiology and improving the quality of life for those afflicted with cardiovascular disease.

The thoughtful contributors to this issue of *Cardiology Clinics* usher readers into the frontiers of nuclear cardiology. They explain how our field provides a comprehensive evaluation and image-guided management to individuals with a range of cardiovascular diseases. They describe how radionuclide myocardial perfusion imaging provides rapid, high-quality, and low-radiation-dose imaging to individuals with known or suspected CAD. They reveal how quantitative imaging of myocardial blood flow can determine the hemodynamic significance of nonobstructive CAD and coronary microvascular dysfunction. They demonstrate how ^{18}F-fluorodeoxyglucose PET provides unique information, in myocardial inflammatory diseases and cardiovascular infections, which cannot be obtained from any other imaging modality. They show how repurposing several molecular imaging tracers (sodium fluoride, ^{99m}Tc-pyrophosphate, ^{18}F-amyloid agents, ^{123}I-metaiodobenzylguanidine-MIBG, and more) may lead to personalized disease evaluation and management of a variety of cardiovascular diseases. Appropriate clinical use of these new techniques and tools has the potential to significantly alleviate the suffering of individuals with a variety of cardiovascular diseases.

We thank Dr Audrey H. Wu for the opportunity to edit this issue on Nuclear Cardiology. It has been a great pleasure to work with each of the authors; we thank each of them for their insightful contributions. Our special thanks to Alison Swety and her team for supporting us and keeping us on track for the issue.

Sharmila Dorbala, MD, MPH, FACC
Brigham and Women's Hospital
70 Francis Street
Shapiro 5th Floor, Room 128
Boston, MA 02115, USA

Piotr Slomka, PhD, FACC
Artificial Intelligence in Medicine Program
Cedars-Sinai Medical Center
North Tower A047
8700 Beverly Boulevard
Los Angeles, CA 90048, USA

E-mail addresses:
sdorbala@partners.org (S. Dorbala)
piotr.slomka@cshs.org (P. Slomka)

Cardiol Clin 34 (2016) xiii
http://dx.doi.org/10.1016/j.ccl.2015.10.001
0733-8651/16/$ – see front matter

Advances in Single-Photon Emission Computed Tomography Hardware and Software

Marina Piccinelli, PhD, Ernest V. Garcia, PhD*

KEYWORDS

- SPECT imaging system • SPECT instrumentation • Image reconstruction
- SPECT hardware and software advances

KEY POINTS

- Nuclear imaging remains today's most reliable modality for the assessment and quantification of myocardial perfusion.
- Nuclear imaging techniques have recently experienced tremendous progress in terms of dedicated cameras for cardiac applications and software techniques, bringing myocardial perfusion imaging (MPI) to the next level.
- Hardware and software advances allow studies to be performed with reduced radiation exposure and acquisition time while providing even better image quality and diagnostic power.

INTRODUCTION

Principles of Nuclear Cardiology Imaging

Nuclear cardiology's signal is a radioactive tracer injected into a patient that emits x-ray or γ-ray photons, and its imaging systems are either single-photon emission computed tomography (SPECT) or positron emission tomography (PET) cameras. This combination has met with remarkable success in clinical cardiology, a success that is the result of sophisticated electronic nuclear instrumentation associated with a highly specific and thus powerful signal—the measured signal is as important as or more important than the imaging systems.

There is a misconception that MRI, echocardiography, and computed tomography (CT) are superior to nuclear cardiology imaging because of their superior spatial resolution. Yet, for efficiently detecting perfusion defects, what is necessary is superior contrast resolution. It is this superior contrast resolution that allows differentiating between normal and hypoperfused myocardium, facilitating the visual and quantitative analysis of nuclear cardiology images. Because the normal myocardium is bright compared with the background, it serves as an excellent signal and has allowed the development over the past decades of software packages for fully automated and objective processing and quantification of nuclear cardiology images, an achievement yet to be reached by other modalities.[1,2]

New Requirements for Nuclear Cardiology

In recent years, both the medical community and the general public have had many concerns regarding the increased use of ionizing radiation to diagnose all types of diseases and its associated risks for patients.[3] In particular, there is a widespread perception that nuclear imaging is associated with high radiation doses. Although

Department of Radiology and Imaging Sciences, Emory University Hospital, Emory University School of Medicine, 1364 Clifton Road Northeast, Atlanta, GA 30322, USA
* Corresponding author.
E-mail address: Ernest.Garcia@emory.edu

Cardiol Clin 34 (2016) 1–11
http://dx.doi.org/10.1016/j.ccl.2015.06.001
0733-8651/16/$ – see front matter

the risk-benefit ratio of performing a nuclear imaging procedure is favorable, the nuclear imaging communities have quickly reacted by implementing a new set of guidelines to decrease patient radiation exposure. The American Society of Nuclear Cardiology (ASNC) has recently published documents[4,5] that encourage laboratories to greatly decrease patient radiation dose and has set a goal of 50% of all myocardial perfusion studies performed with an associated radiation exposure of 9 mSv by 2014 (a combined stress/rest study with conventional instrumentation and reconstruction techniques delivers a radiation dose of 12 mSv to a patient). Additionally, one of the main drawbacks of MPI is the long acquisition time necessary to maintain image quality and contain radiation dose. Long procedures have a further negative impact on patient comfort and laboratory efficiency, thus increasing study costs.

Stimulated by these sociologic, clinical, and financial needs, manufacturers and scientists have begun to break away from standard MPI imaging systems to create innovative designs of dedicated cardiac cameras and to implement new software techniques to bring MPI to the next level. The basic SPECT camera design is 50 years old and the conventional image reconstruction algorithm, the filtered back-projection (FBP), is even older, dating to more than 90 years ago.

In this article, after introduction of the main aspects of conventional SPECT MPI, the most recent hardware and software advances and how they can result in more accurate diagnostic studies with reduced radiation exposure and study time are reviewed. This reduction in radiation dose and study time is being achieved while providing better image quality compared with standard approaches. These new hardware and software tools provide a large degree of flexibility, which eventually will allow for a more patient-centered approach as required by new clinical guidelines. There are several good reviews[6–11] on these issues, which are referred to for additional details; and the authors hope to further emphasize the need for these improvements in devices and techniques.

CONVENTIONAL SINGLE-PHOTON EMISSION COMPUTED TOMOGRAPHY: INSTRUMENTATION AND PRINCIPLES

The main components of SPECT imaging systems are the scintillation camera, the gantry, and the computer systems (including both hardware and software tools). The camera integrates the collimator; the scintillating crystal, traditionally a sodium iodide (NaI) crystal; and the photomultipliers (PMTs). All these components work together to acquire and reconstruct the tomographic images[2] (**Fig. 1**). A γ-ray is emitted from a source within a patient and strikes the crystal. In the crystal, photons are converted into visible light that is further transformed into an electrical signal by the PMTs. Because γ-rays are emitted from a source uniformly in all directions, a photon from any area in the body can theoretically strike any area of the detector. To localize the exact source of the photon, a parallel-hole lead collimator is placed between the patient and crystal. This collimator consists of an array of long narrow parallel holes that exclude all photons except those that are traveling parallel to the direction of the hole.

Collimators are rated by their sensitivity and spatial resolution, 2 of the most important concepts in nuclear image formation and quality.[2] Sensitivity is the number of photons that travel through the collimator in a certain amount of time. Image spatial resolution is the ability of the imaging systems to separate 2 distinct point sources in the object. In the particular case of nuclear images, resolution is affected by collimation because a portion of the photons not traveling in a parallel path can still get through a collimator hole, making the single point source appear fuzzy

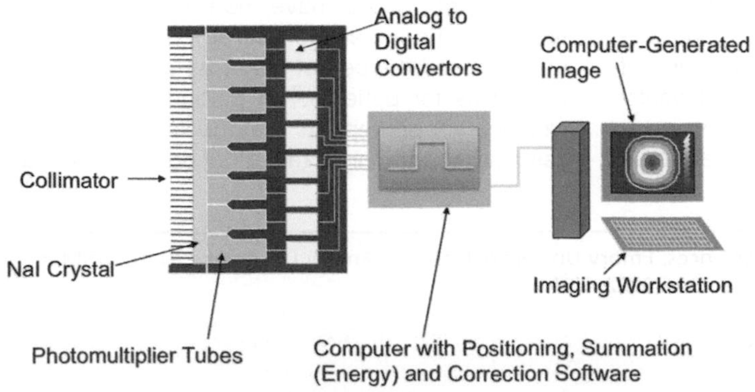

Fig. 1. Traditional SPECT camera instrumentation. (*Courtesy of* James Galt, PhD, Atlanta, GA.)

on the detector. How much the point spreads out, which also determines the system point-spread function (PSF), defines the spatial resolution and depends on the length and width of the collimator holes. General-purpose parallel-hole collimators have short and wide holes and can accept more photons than high-resolution collimators, characterized by longer and/or smaller diameter holes. Increasing the length of the holes increases the spatial resolution by decreasing the angle subtended to the hole and consequently eliminating more photons that do not travel parallel to a specific hole direction. Sensitivity and image resolution are inversely related: a high-sensitivity collimator has low resolution and vice versa.

Another important relationship exists between sensitivity, spatial resolution, and collimator geometry.[2] The amount of radiation from a point source that reaches a generic plane decreases as $1/r^2$, but when a collimator is placed between the source and the detector, this relation no longer holds and the same number of rays travel through the parallel-hole collimator no matter how far the point source is. The crucial difference between a collimator placed near the source and one positioned faraway resides in which hole the γ-rays actually end up passing through. Photons traveling parallel to the collimator correctly go through the hole in line with the source, whereas oblique rays likely pass thorough adjacent holes. In **Fig. 2**A, most of the rays pass through the holes that are nearly in line

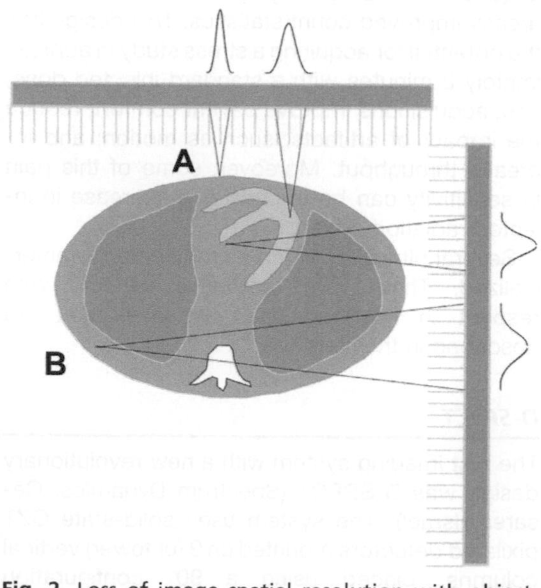

Fig. 2. Loss of image spatial resolution with object-detector distance. (*A*) Most of the rays pass through the collimator holes directly in line with source. (*B*) With increased object-detector distance, more oblique rays pass though holes that are spread around the hole in line with source, widening the PSF.

with that source, even the oblique ones; in **Fig. 2**B, the same number of rays reach the collimator, but the most oblique rays pass through holes that are further away from the one in line with the source. This feature, commonly termed, *detector-response*, or *geometric response*, results in loss of spatial resolution and is exemplified by the larger profile of the PSF.

Once the photons have entered the collimator, the scintillation events generated in the NaI crystal are transformed into electrical signals in the PMTs. Traditional cameras used pulse height analyzers and spatial positioning circuitry to recover the energy and the location of the incident photons, which are successively converted into digital signals using analog-to-digital converters (see **Fig. 1**).

Conventional SPECT systems may have 1 or more scintillation cameras attached to the gantry. The main advantage of multidetector systems is the increase in count sensitivity: doubling the number of heads doubles the number of photons that may be acquired in the same amount of time. As a consequence of this increase in sensitivity, a higher-resolution collimator can be added or a reduction in acquisition time or injected dose can be achieved. In **Fig. 3**A, a common configuration for cardiac applications is depicted with 2 detectors mounted next to each other 90° apart. The full set of projections can be acquired by rotating the gantry only 90° with a consistent reduction in acquisition time. Multiheaded systems with triple detectors are also available although less flexible than single- or double-headed cameras.

HARDWARE ADVANCES: NEW CAMERA DESIGNS

The required improvements both in terms of acquisition time and radiation dose have forced manufacturers to move away from traditional designs to implement dedicated cardiac imaging systems. The new-generation SPECT cameras use detectors constrained to acquire only the cardiac field of view (FOV), cadmium zinc telluride (CZT), or thallium-activated cesium iodide (CsI[Tl]) crystals and solid-state detectors instead of traditional NaI with analog PMTs. Collimators geometry has also been optimized to image the myocardium: new schemes include multi-pinhole or high-sensitivity parallel-hole collimators.

The most beneficial improvement introduced in recent years is use of the CZT[10] detector— a semiconductor that works at room temperatures and can process greater than 10 million photons/s/mm^2. It also exhibits superior energy resolution with respect to traditional crystals (approximately 1.7 × better than thallium-activated NaI[12]). These features

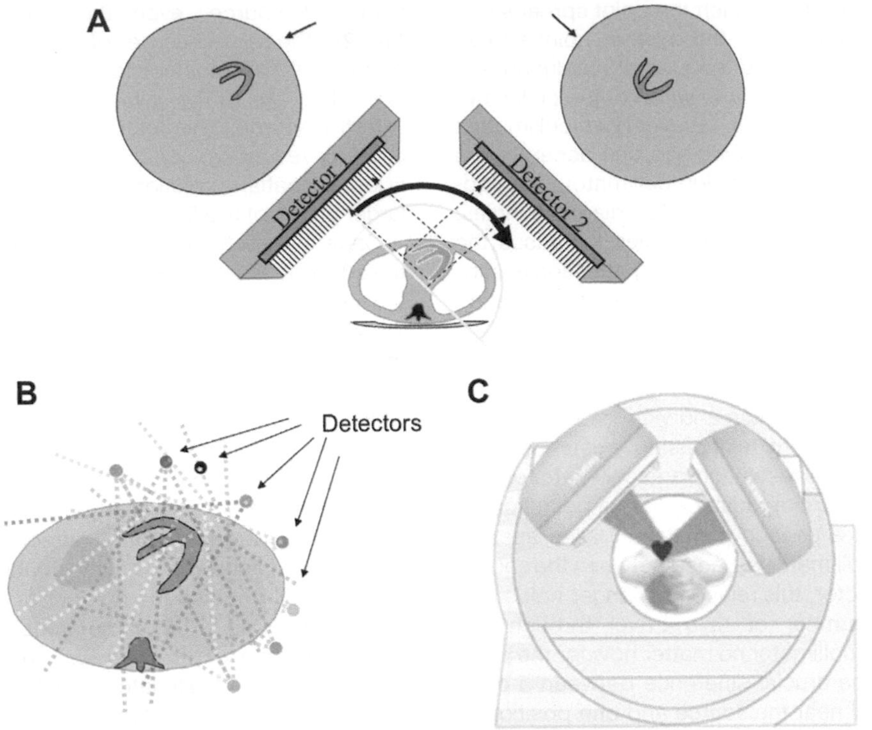

Fig. 3. Camera head configurations. (*A*) Double-headed camera for cardiac applications; the 180° orbit can be achieved by rotating the gantry 90°. (*B*) New camera design concept with stationary detectors acquiring only the heart FOV. (*C*) Diagram of the IQ-SPECT variable focus collimator for increased sensitivity and resolution on the heart FOV.

make it an ideal detector solution for nuclear imaging, although more expensive. Moreover, CZT crystals absorb the γ-ray energy and generate an electrical signal without the need for PMTs. Traditional NaI cameras suffer from inefficient PMTs during the indirect process of conversion of photons to light and to electrical signals (the efficiency of the PMTs cascade approximates 20%) and any loss in visible photon directly results in miscalculation of the energy and the position of the event with consequent blurring of the image and suboptimal spatial resolution. Ultimately, CZT detectors combine the functions of scintillation crystals and PMTs, thus creating smaller and more efficient devices, which may also affect laboratory workflow.

Compared with dual-head traditional Anger cameras, all devices with modern designs and detectors have in common a 5- to 10-fold increase in count sensitivity due to the increased sampling of the FOV at no loss or even gain in spatial resolution.[7,8] Note that **Fig. 3**A shows that much of the crystal in conventional SPECT cameras is not used to image the heart. **Fig. 3**B shows how in the cardiac dedicated cameras, several smaller detectors simultaneously image mostly the heart: the detectors are arranged around the body as to acquire specifically only the cardiac FOV with greatly improved count statistics. This design has the potential for acquiring a stress study in approximately 2 minutes with a standard injected dose. Fast acquisitions improve patient comfort; reduce the impact of artifacts, such as motion; and increase throughput. Moreover, some of this gain in sensitivity can be traded for a decrease in injected radiation dose.

Several ultrafast cameras are already commercialized. Their main innovative aspects with respect to the traditional instrumentation are described in the literature.[6–11]

D-SPECT

The first imaging system with a new revolutionary design was D-SPECT (Spectrum Dynamics, Cesarea, Israel). The system uses solid-state CZT pixilated detectors mounted on 9 (or fewer) vertical columns, placed using a 90° configuration (**Fig. 4**A). Each of the 9 detectors assemblies is equipped with a tungsten, square, parallel-hole collimator. Each hole measures 2.46 mm on its side, larger in comparison with traditional collimators geometry, resulting in camera-increased

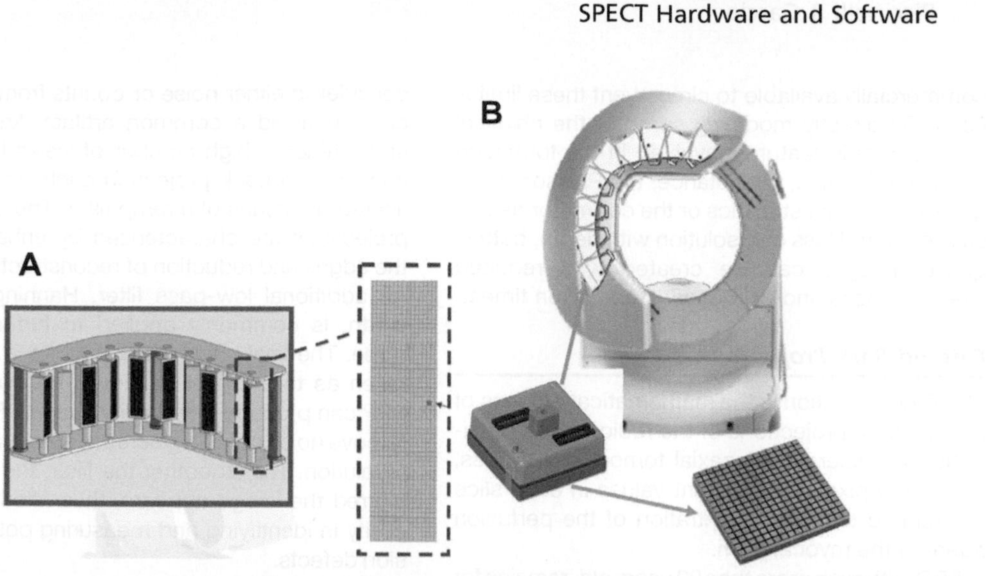

Fig. 4. Ultrafast camera designs. (*A*) D-SPECT. Modified from slides. (*B*) Discovery NM 530c. Modified from slides. (*Courtesy of* [*A*] Spectrum Dynamics, Cesarea, Israel, with permission; and [*B*] GE Healthcare, Haifa, Israel, with permission.)

sensitivity. All detectors move in synchrony and image the heart simultaneously. An initial 1-minute scout acquisition is performed to identify the location of the heart in the FOV and set the limits for the detectors movement during the diagnostic scan.

A modified iterative algorithm implementing resolution recovery (RR) is used for the image reconstruction to compensate for the loss in resolution due to the large collimator hole dimensions (discussed later).

Discovery NM 530c

The second CZT system introduced is the Discovery NM 530c (GE Healthcare, Haifa, Israel), displayed in **Fig.** 4B. The SPECT design uses Alcyone technology, consisting of an array of 19 pinhole collimators, each with 4 solid-state CZT pixilated detectors. All 19 pinholes simultaneously image the heart with no component moving during data acquisition. Nine of the pinhole detectors are oriented perpendicular to the patient's long axis, whereas 5 are angulated above and the remaining 5 below the axis. The use of simultaneously acquired views improves the overall sensitivity and provides all the data necessary for both dynamic studies (promoting the feasibility of absolute flow measurement with SPECT) and reduction of motion artifacts. Breast attenuation artifacts are also minimized because not all the views are imaged through the attenuator, but some from are above and some from below the breast.

Cardius 3 XPO

The Cardius 3 XPO (Digirad, Siemens, Poway, CA, US) also uses solid-state electronics. The system has CsI(Tl) pixilated detectors coupled with individual silicon photodiodes and digital Anger electronics, which improve the efficiency of energy conversion with respect to traditional PMTs. Three detectors are fixed using a 67.5° angular separation and the patient is rotated through an arc of 202.5° while sitting in a chair. Manufacturers of this device claim that up to 38% more count sensitivity compared with conventional dual-head systems while maintaining image quality.

IQ-SPECT

The IQ-SPECT system (Siemens, Munich, Germany) has the virtue of having reintroduced to the field the use of confocal collimators. Two collimators are mounted on a dual-detector SPECT camera, with a 90° configuration and a 180° orbit movement. What makes these collimators peculiar is that their FOVs are most convergent at their center, allowing an increased sensitivity and resolution in the heart FOV, whereas the convergence is relaxed toward the FOV edges where it is less important. In **Fig.** 3C, the IQ-SPECT design is shown with the focused collimation. An advantage of this approach is that it can be used with the existing traditional dual-detector systems by upgrading the collimators design.

SINGLE-PHOTON EMISSION COMPUTED TOMOGRAPHY IMAGE RECONSTRUCTION ALGORITHMS

As discussed previously, several factors can affect the formation of SPECT images, which in turn constrain the ability to decrease acquisition time and injected radiation dose.[2] New software methodologies have been developed and are now commercially available to circumvent these limitations. By directly modeling some of the physical and geometric features involved in the formation of nuclear images, for instance, the Poisson noise due to low-count statistics or the collimator geometry to control loss of resolution with depth, better-quality images can be created with reduced injected doses and/or reduced acquisition times.

Filtered Back-Projection

MPI reconstruction is the mathematical process of using planar projections of the radionuclide distribution to generate transaxial tomographic slices, where the pixel (voxel) count values in each slice are related to the concentration of the perfusion agent in the myocardium.

FBP, although more than 90 years old, remains for a majority of nuclear laboratories the most commonly used image reconstruction method. FBP is an analytical method for image reconstruction combining back-projection and filtering theories. Each row of the acquired projection contains counts that originate from the entire transverse plane. The count profile is then projected back by setting all the image pixels along the ray pointing to each profile sample to the same value. FBP assumes that the photons acquired at a voxel over a collimator's parallel hole were originated from a radioactive source positioned along a straight line from the detector (**Fig. 5**); all other photons are considered either noise or counts from other sources. To avoid a common artifact, known as the star artifact, a high number of views is necessary and prior to back-projection each view has to be filtered by means of a ramp filter. The ramp-filtered projections are characterized by enhancement of the edges and reduction of reconstruction artifacts. An additional low-pass filter, Hanning or Butterworth, is commonly applied to further decrease noise. The final back-projected image is ultimately taken as the sum of all views. Although efficient, FBP can produce low-quality images. Filtering may remove noise but also decrease spatial and contrast resolution. The smoother the filter, the increasingly blurred the image appears, thus affecting the reliability in identifying and measuring potential perfusion defects.

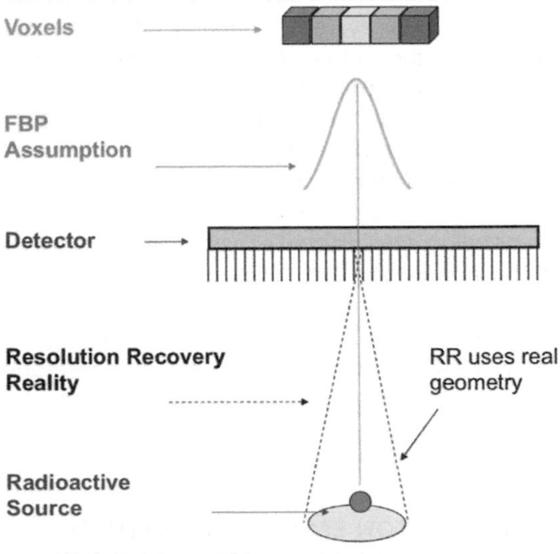

Fig. 5. Differences between FBP assumption and RR techniques. FBP assumes that photons counted in a voxel over a collimator's holes were emitted in straight line with the hole. RR techniques take into account the depth-dependent loss of spatial resolution depicted here by the dashed cone. By incorporating the geometry of the imaging system and the collimator, RR can be achieved.

Iterative Reconstruction Techniques

Due to the advances in computational techniques, iterative methodologies have rapidly become the state-of-the-art reconstruction techniques, although not always implemented by nuclear laboratories. Although more expensive from the computational time standpoint, iterative reconstructions (IRs) allow incorporating corrections for the factors that degrade image quality by modeling the imaging systems and the emission/detection processes.

As shown in **Fig. 6**, IR starts by providing an initial predicted image of the object being acquired. It can be a simple uniform flood field or a better estimation of the configuration of the heart. This volumetric image is used to obtain predicted projections that are compared with the actual measured SPECT projections. Depending on the difference between predicted and acquired profiles, the predicted projections are updated and this process is continued until the reconstruction is such that the predicted projections match the actual ones within an error margin. One of the first IR techniques introduced was based on maximum likelihood expectation maximization (MLEM),[13,14] followed by a similar but faster method, the ordered subsets expectation maximization (OSEM).[15] The primary differences between various iterative methods are how the predicted reconstructions and projections are created and how they are modified at each step. The more theoretically accurate the iterative technique is, the more time consuming the process. The OSEM technique was developed as a shortcut for the more computationally intensive MLEM: during each iteration only a subset of the projections is used rather than the entire set. Given its flexibility and efficiency, OSEM is commonly implemented into most of new imaging systems software.

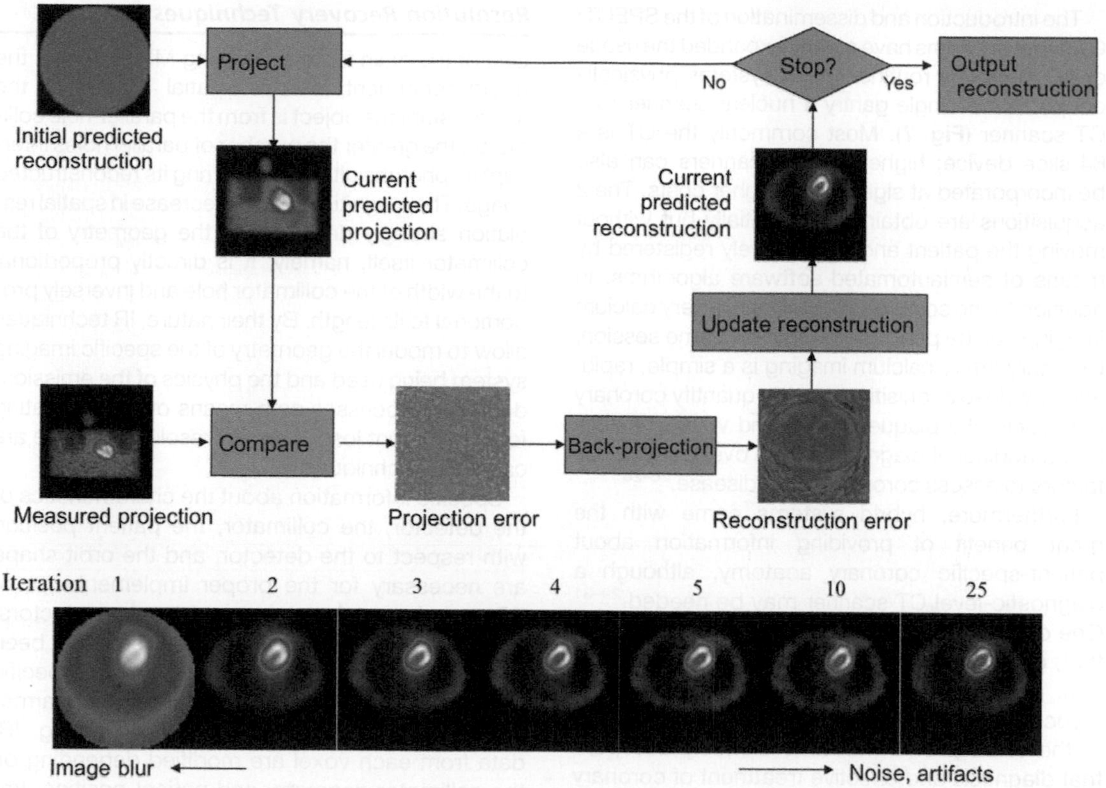

Fig. 6. Principle of IR algorithms. IR starts with an initial predicted image to obtain predicted projections. Actual measured projections and predicted ones are compared and a projection error is computed. By means of this error the image is updated and the procedure continued until convergence is reached. At the bottom of the image an example of IR by means of MLEM is shown with different number of iterations. There is no common rule to stop the iterative process, but, importantly, as the number of iterations increases so do noise and artifacts.

Myocardial perfusion SPECT images reconstructed with OSEM are of better quality with respect to images reconstructed with FBP. This difference between the 2 reconstruction modalities may not be crucial in cases of high-count density scans, but it becomes clinically relevant for images with low counts.[9] As a result, the improvements achieved by means of IR techniques can be traded for shorter protocols or decreased radiation dose without measurable loss in image quality. This is particularly true when additional corrections are incorporated into IRs.

Attenuation Correction and Single-Photon Emission Computed Tomography/Computed Tomography Hybrid Systems

Attenuation of emitted photons by soft tissue is another important shortcoming of SPECT imaging.[16] This soft tissue attenuation is what commonly gives rise to reduced counts in the anterior and/or lateral walls in women due to breast attenuation and reduced counts in the inferior wall in men due to preferential diaphragmatic attenuation.[17] Attenuation correction (AC) means the compensation during iterative image reconstruction for those absorbed photons. Several comparative studies of SPECT MPI[16,18–25] have shown that AC increases diagnostic performance by significant increases in specificity usually at no significant loss of sensitivity for detecting CAD. In 2002, ASNC released a statement directly addressing the issue and recommending that appropriate hardware and software tools for nonuniform AC be used for an improved image quality and diagnostic accuracy.[18,19] Corrections for photon absorption usually use a CT transmission scan from which attenuation coefficients along the thorax may be measured and used to mathematically correct for the absorption. The improvement is even more significant today with the use of solid-state detectors and with RR and noise regularization techniques (described later). The more each physical phenomenon affecting the image formation process is accounted for and corrected, the more accurate the image formation process becomes.

The introduction and dissemination of the SPECT/CT hybrid systems have greatly expanded the usage of AC in clinical routine. These systems physically couple into a single gantry a nuclear scanner to a CT scanner (**Fig. 7**). Most commonly the CT is a 64-slice device; higher-quality scanners can also be incorporated at significantly higher costs. The 2 acquisitions are obtained sequentially but without moving the patient and successively registered by means of semiautomated software algorithms. In addition to the scan for AC, coronary artery calcium imaging can be performed within the same session. Coronary artery calcium imaging is a simple, rapid, and low-dose acquisition used to quantify coronary atherosclerotic plaque burden and with an established additional diagnostic value over general risk factors to assess coronary artery disease.[26–28]

Furthermore, hybrid systems come with the great benefit of providing information about patient-specific coronary anatomy, although a diagnostic-level CT scanner may be needed.[29–31] One of the main drawbacks of nuclear imaging is that, given the lack of specific anatomic information, it relies on standard separation of the LV myocardium in vascular territories or according to the 17-segments model. It is widely accepted that diagnosis and effective treatment of coronary artery disease often require the integration of the 2 types of information, anatomy and function. By means of multimodality image fusion, a more comprehensive picture of patient status can be derived with established additional diagnostic and prognostic value. A large literature exists on the subject for a more detailed description of the field.[32–36] Although each acquisition, in particular a diagnostic one, increments the combined radiation dose, the continuous technical improvements of devices and protocols have greatly decreased the dose administered by each modality.[37,38] A diagnostic computed tomography (CT) angiogram can now be performed with less than 1 mSv.

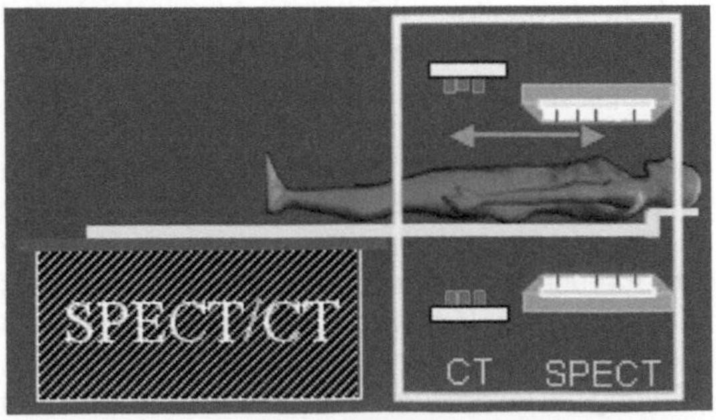

Fig. 7. Common configuration of SPECT/CT hybrid system. (*Courtesy of* James Galt, PhD, Atlanta, GA.)

Resolution Recovery Techniques

One of the main factors affecting MPI quality is the depth-dependent loss of spatial resolution: the more distant the object is from the parallel-hole collimator, the greater the number of parallel holes intercept its photons ultimately blurring its reconstructed image. The magnitude of this decrease in spatial resolution strongly depends on the geometry of the collimator itself, namely, it is directly proportional to the width of the collimator hole and inversely proportional to its length. By their nature, IR techniques allow to model the geometry of the specific imaging system being used and the physics of the emission/detection processes as a means of compensating for the inherent loss in spatial resolution. These are called RR techniques.[6–11]

Specific information about the characteristics of the detector, the collimator, the patient position with respect to the detector, and the orbit shape are necessary for the proper implementation of RR techniques. A database of known detectors' characteristics and collimator designs has been derived and is used depending on each specific combination of acquisition system, radiopharmaceutical, and protocol. Particularly during IR, data from each voxel are modified depending on the collimator geometry and patient position. Image pixels weights are analytically computed, taking into account the solid angles subtended by the collimator between each detector pixel and each body voxel (see **Fig. 5**). Additional parameters, such as center of rotation of the imaging system and detector-patient distances, are necessary at each iteration and projection. Newer cameras usually can provide these distances; if this is not the case, simple segmentation algorithms applied to each projection can be used to efficiently estimate body-detector distances.

Noise Compensation Techniques

Nuclear images are known to be inherently noisy due to the low-count statistics. Low-count density SPECT images are characterized by noise levels that appear at similar or higher frequencies with respect to the actual myocardial signal. As discussed previously, FBP reduces noise by reducing the high-frequency portion of the data. This results in blurring of the images and decreased image contrast, image resolution, and diagnostic power in detecting perfusion defects and wall motion abnormalities. At the same time RR is performed, noise compensation techniques allow also noise to be regularized and modeled in the reconstruction process. **Fig. 8** graphically depicts this concept. Jagged high-frequency noise in the count profile is removed just as it is removed

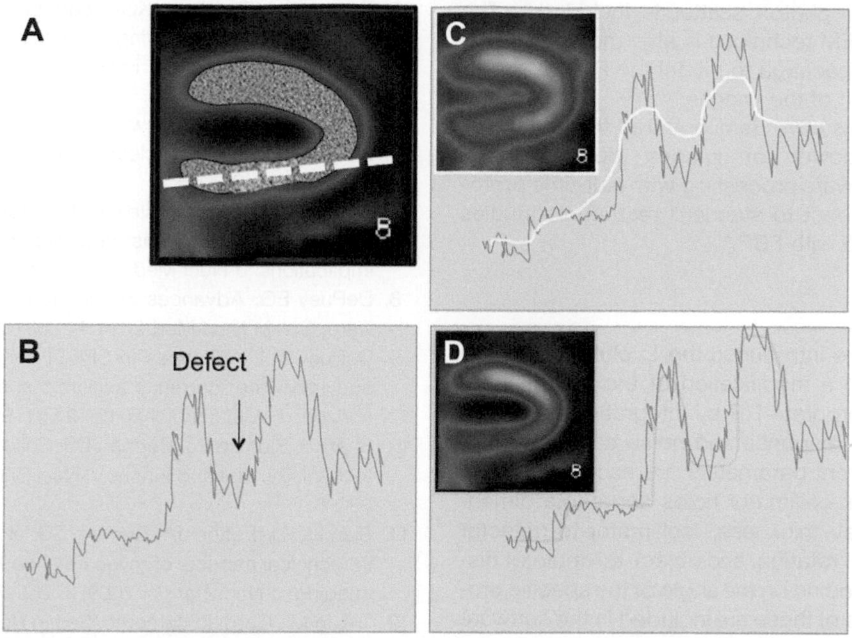

Fig. 8. Rationale for noise compensation techniques. (*A*) Perfusion defect in the inferior wall. (*B*) Count profile as obtained from original image along the dashed line depicted in (*A*) with common high-frequency noise. (*C*) Smoothing by means of traditional low-pass filters reduces high-frequency noise and also image contrast and ability to detect the defect. (*D*) By means of noise regularization techniques, high-frequency noise is removed while maintaining image contrast and perfusion defect appearance.

with low-pass filtering. What is different from conventional low-pass filtering is that the modeling process preserves the original defect contrast, thus making it possible to reduce noise without compromising image contrast.

Manufacturers of new SPECT cameras have all incorporated into their devices these advanced software methods, including IR, RR, and noise compensation techniques. Some of the most common software packages are briefly presented.

Wide Beam Reconstruction

UltraSpect (UltraSPECT Inc, Haifa, Israel) developed for its stand-alone workstation the patented algorithm, Wide Beam Reconstruction (WBR).[39] The algorithm includes both RR and noise compensation techniques. As described previously, the geometry of the imaging system and the dimensions of the collimator are used within IRs to perform RR. This method can be implemented in both old and newer cameras provided that information about the various scintillation systems is given. By modeling the Poisson distribution of emission process in the creation of nuclear images, noise compensation is also achieved. The objective function implemented in the reconstruction procedure includes both a Poisson and a gaussian component. By differently weighting the 2 components, high-frequency data are either enhanced or smoothed.

It has been reported that SPECT MPI may be performed with the WBR RR algorithm using half the conventional scan time without compromising imaging results.[39] Other studies showed that 2 different implementations of these RR algorithms applied to half-time ECG-gated MPI SPECT acquisitions compare favorably with FBP of full-time acquisitions, although systematic offsets in end-diastolic and systolic volumes and ejection fraction were reported due to the increase in image contrast over FBP images.[40,41] Another clinical trial showed that adaptive noise control with WBR improves uniformity of myocardium comparing to FBP techniques and results in improved diagnostic certainty while preserving normalcy and accuracy.[42]

Astonish

The Astonish algorithm (Philips) includes an OSEM reconstruction technique and corrections for the main factors degrading SPECT images, specifically introduced to shorten MPI protocols without compromising image quality. RR is achieved by including information about the collimator geometry in the IR during both the forward and back-projection parts of the algorithm. Additional correction for photon scatter is included.[43] The standard OSEM technique is also modified within the Astonish package to model the Poisson noise in the creation of the images.[44]

Clinical trials have demonstrated the equivalent diagnostic power of images obtained with Astonish software processing with half-time protocols with respect to standard rest/stress studies reconstructed with FBP.[45]

Evolution

GE Healthcare introduced the Evolution software package with a modification of the OSEM technique to incorporate RR by integrating collimator and detector response and noise compensation. Several different parameters are accounted for in the algorithm: collimator holes and septa dimensions, crystal thickness, collimator-to-detector gap, center of rotation, and object-to-detector distances, depending on the angle of the specific projection. Some of these are included in the software as look-up tables; others are directly retrieved from the raw projection data. Implementation details about the algorithm can be found in Refs.[40,46,47]

SUMMARY

Nuclear cardiology's inherent basic attributes have established it as a modality that has withstood the test of times. This article reviews recent advances in hardware and software techniques for MPI SPECT. These developments have been carefully studied and documented in the literature as to how they may be used in the diagnosis, prognosis, and treatment of heart disease. Challenges are mostly socioeconomic in nature but require focusing on reducing radiation exposure, maintaining high study quality, and increasing study value. Documenting progress needs to be continued in these areas.

REFERENCES

1. Garcia EV. Quantitative nuclear cardiology: we are almost there! J Nucl Cardiol 2012;19:424–37.
2. Garcia EV, Galt R, Faber TL, et al. Principles of nuclear cardiology imaging. In: Dilsizian V, Narula J, editors. Atlas of nuclear cardiology. 4th edition. New York: Springer; 2013. p. 1–53.
3. Sadehi MM, Schwartz RG, Beanlands RS, et al. Cardiovascular nuclear imaging. Balancing proven clinical value and potential radiation risk. J Nucl Med 2011;52:1162–4.
4. DePuey EG, Mahmarian JJ, Miller TD, et al. Patient-centered imaging. J Nucl Cardiol 2012;19:185–215.
5. Cerqueira MD, Allman KC, Ficaro EP, et al. Recommendations for reducing radiation exposure in myocardial perfusion imaging. J Nucl Cardiol 2010;17:709–18.
6. Garcia EV, Faber TL. New trends in camera and software technology in nuclear cardiology. Cardiol Clin 2009;27:227–36.
7. Garcia EV, Faber TL, Esteves FP. Cardiac dedicated ultrafast SPECT cameras: new designs and clinical implications. J Nucl Med 2011;52:210–7.
8. DePuey EG. Advances in cardiac processing software. Semin Nucl Med 2014;44:252–73.
9. DePuey EG. Advances in SPECT camera software and hardware: currently available and new on the horizon. J Nucl Cardiol 2012;19:551–81.
10. Sharir T, Slomka PJ, Berman DS. Solid-State SPECT technology: fast and furious. J Nucl Cardiol 2010;17:890–6.
11. Slomka PJ, Patton JA, Berman DS, et al. Advances in technical aspects of myocardial perfusion SPECT imaging. J Nucl Cardiol 2009;16:255–76.
12. Travin MI. Cardiac cameras. Semin Nucl Med 2011;41:182–201.
13. Shepp LA, Vardi Y. Maximum likelihood reconstruction for emission tomography. IEEE Trans Med Imaging 1982;1:113–22.
14. Lange K, Carson R. EM reconstruction algorithms for emission and transmission tomography. J Comput Assist Tomogr 1984;8:306–16.
15. Hudson HM, Larkin RS. Accelerated image reconstruction using ordered subsets of projection data. IEEE Trans Med Imaging 1994;13:601–9.
16. Garcia EV. SPECT attenuation correction: an essential tool to realize nuclear cardiology's manifest destiny. J Nucl Cardiol 2007;14:16–24.
17. DePuey EG, Garcia EV. Optimal specificity of Thallium-201 SPECT through recognition of imaging artifacts. J Nucl Med 1989;30:441–9.
18. Hendel RC, Corbett JR, Cullom SJ, et al. The value and practice of attenuation correction for myocardial perfusion SPECT imaging: a joint position statement from the American Society of Nuclear Cardiology and the Society of Nuclear Medicine. J Nucl Cardiol 2002;9:135–43.
19. Heller GV, Links J, Bateman TM, et al. American Society of Nuclear Cardiology and Society of Nuclear Medicine joint position statement: attenuation correction of myocardial perfusion SPECT scintigraphy. J Nucl Cardiol 2004;11:229–30.
20. Heller GV, Bateman TM, Johnson LL, et al. Clinical value of attenuation correction in stress-only Tc-99m sestamibi SPECT imaging. J Nucl Cardiol 2004;11:273–81.
21. Ficaro EP, Fessler JA, Achermann RJ, et al. Simultaneous transmission-emission thallium-201 cardiac SPECT: effect of attenuation correction on myocardial tracer distribution. J Nucl Med 1995;36:921–31.

22. Grossman GB, Garcia EV, Bateman TM, et al. Quantitative Tc-99m sestamibi attenuation corrected SPECT: development and multicenter trial validation of myocardial perfusion stress gender-independent normal database in an obese population. J Nucl Cardiol 2004;11:263–72.
23. Prvulovich EM, Lonn AH, Bomanji JB, et al. Effect of attenuation correction on myocardial thallium-201 distribution in patients with a low likelihood of coronary artery disease. Eur J Nucl Med 1997;24:266–75.
24. Kluge R, Sattler B, Seese A, et al. Attenuation correction by simultaneous emission-transmission myocardial single-photon emission tomography using a technetium-99m-labelled radiotracer: impact on diagnostic accuracy. Eur J Nucl Med 1997;24:1107–14.
25. Ficaro EP. Should SPET attenuation correction be more widely employed in routine clinical practice? Eur J Nucl Med Mol Imaging 2002;29:409–12.
26. Arad Y, Goodman KJ, Roth M, et al. Coronary calcification, coronary disease risk factors, C-reactive protein, and atherosclerotic cardiovascular disease events: the St. Francis Heart study. J Am Coll Cardiol 2005;46:158–65.
27. Shaw LJ, Raggi P, Schisterman E, et al. Prognostic value of cardiac risk factors and coronary artery calcium screening for all-cause mortality. Radiology 2003;228:826–33.
28. Greenland P, LaBree L, Azen SP, et al. Coronary artery calcium score combined with Framingham score for risk prediction in asymptomatic individuals. J Am Med Assoc 2004;291:210–5.
29. Gaemperli O, Saraste A, Knuuti J. Cardiac hybrid imaging. Eur Heart J 2012;13:51–60.
30. van der Hoeven BL, Schalij MJ, Delgrado V. Multimodality imaging in interventional cardiology. Nat Rev Cardiol 2012;9:333–46.
31. Kramer CM, Narula J. Fusion images: more informative than the sum of individual images? JACC Cardiovasc Imaging 2010;3:985–6.
32. Santana CA, Garcia EV, Faber TL, et al. Diagnostic performance of fusion myocardial imaging (MPI) and computed tomography angiography. J Nucl Cardiol 2009;16:201–11.
33. Piccinelli M, Garcia E. Multimodality image fusion for diagnosing coronary artery disease. J Biomed Res 2013;27:439–51.
34. Faber TL, Santana CA, Garcia EV, et al. Three-dimensional fusion of coronary arteries with myocardial perfusion distribution: clinical validation. J Nucl Med 2004;45:745–53.
35. Faber TL, Santana CA, Piccinelli M, et al. Automatic alignment of myocardial perfusion images with contrast-enhanced cardiac computed tomography. IEEE Trans Nucl Sci 2011;58:2296–302.
36. Slomka PJ. Software approaches to merging molecular with anatomic information. J Nucl Med 2004;45:36S–45S.
37. Thompson RC, Cullom SJ. Issues regarding radiation dosage of cardiac nuclear and radiography procedures. J Nucl Cardiol 2006;13:19–23.
38. Flotats A, Knuuti J, Gutberlet M, et al. Hybrid cardiac imaging: SPECT/CT and PET/CT. A joint position statement by the European Association of Nuclear Medicine (EANM), the European Society of Cardiac Radiology (ESCR) and the European Council of Nuclear Cardiology (ECNC). Eur J Nucl Med Mol Imaging 2011;38:201–12.
39. Borges-Neto S, Pagnanelli RA, Shaw LK, et al. Clinical results of a novel wide beam reconstruction method for shortenings can time of Tc-99m cardiac SPECT perfusion studies. J Nucl Cardiol 2007;14:555–65.
40. DePuey EG, Gadraju R, Clark J, et al. Ordered subset expectation maximization and wide beam reconstruction "half-time" gated myocardial perfusion SPECT functional imaging: a comparison to "full-time" filtered backprojection. J Nucl Cardiol 2008;15:547–63.
41. DePuey EG, Bommireddipalli S, Clark J, et al. Wide beam reconstruction "quarter-time" gated myocardial perfusion SPECT functional imaging: a comparison to "full-time" ordered subset expectation maximum. J Nucl Cardiol 2009;16:736–52.
42. Druz RS, Phillips LM, Chugkowski M, et al. Wide-beam reconstruction half-time SPECT improves diagnostic certainty and preserves normalcy and accuracy: a quantitative perfusion analysis. J Nucl Cardiol 2011;18:52–61.
43. Kadrmas DJ, Frey EC, Karimi SS, et al. Fast implementation of reconstruction-based scatter compensation in fully 3D SPECT image reconstruction. Phys Med Biol 1998;43:857–73.
44. Ye J, Song X, Zhao Z, et al. Iterative SPECT reconstruction using matched filtering for improved image quality. IEEE Nucl Sci Symp Conf Rec (1997) 2006.
45. Venero CV, Ahlberg AW, Bateman TM, et al. Enhancement of nuclear cardiac laboratory efficiency - multicenter evaluation of a new post-processing method with depth-dependent collimator resolution applied to full and half-time acquisitions. J Nucl Cardiol 2008;15:S4.
46. Tsui BMW, Hu HB, Gilland DR, et al. Implementation of simultaneous attenuation and detector response correction in SPECT. IEEE Trans Nucl Sci 1988;35:778–83.
47. Tsui BMW, Gullberg GT. The geometric transfer-function for cone and fan beam collimators. Phys Med Biol 1990;35:81–93.

Technical Aspects of Cardiac PET Imaging and Recent Advances

Guido Germano, PhD[a,b,*], Daniel S. Berman, MD[a,b], Piotr Slomka, PhD[a,b]

KEYWORDS

• PET • Attenuation correction • PET detectors • Time-of-flight • PET reconstruction
• Myocardial perfusion PET • Respiratory gating

KEY POINTS

- Cardiac PET is currently often performed on 3-dimensional PET/computed tomography (CT) systems, which have different imaging characteristics compared with traditional 2-dimensional PET systems.
- Time-of-flight imaging has been incorporated into commercial PET/CT systems and may allow image contrast improvement in cardiac imaging, especially when combined with resolution recovery.
- Digital photon detectors have been proposed for PET imaging, and is likely to lead to a better count rate and better overall imaging performance.
- Cardiac PET attenuation correction is most often performed with CT; care must be taken to ensure appropriate registration of the CT attenuation maps.

As the number of myocardial perfusion single photon emission compute tomography (SPECT) studies performed in the United States has steadily declined over the past several years, an opposite trend can be seen for myocardial perfusion PET (**Fig. 1**). One of the reasons for this discrepancy (in addition to clinical, technical, and reimbursement considerations) is increasing public awareness of the potential dangers of radiation exposure, with regard to which PET radiopharmaceuticals compare favorably with SPECT radiopharmaceuticals, mainly because of the shorter half-life of the related radioisotopes (**Fig. 2**). New SPECT cameras and software approaches have been and are being developed to decrease the radiation dose and improve study efficiency in the SPECT world, as described by Piccinelli M and Garcia EV.[1] This article focuses on technical aspects peculiar to PET imaging, as well as hardware and software approaches that maximize the quality and efficiency of cardiac PET.

RADIOISOTOPES FOR MYOCARDIAL PERFUSION PET

Although one of the most interesting characteristics of PET is its minimal interference with the biologic processes it sets out to measures (through the use of positron-emitting isotopes of elements naturally occurring in the human body, like ^{15}O, ^{13}N, ^{11}C, and ^{18}F, the latter being an analog of hydrogen), the radioisotopes in clinical use for the practical purpose of measuring myocardial perfusion are ^{82}Rb, ^{13}N, and ^{18}F. A summary of relevant properties for these 3 radioisotopes is shown in **Table 1**. The energy with which positrons are emitted depends on the radioisotope and, because a positron needs to dissipate its

[a] Departments of Imaging and Medicine, Cedars-Sinai Medical Center, 8700 Beverly Boulevard, Los Angeles, CA 90048, USA; [b] David Geffen School of Medicine at UCLA, Los Angeles, CA, USA
* Corresponding author. Artificial Intelligence in Medicine Program, 8700 Beverly Boulevard, Suite A047N, Los Angeles, CA 90048.
E-mail address: guido.germano@cshs.org

Cardiol Clin 34 (2016) 13–23
http://dx.doi.org/10.1016/j.ccl.2015.07.015
0733-8651/16/$ – see front matter

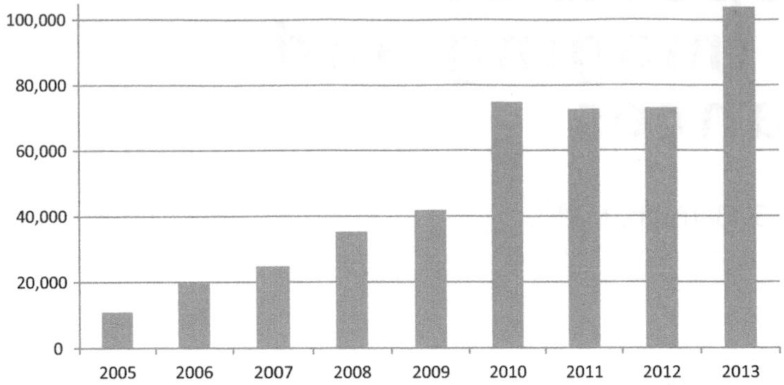

Fig. 1. Annual myocardial perfusion PET studies performed in the United States (Medicare Part B utilization data, Current Procedural Terminology code 78492, multiple studies at rest and/or stress). (*Data from* Wheaton Partners, LLC. CodeMap. Available at: https://www.codemap.com/. Accessed July 15, 2015.)

energy through multiple impacts before annihilating with an electron, there is a "positron range" connected with the difference between the location of emission and that of annihilation—the greater the energy, the greater the uncertainty about where the emission actually occurred, and ultimately, the lesser the PET image resolution. Positron range distributions or "line-spread functions" are not well-described by Gaussian curves owing to their long "tails,"[2] and therefore both their full-width half maximum and full-width tenth maximum are reported in **Table 1**, showing that the highest quality PET imaging is theoretically achieved using ^{18}F, followed by ^{13}N and, much lower, ^{82}Rb. Of note, ^{82}Rb is the only generator-produced myocardial perfusion PET radioisotope, and this has contributed greatly to its diffusion in sites for which it is not possible, convenient, or economical to use cyclotron-produced alternatives. For the future, it is reasonable to conjecture that improvements in image quality will be associated with advances in the development and availability of ^{18}F-based perfusion radiopharmaceuticals.

COINCIDENCE DETECTION

The result of a positron's annihilation is the simultaneous emission of two 511-keV photons (γ-rays), which for practical purposes can be considered to be collinear and traveling in opposite directions (to be accurate, the angle between them is a Gaussian curve peaked at 180° and with an full-width half maximum of 0.3°). Consequently, a line of response (LOR) is defined as the result of each annihilation, and the use of a physical collimator is not strictly necessary in PET, because collimation is achieved electronically by setting an acceptance time window (to account for time of flight and timing inaccuracies) on γ-rays detected by directly opposing detectors. Moreover, the total attenuation for the 2 photons is constant for a given LOR through the patient, no matter how deep within the patient the annihilation occurred. This allows the use of a radiation source external to the patient (eg, obtained by CT) to measure accurately the attenuation along all the LORs of interest, and determine the appropriate correction factors; by comparison, attenuation correction (AC) in SPECT is a more complex problem. The goal in PET data acquisition is that of accurately identifying, temporally and spatially, the γ-rays produced by positron annihilation in the object being scanned. Each 511-keV photon that dissipates part or all of its energy in a detector corresponds with a single event ("event"). The pair of single events produced by the same annihilation

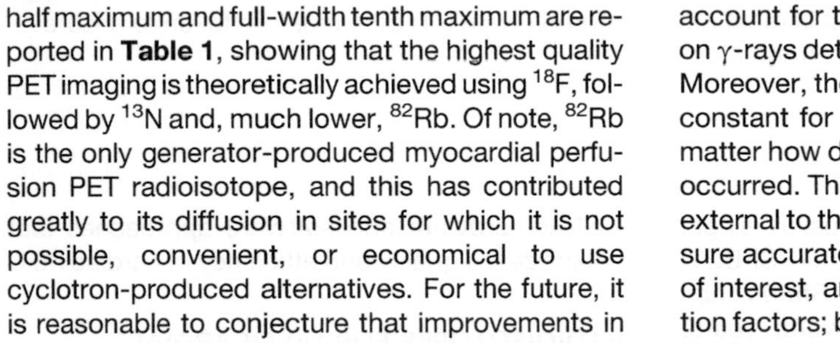

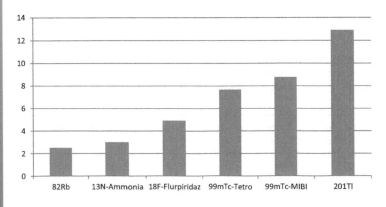

Fig. 2. Effective dose delivered to an adult patient for typical injected activities in myocardial perfusion PET and single photon emission CT stress studies (standard cameras/protocols). Activities are 50 mCi for ^{82}Rb, 30 mCi for ^{13}N-ammonia, 7 mCi for ^{18}F-flurpiridaz, 30 mCi for 99mTc-tetrofosmin, or 99mTc-MIBI, 2.5 mCi for 201Tl.[44–49] A new PET radiopharmaceutical, ^{18}F-rhodamine 6G, has been reported to deliver a dose of only 1.04 mSv for a 10-mCi injection.[50] (*Data from* Refs.[44–50])

Table 1
Common radioisotopes used in myocardial perfusion PET

Radioisotope	Source	Half-Life (min)	Max β^+ Energy (MeV)	FWHM (mm)	FWTM (mm)
^{18}F	Cyclotron	109.70	0.635	0.22	1.09
^{13}N	Cyclotron	9.96	1.19	0.60	2.80
^{82}Rb	Generator	1.25	3.35	2.60	13.20

The full-width half maximum (FWHM) and full-width tenth maximum (FWTM) of the LSF owing to the positron range are reported.

is defined as a true coincidence event ("true event"), in that it ideally identifies the true LOR. In practice, 1 or 2 of the γ-rays may have been scattered, thus producing a scattered coincidence event ("scattered event"), where the apparent LOR deviates from the true LOR. If 1 of the 2 γ-rays is scattered outside the plane where the real LOR lies, only a single event is recorded. If 2 single events from unrelated annihilations are detected simultaneously, they may seem to be a true coincidence event, but really represent a random coincidence event ("random event"). The number of random events is directly related to the resolving time of the system, or the time window chosen to define the simultaneity of detection. A graphical explanation of the genesis of single, true coincidence and scattered coincidence events is shown in **Fig. 3** for a simple, 2-detector configuration. The goal, of course, is that of maximizing the amount of true events collected, at the same time decreasing as much as possible the contribution of other types of events to the cardiac PET images.

FIELD OF VIEW AND SINOGRAMS

Detectors are generally arranged in a ring in modern PET systems, and the field of view of an acquisition is determined by the number of detectors that are electronically enabled to be in coincidence with an opposing detector (**Fig. 4**). This number is limited to avoid artifacts associated with interdetector penetration and scatter,[2] and the overlapping portion of the intersecting "fans" of LORs for all detectors in the ring defines the field of view.

Under these assumptions, many LORs are parallel (**Fig. 5**). All parallel LORs define a direction (also termed projection, or angle). Each LOR in a parallel set is named a position, or sample, and each sample in a given direction set gives information on the amount of activity encountered by traversing the scanned object along that specific LOR. The data from all the different angles and positions can be conveniently collected and displayed in a sinogram (**Fig. 6**), or a matrix whose rows (each identifying a direction or angle) represent the data profiles across the object along those angles.

As **Fig. 7** shows, sinograms are directly related to projection images, and 1 set can be easily derived from the other. This is important because sinograms are the basic (raw) building blocks of PET images, much like projection images are for SPECT images, and their interchangeability makes it easy to apply similar reconstruction and image recovery techniques to data acquired using either of the 2 modalities.

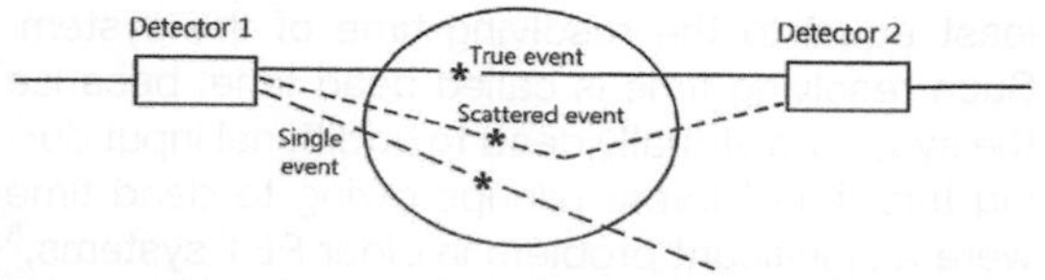

Fig. 3. Single event, true coincidence, and scattered coincidence events exemplified in a 2-detector configuration.

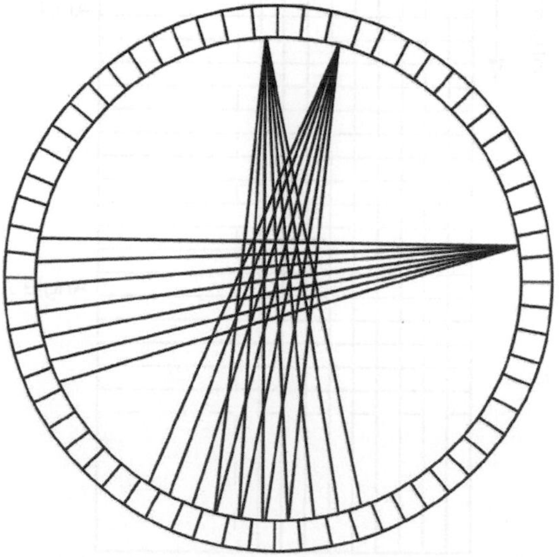

Fig. 4. Fans of lines of response connecting a detector with its directly opposed detector plus 6 other detectors, 3 to the left and 3 to the right of it. The greater the number of detectors with which a detector is in coincidence, the greater the effective field of view of the system.

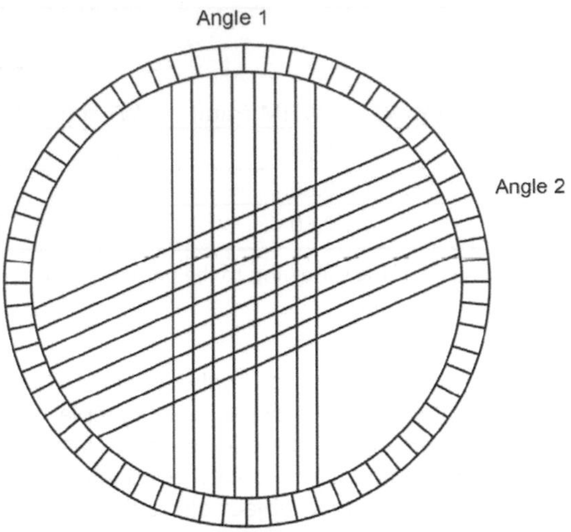

Fig. 5. Parallel sets of lines of response (LORs), each set defining a direction or angle. Within a set, each LOR represents a position, or sample.

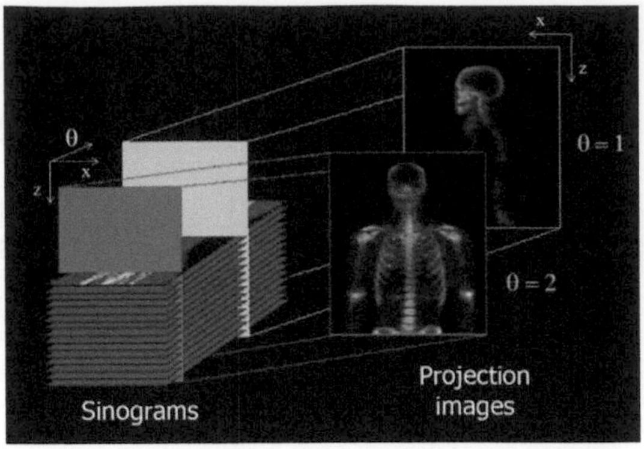

Fig. 7. Relationship between sinograms and projection images. If sinograms corresponding with adjacent detector rings (along the *z* direction, or patient long axis) are stacked on top of one another, projection images can be extracted from the sonogram stack by cutting through it perpendicularly. (*Courtesy of* Magnus Dahlbom, PhD, Los Angeles, CA.)

TWO- VERSUS 3-DIMENSIONAL PET

As mentioned, coincidence detection makes it unnecessary to use an "in-plane" collimator for PET, thus increasing count sensitivity compared with SPECT. Removing the interplane septa that physically separate detector rings along the axial dimension allows to further improve count collection, by enabling interplane or cross-ring LORs (**Fig. 8**). Of note, the individual detectors shown in **Figs. 4**, **5**, and **8** are actually detector matrixes and therefore define more than 1 axial plan, but for the sake of discussion the simplified setups shown shall suffice.

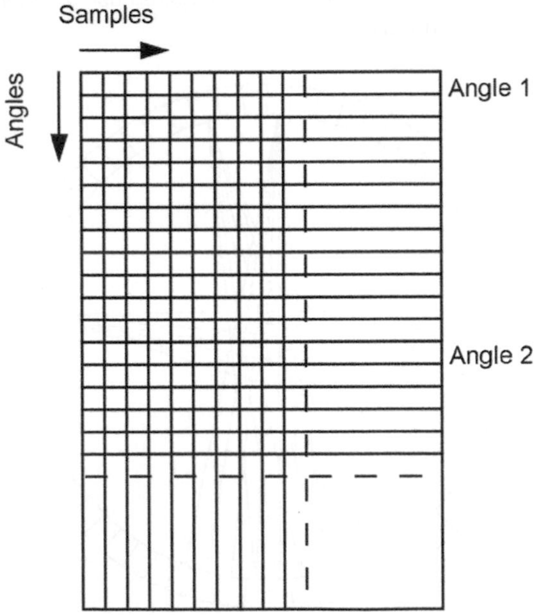

Fig. 6. Sinogram in PET. Each sample (*pixel*) represents the activity distribution in the object of interest, integrated along a line of response (LOR) connecting 2 detectors. All LORs contributing to the same sinogram row are parallel, thus identifying a direction or an angle.

Operating in 3D mode, without the interplane septa, results in greater photon sensitivity by a factor of 4 to 6 compared with 2D mode. The downside of 3D acquisitions is that the number of scattered events detected as a percentage of all coincidence events, also called scatter fraction, increases from 10% to 15% to 30% to 40%.[3] The number of single events also greatly increases, and consequently so does the number of multiple coincidence events ("multiple events"), which are produced primarily by the simultaneous occurrence of a true coincidence event and a single event in 3 detectors, and secondarily by the simultaneous occurrence of 3 single events in 3 individual detectors (see **Fig. 3**). It is intuitive that the simultaneous occurrence of many events, whether single or coincidence, creates problems for the PET system, which must count, time, and characterize the events. This is a consequence of the fact that, for any counting system to be able to differentiate between 2 consecutive events, those events must be separated in time by an interval at least equal to the resolving time of the system. Such resolving time is called dead time, because the system is virtually dead to additional input during this time.[4] Event pileups owing to dead time were a significant problem in older PET systems,[5] but the use of newer detector materials and techniques has allowed all modern PET and PET/CT systems to operate in 3D mode, with substantial

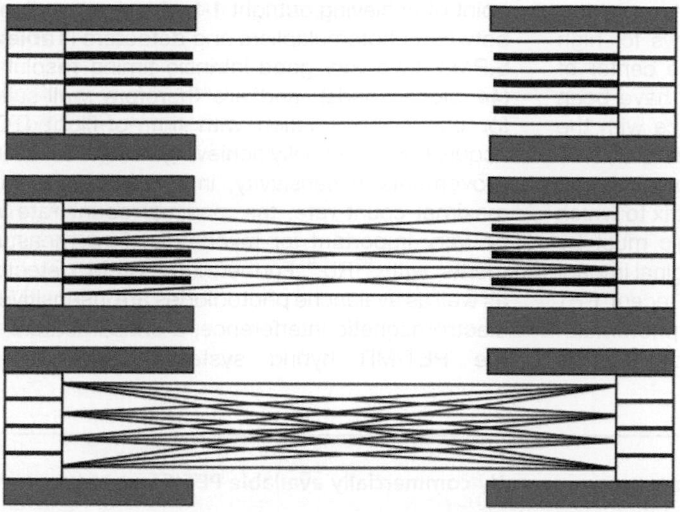

Fig. 8. Axial section of a simplified, 4-ring PET system with and without septa to separate imaging planes. Coincidence detection can be (*A*) strictly 2-dimensional (2D), allowing only "in-plane" lines of response (LORs); (*B*) in modified 2D fashion, including "cross-plane" LORs between adjacent rings; (*C*) fully 3-dimensional, removing the septa and allowing LORs between any ring pair.

improvements in photon sensitivity compared with 2D PET.

PET DETECTORS

There are several ways in which the choice of PET scintillating detector material affects image quality. The denser the material, the higher its photoelectric fraction, or its ability to stop the incoming 511-keV radiation completely on the first interaction, and consequently the lower the interdetector scatter. In addition, high luminosity or light yield (expressed as the number of light photons emitted for each MeV of energy absorbed) is desirable for signal-to-noise considerations. Finally, the speed at which a detector emits light after absorbing a 511-keV γ-ray is directly proportional to its count rate capability, which is important in 3D acquisitions. The decay time is defined as the time needed for the detector's light output pulse to decrease to 1/e of its maximum amplitude value, and a low decay time is virtually essential for time of flight imaging. **Table 2** shows the characteristics of 2 historically relevant PET scintillator materials, bismuth germanate oxide ($Bi_4Ge_3O_{12}$ or BGO) and cerium-doped gadolinium oxyorthosilicate (Gd_2SiO_5(Ce), or GSO), together with a newer and widely used material, cerium-doped lutetium oxyorthosilicate (Lu_2SiO_5(Ce) or LSO), which combines high density with low decay time and a light output that come closest to the NaI(Tl) standard. A variant of LSO in which lutetium is in part replaced by yttrium has been incorporated more recently in commercially available PET/CT scanners, and active research continues with regard to developing new PET detector materials.

The size of the individual elements in a matrix (block) PET detector has not changed substantially over the past 20 years (from 5.6 × 5.6 mm^2 in a CTI/Siemens ECAT 851/951 to about 4 × 4 mm^2 in current PET systems), owing to

Table 2
Characteristics of inorganic scintillating materials used in PET compared with conventional NaI(Tl) for SPECT

Material	Density (G/cm^3)	Effective Atomic # (Z)	Light Yield [% NaI(Tl)]	Decay (ns)
NaI(Tl)	3.67	51	100	230
BGO	7.13	74	8	300
GSO	6.71	59	16	60
LSO	7.4	66	75	40

Abbreviations: BGO, bismuth germanate oxide; GSO, cerium-doped gadolinium oxyorthosilicate; LSO, cerium-doped lutetium oxyorthosilicate.

Data from Derenzo S, Boswell M, Weber M, et al. Scintillation properties. Available at: http://scintillator.lbl.gov/. Accessed July 15 2015; and Dahlbom M, MacDonald L, Ericsson L, et al. Performance of a YSO/LSO phoswich detector for use in a PET/SPECT system. IEEE Trans Nucl Sci 1997;44:1114–19.

detection efficiency and interdetector scatter considerations. Although this still allows for high spatial resolution of 4 to 5 mm in the center of the field of view, great improvements have been achieved in the way detectors interface with the scanner's front end electronics. Traditional PET scanners use photomultiplier tubes much larger than the individual detectors in the matrix to which the tubes are coupled, so Anger logic must be used to estimate the location of the original impact of the γ-ray. By contrast, some very recent PET designs feature smaller silicon digital photomultipliers (SiPM)[6] or avalanche photodiodes,[7] to the point of achieving outright 1-to-1 correspondence between photomultipliers and detectors (**Table 3**). SiPMs have very good intrinsic timing resolution (44 picoseconds), and are therefore well-suited for use in conjunction with time-of-flight (TOF) acquisition, potentially achieving simultaneous improvements in sensitivity, image resolution, and maximal count rate; the maximal count rate will be very important for myocardial flow measurements with ^{82}Rb.[8] Furthermore, SiPM detectors as well as avalanche photodiodes are insensitive to electromagnetic interference, a critical feature for the PET/MR hybrid systems described by

Table 3
Specifications and key parameters for modern, recently commercially available PET/CT systems

PET/CT Model	Ingenuity TF	Discovery 710	Biograph mCT Flow	Vereos
Patient port (cm)	70 OpenView	70	78	70
CT (slices)	64, 128	16, 64, 128	20, 40, 64, 128	64, 128
Patient scan range (cm)	190	200	195	190
Maximum patient weight, kg (lb)	195 (430)	226 (500)	226 (500)	195 (430)
Acquisition modes	3D S&S	3D S&S	3D S&S, continuous	3D S&S
No. of image planes	45 or 90	47	109	72
Plane spacing (mm)	2 or 4	3.27	2	1, 2, or 4
Crystal size (mm)	4 × 4 × 22	4.2 × 6.3 × 25	4 × 4 × 20	4 × 4 × 22
No. of crystals	28,336	13,824	32,448	23,040
No. of photomultipliers	420	256	768	23,040 SiPMs
Physical axial field of view (cm)	18	15.7	21.8	16.3
Detector material	LYSO	LYSO	LSO	LYSO
System sensitivity 3D, (%)[a]	0.74	0.75	0.95	>1.0
Transaxial resolution @ 1 cm (mm)[a]	4.7	4.9	4.4	4.0
Transaxial resolution @ 10 cm (mm)[a]	5.2	5.5	4.9	4.5
Axial resolution @ 1 cm (mm)[a]	4.7	5.6	4.5	4.0
Axial resolution @ 10 cm (mm)[a]	5.2	6.3	5.9	4.5
Peak NECR (kcps)	120 @19 kBq/mL	130 @29.5 KBq/mL	175 @28 kBq/mL	650 @50 kBq/mL
Time-of-flight resolution (picoseconds)	591	544	540	307
Time-of-flight localization (cm)	8.9	8.2	8.1	4.6
Coincidence window (nanoseconds)	4.5	4.9	4.1	1.5

Systems are by Philips (ingenuity TF and Vereos), GE (Discovery 710), and Siemens (Biograph mCT Flow).

Abbreviations: 3D, 3-dimensional; BGO, bismuth germanate oxide; CT, computed tomography; GSO, cerium-doped gadolinium oxyorthosilicate; LSO, cerium-doped lutetium oxyorthosilicate; LYSO, lutetium yttrium orthosilicate; NECR, noise equivalent count rate; S&S, step and shoot.

[a] NEMA 2001.

LaForest R and colleagues.[9] **Fig. 9** shows a comparison of photon detection using conventional photomultipliers and digital silicon photomultipliers with 1:1 detector coupling.

As shown in **Table 3**, the axial coverage of 16 to 22 cm in modern PET/CT systems should allow full coverage of the myocardium at 1 bed position. For cardiovascular applications, where more than 1 bed position is required, it is possible to achieve more uniform axial noise sensitivity by continuously moving the patient through the detection system and rebinning the data appropriately in real time,[10] as opposed to using a standard approach.

TIME-OF-FLIGHT IMAGING

The picosecond timing resolution achievable by combining the fast decay time of LSO and lutetium yttrium orthosilicate detectors with fast coincidence electronics has made it possible to implement TOF imaging in modern clinical PET scanners. The concept of TOF PET had actually been proposed decades ago,[11] but until recently its realization had been limited to research PET scanners. In brief, if Δt is the difference in the detection times of 2 photons from the same coincidence event and c is the velocity of light (3×10^{11} mm/s), the exact annihilation location along the LOR can be determined with an uncertainty Δd (depth resolution) expressed by the following formula:

$$\Delta d = \frac{\Delta t \times c}{2}$$

The faster the detector and front-end electronics, the smaller the Δt that can be measured, and consequently the smaller the portion of the LOR, where we can say the annihilation occurred (**Fig. 10**). The iterative reconstruction algorithm used to generate tomographic PET images from sonograms can incorporate this depth resolution information, resulting in an improved signal-to-noise ratio, particularly in large patients.[12] It has been shown that TOF imaging results in contrast improvement and increased uptake in the lateral wall for N-13 ammonia myocardial perfusion PET imaging.[13]

It is expected that the use of digital SiPM can further improve the TOF performance of PET systems. Making reference to the equation, if Δt equals SiPMs' timing resolution of 4.4×10^{-11} s, the Δd would be about 6 mm, resulting in substantial improvement in the quality of the final images.

IMAGE RECONSTRUCTION

Most current PET/CT systems employ a fully 3D iterative PET reconstruction, which allows the incorporation of CT attenuation maps as well as corrections for scatter, random events, spatial system response, and dead time. An accelerated type of iterative reconstruction, 3D ordered subset expectation maximization can be implemented on all systems to reduce reconstruction time. Despite such implementation, 3D iterative reconstruction can still pose significant limitations with respect to processing speed in standard workstations, particularly for cardiac PET imaging using dynamic and gated protocols.

When performing 3D PET imaging with ^{82}Rb, attention must be paid to the approximately 13% of nuclear decays associated with a 776-keV prompt-γ emission, which can downscatter into the 511-keV PET energy window. Prompt-γ

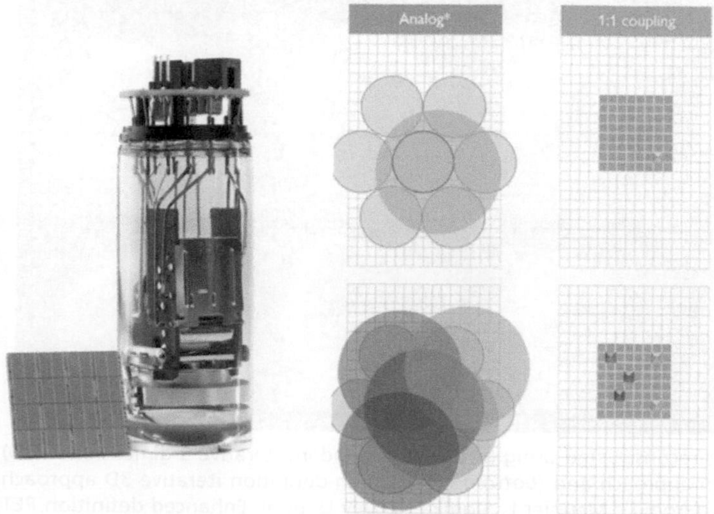

Fig. 9. Comparison of photon detection using conventional photomultipliers (*left*) and digital silicon photomultipliers with 1:1 detector coupling (*right*). The digital approach results in higher spatial resolution and faster timing resolution. (*Courtesy of* Philips Healthcare, Eindhoven, The Netherlands; with permission.)

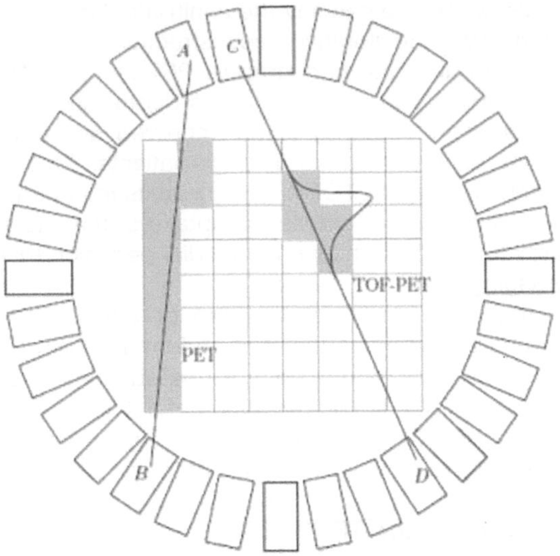

Fig. 10. Principle of time-of-flight (TOF) imaging in PET. In standard PET, a coincidence event detected by detectors *A* and *B* identifies an annihilation that can be located anywhere along the line of response (LOR) connecting *A* and *B*. In TOF-PET, a similar coincidence event detected by detectors *C* and *D* can be more accurately related to an annihilation that occurred in a subsection of the LOR connecting *C* and *D*. (*From* Sitek A. Data analysis in emission tomography using emission-count posteriors. Phys Med Biol 2012;57(21):6779; with permission.)

corrections have been developed[14] and can be incorporated in the 3D reconstruction process together with corrections for standard scattered events; this adjustment was not necessary for 2D PET imaging, but is very important for cardiac 3D PET ^{82}Rb imaging with new-generation scanners.

Another recently introduced feature of 3D iterative reconstruction algorithms is the 3D modeling of scanner-specific point spread function maps, which are used subsequently to predict the input signal during reconstruction.[15] This resolution recovery method has been equivalently termed point spread function or high-definition reconstruction, and is currently offered by all commercial PET vendors. Effective tomographic image resolution as low as 2 mm and significant improvements in image contrast have been achieved using resolution recovery[16]; better definition of subtle myocardial perfusion defects have been reported in clinical settings with the use of this approach[17] (**Fig. 11**). The combination of TOF reconstruction and point spread function correction has also been shown to improve image quality.[18,19] Overall, it can be stated that the advanced image reconstruction techniques utilized for 3D PET are significantly different from those previously used in 2D PET. Therefore, 3D PET imaging is not equivalent to 2D PET.

ATTENUATION CORRECTION AND HYBRID PET/COMPUTED TOMOGRAPHY

AC has been used in cardiac PET imaging ever since the introduction of the first PET scanners, but was originally based on radionuclide transmission rod sources circling around the patient to collect photon attenuation maps. With the advent of hybrid PET/CT systems, it became apparent that CT-based AC could offer the advantages of low-noise attenuation maps, fast data acquisition, and elimination of bias from emission contamination of postinjection transmission scans.[20] Disadvantages of CT-based AC

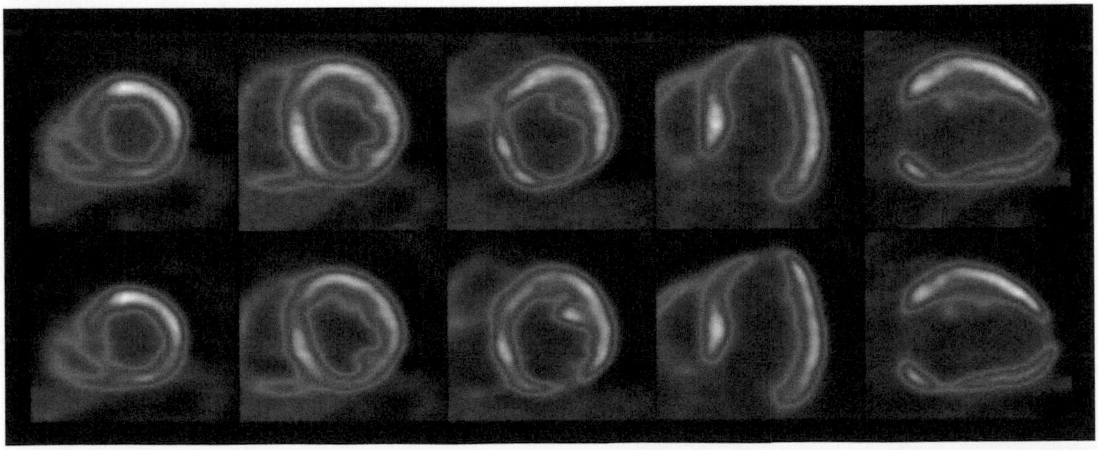

Fig. 11. ^{18}F-FDG viability PET scan images reconstructed using (*top row*) a standard iterative 3-dimensional (3D) ordered subset expectation maximization approach and (*bottom row*) a high-definition iterative 3D approach incorporating image resolution recovery. (*From* Le Meunier L, Slomka PJ, Dey D, et al. Enhanced definition PET for cardiac imaging. J Nucl Cardiol 2010;17:424; with permission.)

are related to the additional radiation dose for the patient and to metal-induced artifacts from pacemakers or implantable cardioverter–defibrillators. CT-based AC for PET has also proven challenging because of the misalignment between CT and PET images, mostly owing to respiratory motion,[21] a particularly important factor in myocardial perfusion imaging.[22,23] Because CT has a temporal resolution of less than 1 second, as opposed to 1 full respiratory cycle for PET, the mismatch has been reported to cause false-positive results in about 40% to 60% of all studies.[23–25] It has also been shown that there are significant differences between traditional transmission source-based AC (using Ge-68 or Cs-137) and CT-based AC, which may remain even after alignment of the CT maps to the emission data[23,26]; therefore, careful visual verification of the alignment is needed to minimize misregistration artifacts. Methods for the automatic registration of CT and PET maps to reduce these artifacts have been developed,[27] but are not yet applied routinely in clinical practice.

Alternatively, averaging the cine CT data acquisition over 1 breath cycle (about 4–5 s) to match the temporal resolutions of CT and PET has been proposed, and even implemented in some commercially available scanners. It has been reported that this approach could reduce the rate and magnitude of misregistration between CT and PET,[23] at the cost of an increase in radiation dose of 0.4 mSv[28] compared with the 0.8 mSv associated with helical CT protocols. However, current implementations require a respiratory gating device to generate the average CT images, which introduces an additional element of complexity to the study.[29] Of note, researchers have proposed using CT calcium scans for AC purposes,[30] and it may be also possible to estimate coronary calcium from nongated low-dose CT attenuation maps.[31,32]

The maximum number of slices for the CT scanner component of a hybrid PET/CT is 128, and the largest detector coverage is 4 cm in the axial direction, enabling coronary artery CT imaging in about 5 to 6 seconds. To minimize radiation dose, automatic tube current control techniques are an integral part of most multislice PET/CT systems. Moreover, approaches have been developed to "virtually" double the number of simultaneously acquired slices in the axial dimension without reducing the detector size; 1 such approach relies on periodically moving the focal spot (z-flying focal spot) along the axial direction, increasing sampling and achieving high-resolution CT imaging with 0.3-mm isotropic resolution.

A 64-slice CT component with gantry rotation of 0.33 to 0.35 s, as available in the latest PET/CT, permits to combine, in 1 scanning session, high-quality coronary CT angiography with myocardial perfusion PET.[33,34] It should be noted that cardiac PET and coronary CT angiography images obtained on a hybrid PET/CT scanner are not truly simultaneous, because they are obtained in different breathing patterns. This difference may result in significant misalignments between PET and CT data, requiring software registration.[25] The 16-slice CT is sufficient to perform CT calcium scans, which could then be incorporated into routine hybrid PET/CT clinical imaging.[35]

RESPIRATORY GATING

Image blurring and CT–AC misregistration artifacts caused by the movement of the heart during breathing potentially could be corrected by respiratory gating.[36,37] Breathing motion can be detected by an infrared camera registering the movement of an infrared reflective marker on the patient's abdomen, or by an inductive respiration monitor with an elastic bellows/pressure sensor around the patient's chest (spirometry),[38–40] both hardware setups being provided by PET/CT scanners' vendors. These external breathing signals are then used as triggers to assign the PET events into appropriate respiratory phases during image reconstruction. Respiratory gating can also be used for correction of the upward creep of the heart, a frequent occurrence during exercise stress imaging.[41] Simultaneous acquisition of both respiratory and cardiac gating signals using bioimpedance techniques and signals obtained from standard ECG electrodes during cardiac PET[42] and techniques based on accelerometers[43] have been proposed recently, and have the potential to simplify the challenging logistics of dual gating for cardiac imaging. In addition, "self-gating" methods have been developed that derive the respiratory-gating signal retrospectively, from the raw list-mode PET data, rather than by using an external device (self-gating or data-driven gating).[36] Nevertheless, currently respiratory gating is not used in routine cardiac PET imaging, owing to the need for external hardware and complexity of acquisition.

REFERENCES

1. Piccinelli M, Garcia EV. Advances in Single-Photon Emission Computed Tomography Hardware and Software. Cardiol Clin 2016, in press.
2. Cherry S, Sorenson JA, Phelps ME. Physics in nuclear medicine. 3rd edition. Philadelphia: Saunders; 2003.
3. Fahey FH. Data acquisition in PET imaging. J Nucl Med Technol 2002;30:39–49.

4. Germano G, Hoffman EJ. A study of data loss and mispositioning due to pileup in 2-D detectors in PET. IEEE Trans Nucl Sci 1990;37:671–5.
5. Germano G, Hoffman EJ. An investigation of methods of pileup rejection for 2-D array detectors employed in high resolution PET. IEEE Trans Med Imaging 1991;10:223–7.
6. van Dam HT, Seifert S, Schaart DR. The statistical distribution of the number of counted scintillation photons in digital silicon photomultipliers: model and validation. Phys Med Biol 2012;57:4885–903.
7. Pichler B, Boning C, Lorenz E, et al. Studies with a prototype high resolution PET scanner based on LSO-APD modules. IEEE Trans Nucl Sci 1998;45:1298–302.
8. Klein R, Beanlands RS, deKemp RA. Quantification of myocardial blood flow and flow reserve: technical aspects. J Nucl Cardiol 2010;17:555–70.
9. LaForest R, Woodard PK, Gropler RJ. Cardiovascular PET/MR: Challenges and Opportunities. Cardiol Clin 2016, in press.
10. Available at: http://www.Google.Com/patents/us8314380. Accessed August 21, 2015.
11. Mullani N, Markham J, Ter-Pogossian M. Feasibility of time-of-flight reconstruction in positron emission tomography. J Nucl Med 1980;21:1095–7.
12. Lois C, Jakoby BW, Long MJ, et al. An assessment of the impact of incorporating time-of-flight information into clinical PET/CT imaging. J Nucl Med 2010;51:237–45.
13. Tomiyama T, Ishihara K, Suda M, et al. Impact of time-of-flight on qualitative and quantitative analyses of myocardial perfusion PET studies using 13n-ammonia. J Nucl Cardiol 2014;1–10.
14. Esteves FP, Nye JA, Khan A, et al. Prompt-gamma compensation in rb-82 myocardial perfusion 3d PET/CT. J Nucl Cardiol 2010;17:247–53.
15. Jakoby BW, Bercier Y, Conti M, et al. Physical and clinical performance of the MCT time-of-flight PET/CT scanner. Phys Med Biol 2011;56:2375–89.
16. Panin VY, Kehren F, Michel C, et al. Fully 3-D PET reconstruction with system matrix derived from point source measurements. IEEE Trans Med Imaging 2006;25:907–21.
17. Le Meunier L, Slomka PJ, Dey D, et al. Enhanced definition PET for cardiac imaging. J Nucl Cardiol 2010;17:414–26.
18. Akamatsu G, Ishikawa K, Mitsumoto K, et al. Improvement in PET/CT image quality with a combination of point-spread function and time-of-flight in relation to reconstruction parameters. J Nucl Med 2012;53:1716–22.
19. Bettinardi V, Presotto L, Rapisarda E, et al. Physical performance of the new hybrid PET/CT discovery-690. Med Phys 2011;38:5394–411.
20. Zaidi H. Is radionuclide transmission scanning obsolete for dual-modality PET/CT systems? Eur J Nucl Med Mol Imaging 2007;34:815–8.
21. Pan T, Mawlawi O, Nehmeh SA, et al. Attenuation correction of PET images with respiration-averaged CT images in PET/CT. J Nucl Med 2005;46:1481–7.
22. Bacharach SL. PET/CT attenuation correction: breathing lessons. J Nucl Med 2007;48:677–9.
23. Gould KL, Pan T, Loghin C, et al. Frequent diagnostic errors in cardiac PET/CT due to misregistration of CT attenuation and emission PET images: a definitive analysis of causes, consequences, and corrections. J Nucl Med 2007;48:1112–21.
24. Klingensmith WC 3rd, Noonan C, Goldberg JH, et al. Decreased perfusion in the lateral wall of the left ventricle in PET/CT studies with 13n-ammonia: evaluation in healthy adults. J Nucl Med Technol 2009;37:215–9.
25. Slomka P, Diaz M, Dey D, et al. Automatic registration of misaligned CT attenuation correction maps in rb-82 PET/CT improves detection of angiographically significant coronary artery disease. J Nucl Cardiol 2015. [Epub ahead of print].
26. Slomka PJ, Le Meunier L, Hayes SW, et al. Comparison of myocardial perfusion 82rb PET performed with CT- and transmission CT-based attenuation correction. J Nucl Med 2008;49:1992–8.
27. Bond S, Kadir T, Hamill J, et al. Automatic registration of cardiac PET/CT for attenuation correction. Paper presented at Nuclear Science Symposium Conference Record, 2008. NSS'08. IEEE. Dresden (Germany), October 19–25, 2008.
28. Pan T, Mawlawi O, Luo D, et al. Attenuation correction of PET cardiac data with low-dose average CT in PET/CT. Med Phys 2006;33:3931–8.
29. Alessio AM, Kohlmyer S, Branch K, et al. Cine CT for attenuation correction in cardiac PET/CT. J Nucl Med 2007;48:794–801.
30. Burkhard N, Herzog BA, Husmann L, et al. Coronary calcium score scans for attenuation correction of quantitative PET/CT 13n-ammonia myocardial perfusion imaging. Eur J Nucl Med Mol Imaging 2010;37:517–21.
31. Einstein AJ, Johnson LL, Bokhari S, et al. Agreement of visual estimation of coronary artery calcium from low-dose CT attenuation correction scans in hybrid PET/CT and SPECT/CT with standard agatston score. J Am Coll Cardiol 2010;56:1914–21.
32. Mylonas I, Kazmi M, Fuller L, et al. Measuring coronary artery calcification using positron emission tomography-computed tomography attenuation correction images. Eur Heart J Cardiovasc Imaging 2012;13:786–92.
33. Danad I, Raijmakers PG, Appelman YE, et al. Hybrid imaging using quantitative h215o PET and CT-based coronary angiography for the detection of coronary artery disease. J Nucl Med 2013;54:55–63.

34. Di Carli MF, Dorbala S, Hachamovitch R. Integrated cardiac PET-CT for the diagnosis and management of cad. J Nucl Cardiol 2006;13:139–44.
35. Hong C, Becker CR, Schoepf UJ, et al. Coronary artery calcium: absolute quantification in nonenhanced and contrast-enhanced multi-detector row CT studies. Radiology 2002;223:474–80.
36. Buther F, Dawood M, Stegger L, et al. List mode-driven cardiac and respiratory gating in PET. J Nucl Med 2009;50:674–81.
37. Martinez-Möller A, Zikic D, Botnar R, et al. Dual cardiac–respiratory gated PET: implementation and results from a feasibility study. Eur J Nucl Med Mol Imaging 2007;34:1447–54.
38. Li XA, Stepaniak C, Gore E. Technical and dosimetric aspects of respiratory gating using a pressure-sensor motion monitoring system. Med Phys 2006;33:145–54.
39. Nehmeh S, Erdi Y, Pan T, et al. Quantitation of respiratory motion during 4d-PET/CT acquisition. Med Phys 2004;31:1333–8.
40. Zhang T, Keller H, O'Brien MJ, et al. Application of the spirometer in respiratory gated radiotherapy. Med Phys 2003;30:3165–71.
41. Friedman J, Van Train K, Maddahi J, et al. "Upward creep" of the heart: a frequent source of false-positive reversible defects during thallium-201 stress-redistribution SPECT. J Nucl Med 1989;30:1718–22.
42. Koivumaki T, Nekolla SG, Furst S, et al. An integrated bioimpedance–ECG gating technique for respiratory and cardiac motion compensation in cardiac PET. Phys Med Biol 2014;59:6373–85.
43. Jafari Tadi M, Koivisto T, Pankaala M, et al. Accelerometer-based method for extracting respiratory and cardiac gating information for dual gating during nuclear medicine imaging. Int J Biomed Imaging 2014;2014:690124.
44. Maddahi J, Czernin J, Lazewatsky J, et al. Phase I, first-in-human study of bms747158, a novel f-18-labeled tracer for myocardial perfusion PET: dosimetry, biodistribution, safety, and imaging characteristics after a single injection at rest. J Nucl Med 2011;52:1490–8.
45. Maddahi J, Packard RRS. Cardiac PET perfusion tracers: current status and future directions. Semin Nucl Med 2014;44:333–43.
46. Stabin MG. Proposed revision to the radiation dosimetry of (Rb)-r-82. Health Phys 2010;99:811–3.
47. Ann ICRP. Radiation dose to patients from radiopharmaceuticals. Addendum 3 to ICRP publication 53. ICRP publication 106. Approved by the commission in October 2007. ICRP 2008;38:1–197.
48. Ann ICRP. Radiation dose to patients from radiopharmaceuticals. ICRP publication 53. ICRP 1988;18:1–4.
49. Ann ICRP. Radiation dose to patients from radiopharmaceuticals (addendum to ICRP publication 53). ICRP publication 80. ICRP 1998;28:1–126.
50. Akurathi V, Zhang S, Treves S, et al. Preliminary radiation dosimetry estimates for 18f-rhodamine 6g, a potential PET myocardial perfusion agent [abstract]. J Nucl Med 2013;54:1033.

Cardiovascular PET/MRI
Challenges and Opportunities

Richard LaForest, PhD, Pamela K. Woodard, MD, Robert J. Gropler, MD*

KEYWORDS

- Positron Emission Tomography (PET) • Magnetic Resonance Imaging (MRI) • PET/MRI
- Cardiovascular • Myocardium • Atherosclerosis

KEY POINTS

- The main advantages of PET/MRI over PET/computed tomography (CT) are the improved soft tissue contrast with MRI obtained without ionizing radiation and the potential for simultaneous acquisition of the PET and magnetic resonance images.
- The complexity of PET/MRI poses some significant technical challenges, which can be broadly characterized as accurate attenuation measurement, motion correction, and streamlining laboratory workflow.
- Clinical acceptance of PET/MRI requires the identification of clinical scenarios in which it has been found that simultaneously acquired information from PET and MRI is required.
- Numerous potential scenarios exist, including combined coronary angiography with measurements of perfusion and function and detection of atherosclerotic plaque and various myocardial diseases.
- Success of PET/MRI will depend in large part on the development of molecular imaging probes that exploit its strengths.

INTRODUCTION

Since its introduction in the early 2000, the hybridization of PET/CT has revolutionized medical imaging by the juxtaposition of functional PET images with high-resolution anatomic CT images. In the clinical setting, this colocalizing capability has been primarily exploited for oncologic purposes in which accurate attribution of biological activity specifically to tumor is of critical importance. In contrast, the colocalization capabilities of PET/CT have not been used to a large extent in cardiovascular (CV) disease, with CT attenuation correction of the PET images being the notable exception. This lack of use is the result of several factors, including the dearth of clinical indications in which the in-depth anatomic information afforded by CT is needed relative to the PET images (and vice versa), the complexities imparted by cardiac and respiratory motion on accurate colocalization, the logistical challenges to laboratory work flow imposed by sequential acquisition of the PET and CT images, and concerns for the risks associated with exposure to low-dose γ radiation and intravenous contrast.

More recently, systems combining PET and MRI have appeared on the market. The 2 main advantages of these systems over PET/CT are the improved soft tissue contrast with MRI obtained without ionizing radiation and the potential for simultaneous acquisition of the PET and MRI. However, its clinical acceptance has been slow for several reasons. Most notable is the high price of these systems in an environment in which reimbursement for using the technology is unclear. The

Conflict of Interest: Washington University has a Biograph mMR System and a Research Agreement with Siemens.

Mallinckrodt Institute of Radiology, Washington University School of Medicine, 4525 Scott Avenue, Suite 1307, St Louis, MO 63110, USA
* Corresponding author.
E-mail address: Groplerr@mir.wustl.edu

Cardiol Clin 34 (2016) 25–35
http://dx.doi.org/10.1016/j.ccl.2015.08.002
0733-8651/16/$ – see front matter

latter reflects the lack of evidence supporting the notion that key clinical information obtained with the simultaneous acquisition of PET and MRI data sets could not be acquired on separate PET and MR examinations. Moreover, significant technical challenges must be overcome from an image acquisition, processing, display, and laboratory workflow perspective for implementing CV PET/MRI on a routine clinical basis. However, the potential is high for PET/MRI to become an important tool in the treatment of the patient with CV disease. This review highlights this potential by discussing the current advantages of MRI versus CT and PET/MRI, the technical challenges in performing PET/MRI and incorporating it into laboratory workflow, and potential clinical scenarios in which PET/MRI might be beneficial in the context of CV imaging.

WHY PET/MRI?

The impetus for the development of PET/MRI reflected the relative advantages of MRI compared with CT (summarized in **Table 1**). Two key advantages for MRI over CT are the higher soft tissue contrast and the lack of radiation reduction exposure to the patient. Although for many applications, such as attenuation correction and coronary angiography, radiation strategies have been used.[1,2] Conversely, the use of electromagnetic fields in MRI generally precludes the imaging of patients with mechanical heart valves, pacemakers, or implantable cardioverter/defibrillators (ICDs). Thus, CT is of critical importance in the treatment of these patients. With respect to the assessment of left ventricular (LV) morphology and function, MRI is considered the gold standard, providing accurate and detailed measurements of LV mass, volume, regional, and global systolic function. Although CT can perform many of these measurements, they come at the cost of significant radiation exposure. Because of its ease of use and speed, CT is widely used for the noninvasive performance of coronary angiography. Moreover, as mentioned above, dose reduction strategies have significantly reduced radiation exposure. Although considerable progress continues for MR angiography, technical challenges still remain, such as the detrimental effects of cardiac, respiratory, and patient motion on image quality and solving the conundrum of attaining high spatial resolution while retaining adequate vessel-to-tissue contrast and signal-to-noise ratio all within an acceptable scanning time. Both MRI and CT require the use of intravenous contrast to enhance imaging for certain applications, however, MRI agents have a better side-effect profile compared with the iodinated CT contrast agents.[3] Moreover, many MRI measurements such as myocardial perfusion (eg, arterial spin labeling) and coronary angiography can be performed without contrast.[4,5] Characterization of tissue properties such as myocardial fiber orientation, the presence of extracellular water, cellular metabolism, and lipid content are possible with various MRI and spectroscopic techniques.[6–9] Tissue characterization with CT is much more limited because the imaging signal is based on differences in x-ray attenuation. Both MRI- and CT-based molecular imaging agents have been developed, with sensitivity being slightly better for MRI ($\sim 10^{-5}$ M) compared with CT ($\sim 10^{-3}$ M). Of note, sensitivity is significantly lower than what can be achieved with PET (10^{-11} to 10^{-12} M).[10] Imaging is faster and easier to perform with CT compared with MRI, which results in higher patent satisfaction and compliance. In addition, the greater complexity of MRI protocols requires greater involvement of highly trained personnel.

Table 1
Relative merits of CT and MRI

Consideration	CT	MRI
Soft tissue contrast	No	Yes
Ionizing radiation	Yes	No
Electromagnetic field	No	Yes
LV structure and function	Fair	Excellent
Angiography	Excellent	Fair
Risk of contrast agents	Low	Very low
Tissue characterization	Low	Excellent
Potential for molecular imaging	Fair	Moderate
Patient comfort	Excellent	Fair

PET/MRI SYSTEMS

Numerous PET/MRI designs have been explored including separate PET and MRI systems connected by an integrated bed system and, more recently, fully integrated PET/MRI systems. The technical specifications and performance characteristics of these systems have been comprehensively reviewed and are be detailed here.[11,12] Most recent development efforts have focused on integrated PET/MRI systems that permit simultaneous (or at least combined) acquisition of all imaging data. To integrate PET into an MRI system, a solution had to be devised to replace photomultiplier tubes, which provide the light read-out of a scintillation event in PET but do not operate in magnetic field because of the action of the Lorentz force electrons propagating in the tube, which prevent them from reaching the anode. The technical breakthrough came with the advent of semiconductor-based light detectors, such as avalanche photodiodes, which convert the scintillation light to electronic pulses.[13] These detectors offer the advantage of insensitivity to magnetic fields, which permits their application inside an MRI magnet and compactness that allows the construction of detectors small enough to be placed within the MRI gantry of an existing MRI magnet. In combined PET/MRI systems, the PET detector ring is installed inside the gradient coil and outside the RF coil. This installation results in a smaller ring diameter compared with PET/CT, which may preclude imaging in very large patients.

TECHNICAL CHALLENGES

The complexity of PET/MRI poses some significant technical challenges, which are broadly characterized as accurate attenuation measurement, motion correction, and streamlining laboratory workflow. The limited space in PET/MRI prevents the use of radioactive transmission sources for attenuation correction; therefore, a solution was sought to use an MRI sequence for this measurement. However, MRI does not provide direct information about the tissue density but about the magnetic properties of the proton spin. The 2-point DIXON MR sequence provides enough information about the tissue that allows segmentation of the body into 4 predefined classes: air, lungs, fat, and water (eg, muscle, organ) with fixed attenuation values.[14] We and others have found that the method works well but can be slightly less accurate in the presence of MR contrast agents because of reduced T1 values and metal objects owing to dephasing artifacts.[15,16]

Another challenge is the different acquisition schemes used by PET and MRI. As pointed out by others, with PET/MRI, the acquisitions are actually in parallel as opposed to truly simultaneous.[11] In the case of PET, volumetric data are acquired over a period of minutes (typically 10–30 min). The acquisition reflects the impact of all forms of motion (eg, cardiac, respiratory, and patient). This information can be time segmented into frames from a few seconds to minutes to generate dynamic data sets for compartmental modeling as well as electrocardiogram-gated to permit LV functional assessments and respiratory gated to correct for ventilatory motion. In contrast, MRI data acquisitions are typically acquired sequentially with acquisition times ranging from milliseconds to those that require several breath holds to complete, all with the goal of minimizing motion. In the case of the latter, this can lead to image artifacts caused by inaccurate image stacking as a result of inconsistent breath holding. Currently in PET/MRI, the ungated PET images are registered with end-systolic MR images that are acquired during breath hold in multiple orthogonal orientations. In addition to being time consuming, the lack of positional information in the PET images limits the potential accuracy of colocalization with the MR images. To circumvent this problem, numerous strategies are being devised ranging from various MRI free-breathing acquisitions to the application of motion correction software that uses the respiratory motion information embedded in the MRI and PET datasets.[17,18]

Finally, the integration to PET/MRI into the workflow of a clinical imaging laboratory is a challenge. Numerous issues still need to be solved, such as devising optimal image acquisition protocols, determining the level of physician oversight during image acquisition, implementing the best reconstruction algorithms, transfer and display of large datasets, and identifying and training the proper mix of physicians with the necessary skill sets for image interpretation. Solutions to these issues are now being developed at centers performing clinical PET/MRI and will continue to evolve with increased clinical use.

CRITERIA FOR CLINICAL ACCEPTANCE

As mentioned previously, clinical acceptance of PET/MRI requires the identification of clinical scenarios in which it has been demonstrated that information from PET and MRI is required and that acquiring the imaging data simultaneously leads to either improved disease detection or reduced risk of imaging that translates into better patient clinical outcomes. Broadly, these scenarios fall into 2 categories: combining different morphologic and biological parameters that characterize a disease to improve its detection or where accurate colocalization of diverse cellular/biological processes are required. Some examples of these scenarios are provided below.

Combining Different Morphologic and Biological Parameters

Combined coronary angiography and myocardial perfusion

One of the more intriguing possibilities of PET/CT is the capability to combine the detection of coronary artery stenoses by CT angiography with assessments of their physiologic significance based on PET measurements of myocardial perfusion. Indeed, combining these measurements suggests that significant improvements can be achieved in the detection of coronary artery disease, particularly multivessel disease, risk stratification, and in the colocalization of individual stenoses with areas of myocardial ischemia.[19,20] However, widespread acceptance of performing these combined measurements has been hampered by several factors including the requirement to perform them sequentially and the logistical difficulties this imposes on patient convenience and laboratory workflow, the increased radiation exposure that occurs when performing both imaging methods, and the risks associated with the use of iodinated contrast. PET/MRI can potentially overcome many of these challenges. The simultaneous acquisition of the morphologic and physiologic information can mitigate the patient convenience and laboratory workflow challenges of deciding on the order of studies, the need for real-time physician interpretation of images to decide if both studies are indicated, and the length of time required for the serial image acquisitions. Moreover, radiation exposure is reduced by the use of MR coronary angiography, and if contrast is needed, the gadolinium-based agents typically exhibit a better side-effect profile than the iodine based agents. As mentioned previously, MRI coronary angiography is not as easy to perform, accurate, or robust as CT coronary angiography. However, the difference in accuracy is less of an issue in the proximal coronary artery tree, which is also the location of coronary artery stenoses of greatest concern, because of its larger size and decreased motion compared with more distal sites.[21,22] One potential protocol that attempts to obtain this combined information is detailed in **Fig. 1**. After MRI measurement of attenuation, vasodilator stress is induced followed by the simultaneous intravenous administration of a gadolinium-based contrast agent and ^{13}N-ammonia. Subsequently, MRI measurements are obtained of the transmural extent relative stress flow abnormalities, the presence of myocardial scar (based on late gadolinium enhancement [LGE]), and presence or absence of stenoses in the proximal coronary arteries. Concurrent with the MRI acquisition are PET measurements of relative and absolute blood flow and regional and global LV function. After allowing for decay of the ^{13}N-ammonia, repeat PET measurements of

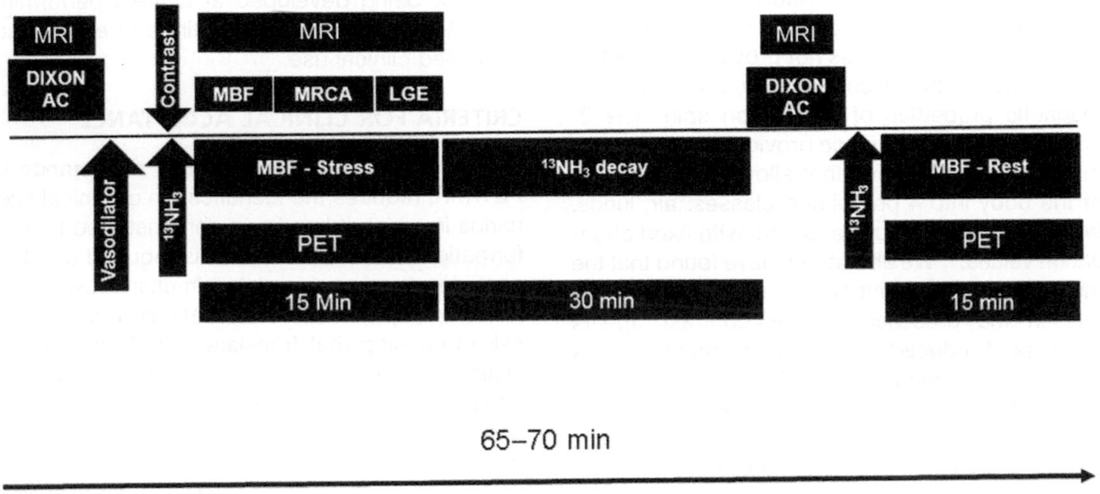

Fig. 1. Potential combined PET/MRI protocol. After attenuation correction with a 2-PT DIXON sequence, a vasodilator is administered intravenously followed by the injection of both gadolinium contrast and ^{13}N-ammonia ($^{13}NH_3$). Stress MR myocardial blood flow (MBF) imaging is performed by using a saturation recovery fast low angle shot (FLASH) sequence with parallel imaging technique. The contrast dose is 0.1 mmol/kg, and additional 0.05 mmol/kg is injected after the completion of the flow imaging for subsequence coronary artery imaging. The flow imaging covers 3 short-axis slices, that is, basal, middle, and apex, as well as a long-axis slice. The typical imaging parameters are repetition time (TR)/echo time (TE), 1.9/0.98 milliseconds; inversion time, 105 milliseconds; field of view (FOV), 380 × 380 mm^2; slice thickness, 8 mm; matrix, 192 × 154; flip angle, 10°; 50 images per slice. MR contrast-enhanced whole-heart coronary artery imaging is performed after the 90-second MR flow imaging and before LGE imaging. The total dose of the gadolinium is 0.15 mmol/kg. This whole-heart imaging is obtained by using a pencil-beam navigator-echo gradient-echo sequence with T2 preparation. The typical imaging parameters are TR/TE, 3.8/1.41 milliseconds; T2prep, 41 milliseconds; FOV, 360 × 247 × 112 mm^3; matrix, 256 × 176 x 80; segment number, 43; flip angle, 15°; scan time, 8 to 10 minutes. During MRI, list mode acquisition of the electrocardiogram-gated $^{13}NH_3$ PET data is performed. After allowing for decay of the $^{13}NH_3$, a repeat DIXON sequence is performed followed by the administration of $^{13}NH_3$ and a subsequent PET data acquisition to measure MBF at rest. The entire study typically takes about 65 to 70 minutes to complete.

relative and absolute blood flow and regional and global LV function are performed at rest. An example of some of the potential information that can be obtained is shown in **Fig. 2**. One of the advantages of PET/MRI is the tremendous flexibility in the imaging protocols that can be devised. An example is shown in **Fig. 3**. In this case, the rest and stress functional assessments are performed with MRI. The relative flow assessments are determined from the stress ^{13}N-ammonia study and the LGE study with the interpretation paradigm being the lack of LGE in a region with a stress perfusion abnormality indicates ischemia, whereas the presence of LGE indicates infarction. Quantitative stress perfusion is still obtained from the ^{13}N-ammonia study. ^{13}N-ammonia is the only radiotracer that used for clinical purposes because the infusion system required for Rb-82 administration is not MRI compatible and ^{15}O-water is not approved for clinical use in the United States. Although requiring further development and validation, such a protocol has the potential to provide all of the key elements for the comprehensive assessment of coronary artery disease, including proximal coronary anatomy, presence or absence of ischemia, quantitative stress blood flow, and LV functional reserve in less than 30 minutes.

Much of this information could be obtained by MRI alone. However, accurate quantitative measurements of blood flow with MRI over the entire LV have proven elusive because of the difficulty in obtaining an accurate arterial input function.[23]

Tumor

Cardiac tumors occur rarely, with most of a secondary nature (eg, metastases) versus primary in origin.[24] In the case of the latter, atrial myxoma in adults and rhabdomyosarcoma in children are the most common. Surgical removal, combined with radiation and chemotherapy in the case of malignancy, is the preferred therapy. Consequently, imaging plays a critical role in preoperative planning by accurate characterization of tumor type and its involvement from both to local and distal sites. After initial evaluation by echocardiography, both MRI and PET/CT are routinely used with MRI, providing exquisite anatomic detail of tumor morphology and its relationship to cardiac and vascular structures and PET/CT with 18F-fluorodeoxyglucose (FDG), adding additional information regarding tumor malignancy and staging.[25] Postoperatively, both of these techniques are used to identify tumor recurrence. Whether preoperative planning or posttherapy surveillance could be improved by obtaining this information simultaneously is unknown. Findings from an initial study of 20 patients with cardiac masses of various etiologies undergoing PET/MRI suggest that the combined information provided by both

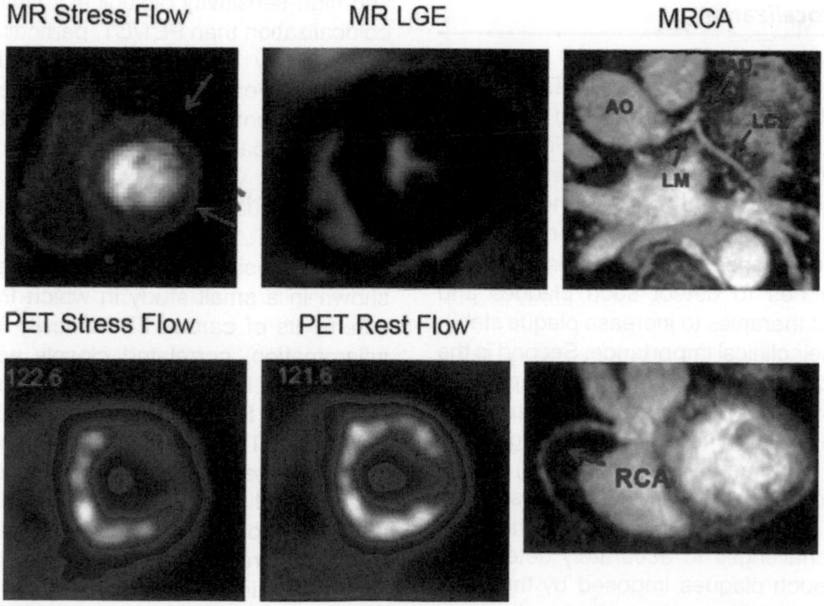

Fig. 2. Images from a study using the protocol in **Fig. 1** show a stress-induced subendocardial myocardial blood flow (MBF) deficit on the MR images and a similar MBF deficit on the PET images. The deficit resolves under resting conditions on the PET images, which is confirmed by the lack of LGE on the MR images. The MR coronary angiogram (MRCA) did not demonstrate significant stenosis, which was confirmed at x-ray angiography. AO, aortic outflow; LM, left main artery; LAD, left anterior descending artery; LCx, left circumflex artery; RCA, right coronary artery.

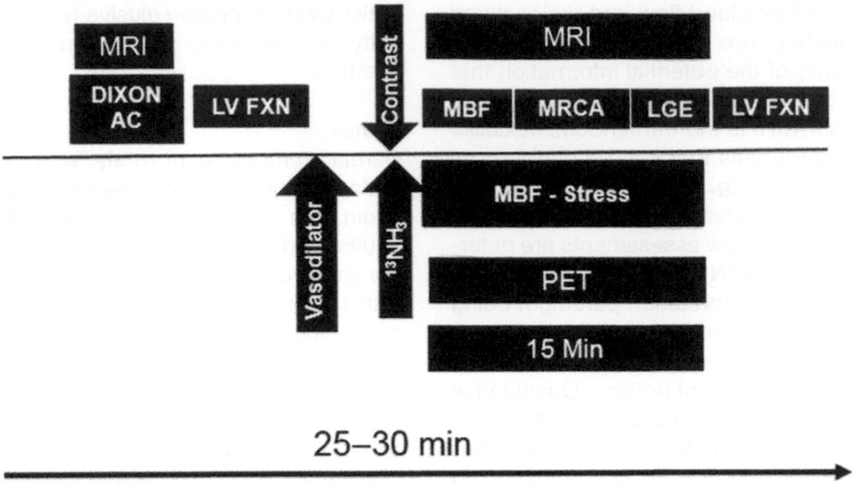

Fig. 3. Modification of protocol 1 that eliminates the rest PET study and adds rest and stress LV function assessments with MRI. Combining the stress PET and LGE permits detection of ischemia and infarction in areas with stress-induced MBF abnormalities measured by PET. The entire examination takes about 25 to 30 minutes to complete.

FDG-PET and MRI is superior to the individual assessments for tumor malignancy.[26] An example is shown in **Fig. 4**. However, given the small size of the study, it is unknown if the results are exportable to the general population and whether there are specific clinical scenarios such as the differentiation of posttherapy inflammation versus tumor recurrence where the PET/MRI acquisition would be beneficial.

Accurate Colocalization

Atherosclerotic plaque

There are many reasons why PET/MRI may be ideally suited for the detection and characterization of atherosclerotic plaque. First is the convincing evidence that the acute complications of atherosclerosis frequently occur in the presence of subclinical nonobstructive but high-risk atherosclerotic plaques. Indeed, the development of imaging approaches to detect such plaques and novel systemic therapies to increase plaque stability highlight their clinical importance. Second is the diverse composition of these high-risk plaques that is characterized by the complex interplay between unique anatomic features (eg, a large lipid-rich necrotic core and thin fibrous cap) and a host of molecular or cellular processes such as inflammation and neovascularization. Third are the imaging challenges to accurately detect and characterize such plaques imposed by the small size of key anatomic components, cardiac and respiratory motion, and the low level of expression of relevant biological signals. Fourth is the increasing evidence to suggest obtaining both PET and MRI parameters of plaque composition/biology (eg, inflammation based on FDG-PET and neovascularization based on delayed contrast enhancement MRI) may provide complementary information regarding plaque progression.[27] Finally, atherosclerosis is a systemic inflammatory process, which, in the future, may require whole-body imaging to either localize affected vascular beds or detect responses to novel anti-inflammatory therapies.[28] Thus, PET/MRI has the potential to provide high-resolution morphologic and high-sensitivity biological imaging with better colocalization than PET/CT, particularly in the coronary artery tree, where motion is most pronounced. Moreover, this is achieved at a lower risk from contrast media and radiation exposure when compared with the need for iodinated contrast for vascular imaging and multiple CT-based attenuation scans for whole-body imaging with PET/CT. The feasibility of PET/MRI to image atherosclerosis in the carotid arteries was recently shown in a small study in which PET/MRI measurements of carotid FDG activity (a measure of inflammation) correlated closely with those obtained with PET/CT.[29] An example is shown is **Fig. 5**. The figure also highlights that compared with PET/CT, the higher soft tissue contrast of MRI facilitates differentiation between the lumen and carotid artery wall, which should permit more complete plaque characterization and perhaps more accurate PET measurements of plaque activity in all vascular beds, particularly when combined with motion correction strategies.

Myocardial disease

There are several examples of where PET/MRI may provide unique information in the evaluation of LV

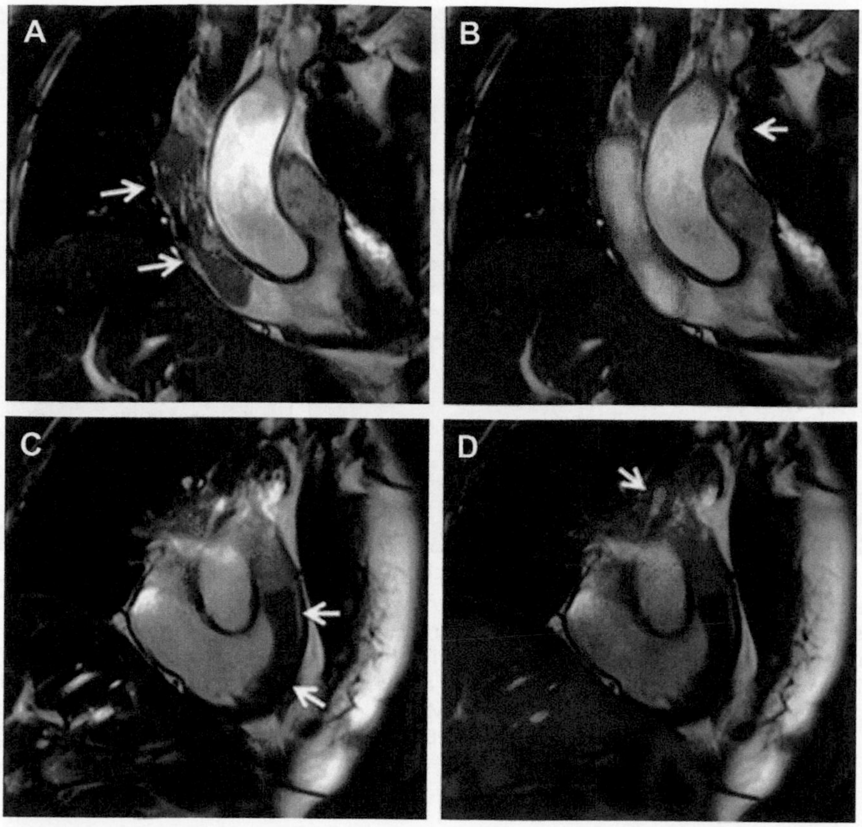

Fig. 4. (*A, B*) Patient with history of breast cancer. (*C, D*) Patient with anal cancer. In both patients, large intracavitary masses were initially found in echocardiography. Arrows in (*A, C*) show MR images of large tubular masses in the superior vena cava and right atrium (*A*) and in the right ventricular outflow tract (*C*). (*B, D*) Fusion images of MR and PET clearly show malignancy in the patient with breast cancer (*B*) and benign mass in the patient with anal cancer (*D*). However, closer inspection of PET images revealed mediastinal lymph node metastases in both patients (*B, D; arrows*). (*From* Nensa F, Tezgah E, Poeppel TD, et al. Integrated F-18 FDG PET/MRI in the assessment of cardiac masses: a pilot study. J Nucl Med 2015;56:258; with permission.)

myocardium in disease. Sarcoidosis is a systemic inflammatory, granulomatous disease of unknown etiology that is characterized histologically by noncaseating, nonnecrotic granulomas with the lymph nodes and lungs the most frequently involved organs. Cardiac involvement is much less frequent but carries a significantly worse prognosis. The clinical manifestations of cardiac sarcoidosis range from asymptomatic, evidence of restrictive cardiomyopathy, conduction abnormalities, to sudden cardiac death. Unfortunately, clinical confirmation of cardiac sarcoidosis has proven elusive because of the nonspecificity of disease manifestations, the lack of a clinical gold standard, and the limitations of endomyocardial biopsy. Both PET and MRI have proven useful in the diagnosis of sarcoidosis. PET and FDG provides information on inflammatory disease activity.[30] Moreover, demonstration of flow abnormalities with PET perfusion imaging suggests myocardial fibrosis.[31] With MRI, early enhancement of sarcoid granulomas on T2-weighted images suggests the presence of inflammation and edema, whereas LGE is consistent with fibrotic changes and scarring.[30] Thus, PET/MRI might provide unique and valuable information in the treatment of these patients. For example, the combined approach could provide confirmatory information regarding inflammation (presence of glucose metabolism and increased edema), which might increase confidence to proceed with anti-inflammatory therapy. In contrast, the presence and location of scar could provide evidence for the prediction for ventricular arrhythmias and guidance for potential ablative therapy or lead placement in the setting of ICD placement.

Increasing evidence shows that the magnitude and duration of the inflammatory response after myocardial infarction is a predictor of adverse LV remodeling and subsequent heart failure.[32] The inflammatory response reflects the release of

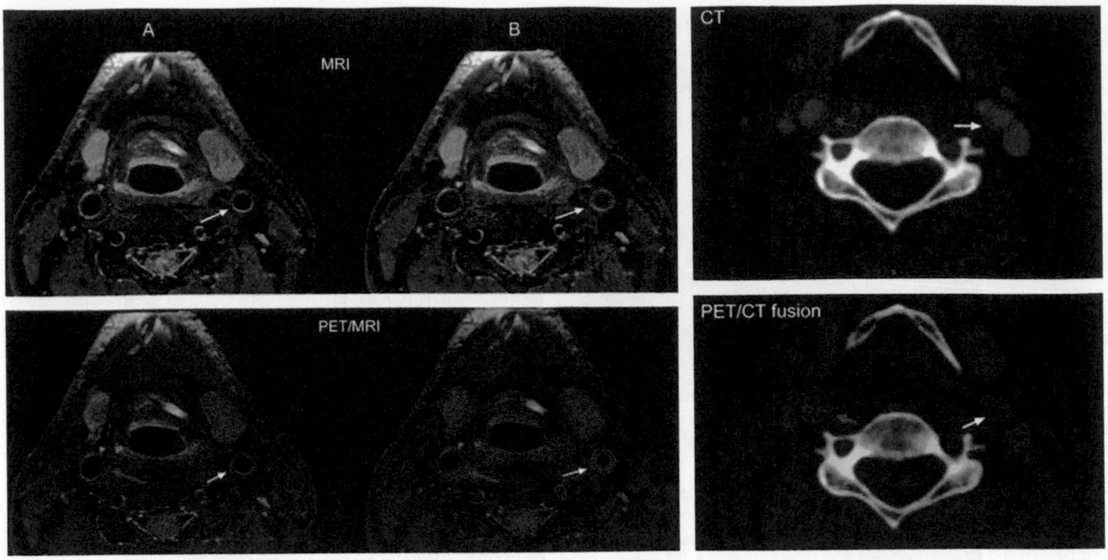

Fig. 5. (*Left*) Example of transverse MRI and fused FDG-PET/MRI at a level with the right common carotid artery (*red arrow*) and the left internal carotid artery (*white arrow*). A region of interest including both the vessel wall and lumen is drawn in column A, and a region of interest including only the vessel wall is drawn in column B. (*Right*) Example of transverse CT and fused FDG-PET/CT. The right common carotid artery is marked by a red arrow and the left internal carotid artery is marked by a white arrow. A region of interest including both the vessel wall and lumen is drawn. (*From* Ripa RS, Knudsen A, Hag AM, et al. Feasibility of simultaneous PET/MR of the carotid artery: first clinical experience and comparison to PET/CT. Am J Nucl Med Mol Imaging 2013;3:364; with permission.)

progenitor cells and proinflammatory cells from the bone marrow and spleen that are delivered to the myocardium.[33] It was recently found that this increased inflammatory response can be detected in myocardium using PET with FDG at the site of infarction delineated by MRI and LGE.[34] Moreover, consistent with the systemic nature of this inflammatory response, both the spleen and bone marrow demonstrate increased FDG uptake, suggestive of activation of proinflammatory cells. Although it requires further study, it seems that PET/MRI could provide a more comprehensive evaluation of post–myocardial infarction remodeling and potentially guide novel immune-modulatory therapeutic strategies.

Sudden cardiac death accounts for up to approximately 360,000 deaths per year with ventricular tachycardia and fibrillation accounting for most.[35] Reduced LV ejection ($\leq$35%) is still the best discriminator of high- and low-risk groups and is the primary criteria for implantation of ICDs for primary prevention. Unfortunately, this criteria underestimates patients at risk given that about 70% of sudden cardiac death patients have an LV ejection fraction of greater than 35%.[35] Thus, more accurate criteria are needed for identification candidates for ICD placement. There are numerous other tissue parameters that may help in this regard including the presence of myocardial scar measured by MRI and LGE, amount of denervated myocardium measured by PET using the neuronal function radiotracer carbon-11 hydroxyephedrine, and the presence of ischemia measured by dobutamine echocardiography.[36–38] Recently, a fluorine-18 neuronal radiotracer has undergone initial human evaluation.[39] Moreover, myocardial ischemia can be detected with PET and FDG.[40] Although requiring further development and validation studies, the likely importance of close juxtaposition of scar, denervated myocardium, and ischemia in the pathogenesis of ventricular arrhythmia suggests PET/MRI could be useful in the assessment of patients being considered for ICD placement or target ablative therapy.

MOLECULAR IMAGING AND THE FUTURE OF CARDIOVASCULAR PET/MRI

In many ways CV PET/MRI is ideally suited for the implementation of new molecular imaging probes. Beyond the high sensitivity and spatial resolution engendered by the hybrid system, the potential for accurate colocalization and sophisticated motion correction will greatly increase the likelihood of noninvasively detecting cellular and molecular

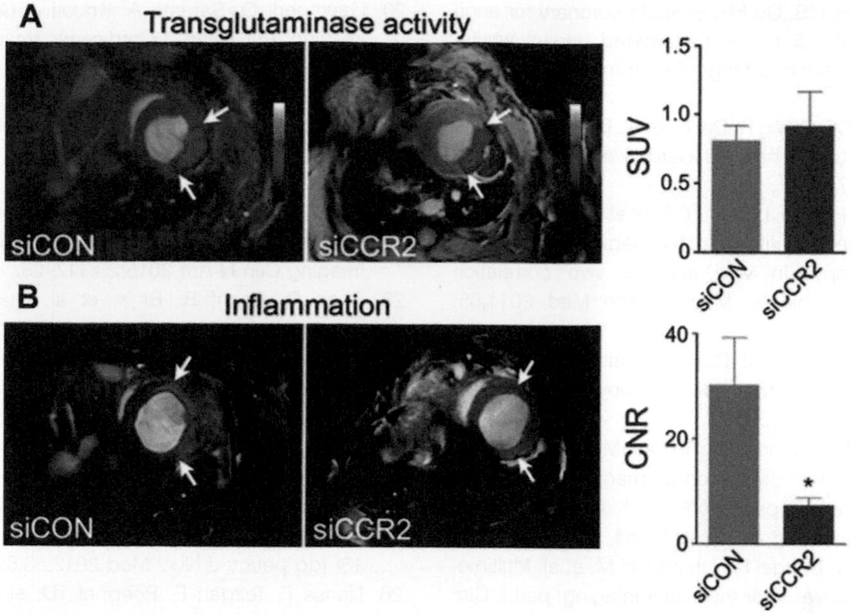

Fig. 6. Dual-target molecular PET/MRI after therapeutic RNA silencing of chemokine C receptor 2 (CCR2). (*A*) Short-axis PET/MR images after respective siRNA treatment. Bar graph of standard uptake value (SUV) shows no difference in fluorine-18–labeled affinity peptide (^{18}F-FXIII) PET signal between treatment groups (n = 5 per group). (*B*) Short-axis MRI shows myeloperoxidase-activatable gadolinium-based MRI agent (MPO-Gd) signal enhancement in siRNA control RNA (siCON)-treated mice and reduced enhancement in siRNA against CCR2 (siCCR2)-treated mice. Arrows indicate infarct area. Bar graph shows contrast-to-noise ratio (CNR). Data are mean ± SEM. [a] $P<.05$. (*From* Majmudar MD, Keliher EJ, Heidt T, et al. Monocyte-directed RNAI targeting CCR2 improves infarct healing in atherosclerosis-prone mice. Circulation 2013;127:2043; with permission.)

signals of interest in humans. Moreover, the ability to detect 2 different signals greatly increases the potential for therapeutically linked molecular imaging or theranostics. For example, one could envision a multifunctional molecular imaging agent that detects a specific process with a targeted PET approach, delivers a therapy to treat that process, and then demonstrates a therapeutic response using an activatable MR probe. An example of this potential is shown in **Fig. 6**. Consequently, the ultimate success of the PET/MRI development will depend in large part on the clinical translation and acceptance of novel molecular imaging probes.

Beyond molecular imaging, the ability to perform whole-body imaging without the need for CT attenuation and vascular imaging without iodinated contrast will facilitate our ability to investigate the systemic nature of most forms of CV disease. In addition, it will provide the opportunity for more complete delineation of responses to novel therapeutics, particularly those that act systemically.

Thus, PET/MRI is slowly being introduced into clinical management schemes of cardiac patients. However, widespread use will require identification and acceptance of those clinical scenarios in which the unique capabilities of PET/MRI are warranted over either PET and MRI or PET/CT. In parallel, solutions need to be devised to address the numerous technical issues (eg, motion correction) and workflow challenges (eg, data management and interpretation) along with the development of the molecular imaging probes designed to exploit this exciting technology.

REFERENCES

1. Fink C, Krissak R, Henzler T, et al. Radiation dose at coronary ct angiography: second-generation dual-source ct versus single-source 64-mdct and first-generation dual-source ct. AJR Am J Roentgenol 2011;196:W550–7.
2. Koepfli P, Hany TF, Wyss CA, et al. Ct attenuation correction for myocardial perfusion quantification using a pet/ct hybrid scanner. J Nucl Med 2004;45:537–42.
3. Weinreb JC. Which study when? Is gadolinium-enhanced mr imaging safer than iodine-enhanced ct? Radiology 2008;249:3–8.
4. Zhang H, Shea SM, Park V, et al. Accurate myocardial t1 measurements: toward quantification of myocardial blood flow with arterial spin labeling. Magn Reson Med 2005;53:1135–42.

5. Jin H, Zeng MS, Ge MY, et al. 3d coronary mr angiography at 1.5 t: Volume-targeted versus whole-heart acquisition. J Magn Reson Imaging 2013;38:594–602.
6. Sosnovik DE, Wang R, Dai G, et al. Diffusion mr tractography of the heart. J Cardiovasc Magn Reson 2009;11:47.
7. O'Connor RD, Xu J, Ewald GA, et al. Intramyocardial triglyceride quantification by magnetic resonance spectroscopy: In vivo and ex vivo correlation in human subjects. Magn Reson Med 2011;65:1234–8.
8. Holloway CJ, Suttie J, Dass S, et al. Clinical cardiac magnetic resonance spectroscopy. Prog Cardiovasc Dis 2011;54:320–7.
9. Ferreira VM, Piechnik SK, Robson MD, et al. Myocardial tissue characterization by magnetic resonance imaging: novel applications of t1 and t2 mapping. J Thorac Imaging 2014;29:147–54.
10. Sinusas AJ, Bengel F, Nahrendorf M, et al. Multimodality cardiovascular molecular imaging, part I. Circ Cardiovasc Imaging 2008;1:244–56.
11. Rischpler C, Nekolla SG, Dregely I, et al. Hybrid pet/mr imaging of the heart: potential, initial experiences, and future prospects. J Nucl Med 2013;54:402–15.
12. Catana C, Guimaraes AR, Rosen BR. Pet and mr imaging: the odd couple or a match made in heaven? J Nucl Med 2013;54:815–24.
13. Pichler B, Lorenz E, Mirzoyan R, et al. Readout of lutetium oxyorthosilicate crystals with avalanche photodiodes for high resolution positron emission tomography. Biomed Tech (Berl) 1997;42(Suppl):37–8 [in German].
14. Coombs BD, Szumowski J, Coshow W. Two-point dixon technique for water-fat signal decomposition with b0 inhomogeneity correction. Magn Reson Med 1997;38:884–9.
15. Vontobel J, Liga R, Possner M, et al. Mr-based attenuation correction for cardiac fdg pet on a hybrid pet/mri scanner: comparison with standard ct attenuation correction. Eur J Nucl Med Mol Imaging 2015;42:1574–80.
16. Lau JM, Laforest R, Sotoudeh H, et al. Evaluation of attenuation correction in cardiac pet using PET/MR. J Nucl Cardiol 2015. [Epub ahead of print].
17. Manber R, Thielemans K, Hutton BF, et al. Practical pet respiratory motion correction in clinical pet/mr. J Nucl Med 2015;56:890–6.
18. Furst S, Grimm R, Hong I, et al. Motion correction strategies for integrated pet/mr. J Nucl Med 2015;56:261–9.
19. Pazhenkottil AP, Nkoulou RN, Ghadri JR, et al. Prognostic value of cardiac hybrid imaging integrating single-photon emission computed tomography with coronary computed tomography angiography. Eur Heart J 2011;32:1465–71.
20. Gaemperli O, Saraste A, Knuuti J. Cardiac hybrid imaging. Eur Heart J Cardiovasc Imaging 2012;13:51–60.
21. Mavrogeni S, Markousis-Mavrogenis G, Kolovou G. Contribution of cardiovascular magnetic resonance in the evaluation of coronary arteries. World J Cardiol 2014;6:1060–6.
22. Ishida M, Sakuma H. Coronary mr angiography revealed: how to optimize image quality. Magn Reson Imaging Clin N Am 2015;23:117–25.
23. Chen D, Sharif B, Bi X, et al. Quantification of myocardial blood flow using non-electrocardiogram-triggered mri with three-slice coverage. Magn Reson Med 2015. [Epub ahead of print].
24. Butany J, Nair V, Naseemuddin A, et al. Cardiac tumours: diagnosis and management. Lancet Oncol 2005;6:219–28.
25. Rahbar K, Seifarth H, Schafers M, et al. Differentiation of malignant and benign cardiac tumors using 18f-fdg pet/ct. J Nucl Med 2012;53:856–63.
26. Nensa F, Tezgah E, Poeppel TD, et al. Integrated 18f-fdg pet/mr imaging in the assessment of cardiac masses: a pilot study. J Nucl Med 2015;56:255–60.
27. Calcagno C, Ramachandran S, Izquierdo-Garcia D, et al. The complementary roles of dynamic contrast-enhanced mri and 18f-fluorodeoxyglucose pet/ct for imaging of carotid atherosclerosis. Eur J Nucl Med Mol Imaging 2013;40:1884–93.
28. Ridker PM, Luscher TF. Anti-inflammatory therapies for cardiovascular disease. Eur Heart J 2014;35:1782–91.
29. Ripa RS, Knudsen A, Hag AM, et al. Feasibility of simultaneous pet/mr of the carotid artery: first clinical experience and comparison to pet/ct. Am J Nucl Med Mol Imaging 2013;3:361–71.
30. Schatka I, Bengel FM. Advanced imaging of cardiac sarcoidosis. J Nucl Med 2014;55:99–106.
31. Osborne M, Kolli S, Padera RF, et al. Use of multimodality imaging to diagnose cardiac sarcoidosis as well as identify recurrence following heart transplantation. J Nucl Cardiol 2013;20:310–2.
32. Maekawa Y, Anzai T, Yoshikawa T, et al. Prognostic significance of peripheral monocytosis after reperfused acute myocardial infarction: a possible role for left ventricular remodeling. J Am Coll Cardiol 2002;39:241–6.
33. Dutta P, Nahrendorf M. Monocytes in myocardial infarction. Arterioscler Thromb Vasc Biol 2015;35:1066–70.
34. Wollenweber T, Bengel FM. Molecular imaging to predict ventricular arrhythmia in heart failure. J Nucl Cardiol 2014;21:1096–109.
35. Chugh SS, Reinier K, Teodorescu C, et al. Epidemiology of sudden cardiac death: clinical and research implications. Prog Cardiovasc Dis 2008;51:213–28.

36. Klem I, Weinsaft JW, Bahnson TD, et al. Assessment of myocardial scarring improves risk stratification in patients evaluated for cardiac defibrillator implantation. J Am Coll Cardiol 2012;60:408–20.
37. Fallavollita JA, Heavey BM, Luisi AJ Jr, et al. Regional myocardial sympathetic denervation predicts the risk of sudden cardiac arrest in ischemic cardiomyopathy. J Am Coll Cardiol 2014;63:141–9.
38. Elhendy A, Chapman S, Porter TR, et al. Association of myocardial ischemia with mortality and implantable cardioverter-defibrillator therapy in patients with coronary artery disease at risk of arrhythmic death. J Am Coll Cardiol 2005;46:1721–6.
39. Sinusas AJ, Lazewatsky J, Brunetti J, et al. Biodistribution and radiation dosimetry of lmi1195: first-in-human study of a novel 18f-labeled tracer for imaging myocardial innervation. J Nucl Med 2014;55:1445–51.
40. Dou KF, Yang MF, Yang YJ, et al. Myocardial 18f-fdg uptake after exercise-induced myocardial ischemia in patients with coronary artery disease. J Nucl Med 2008;49:1986–91.

Radionuclide Tracers for Myocardial Perfusion Imaging and Blood Flow Quantification

Robert A. deKemp, PhD, PEng, PPhys[a,b,*], Jennifer M. Renaud, MSc[a], Ran Klein, PhD[c], Rob S.B. Beanlands, MD, FRCPC[a]

KEYWORDS

• Myocardial blood flow • Coronary flow reserve • Myocardial perfusion imaging

KEY POINTS

- An ideal tracer for quantification of myocardial blood flow (MBF) should have a high extraction fraction (close to 1.0) from blood to tissue.
- Tracer retention fraction is always lower than the extraction fraction, due to the effects of tracer washout.
- Perfusion imaging tracers have extraction and retention fractions that decrease nonlinearly with MBF.
- Tracer retention increases continuously with myocardial blood flow, without any plateau or roll-off at high-flow values.

INTRODUCTION

Stress myocardial perfusion imaging (MPI) can be performed using many different radiolabeled compounds (tracers) with either single-photon emission computed tomography (SPECT) or PET imaging technology. These tracers have different physical and biological properties that determine their ability to identify regions of local ischemia. These tissues are supplied by coronary arteries that are the clinical targets for revascularization by percutaneous coronary intervention (PCI) or coronary artery bypass grafting (CABG).

For many years, invasive coronary angiography has been the accepted gold standard for the detection of obstructive coronary artery disease (CAD), typically defined as a focal narrowing of the arterial lumen greater than 50% to 70% of

Conflicts of Interest: R.A. deKemp and R. Klein receive royalty revenues from rubidium PET technology licensed to Jubilant DraxImage. R.A. deKemp, J.M. Renaud, and R. Klein receive royalty revenues from FlowQuant software licensed to INVIA Medical Imaging. R.A. deKemp, J.M. Renaud, R. Klein, and R.S.B. Beanlands are consultants for Jubilant DraxImage. R.S.B. Beanlands is a consultant for Lantheus Medical Imaging.
This work was supported in part by a medical research grant (Rb-ARMI) from the Canadian Institutes of Health Research (MIS - 100935). R.S.B. Beanlands is a career scientist, supported by the Heart and Stroke Foundation of Ontario, the Vered Chair of Cardiology, and the University of Ottawa Tier 1 Chair in Cardiovascular Imaging Research.
[a] National Cardiac PET Center, Cardiac Imaging Department, University of Ottawa Heart Institute, 40 Ruskin Street, Ottawa, Ontario K1Y 4W7, Canada; [b] Division of Cardiology, Department of Medicine, University of Ottawa Heart Institute, 40 Ruskin Street, Ottawa, Ontario K1Y 4W7, Canada; [c] Division of Nuclear Medicine, Department of Medicine, The Ottawa Hospital, 1053 Carling Avenue, Ottawa, Ontario K1Y 4E9, Canada
* Corresponding author. National Cardiac PET Center, Cardiac Imaging Department, University of Ottawa Heart Institute, 40 Ruskin Street, Ottawa, Ontario K1Y 4W7, Canada.
E-mail address: RAdeKemp@ottawaheart.ca

http://dx.doi.org/10.1016/j.ccl.2015.08.001
0733-8651/16/$ – see front matter

the diameter. Stress MPI relative reductions in tracer uptake (defects) less than 60% to 75% of maximum (outside the normal range) uptake have been shown in many studies to have very good utility for identification of obstructive CAD,[1] with accuracy in the range of 80% for SPECT and 90% for PET.[2]

More recently, the physiologic significance of epicardial coronary lesions is also assessed using invasive measurements of fractional flow reserve (FFR) to identify and treat disease associated with myocardial ischemia, defined as FFR less than 0.75 to 0.80 (75%–80% of unobstructed coronary flow).[3] Ischemic myocardium associated with focal flow-limiting disease can be identified noninvasively as regions with reversible perfusion defects (abnormal at stress, normal at rest) by relative MPI. In patients with multivessel or microvascular disease, the sensitivity and prognostic value can be improved using absolute quantification of myocardial blood flow (MBF) at rest and stress to identify abnormal stress/rest myocardial flow reserve (MFR) less than 2.0 to 2.5.[4–7]

This review describes the important tracer properties for stress MPI and blood flow quantification, as required for the identification of CAD and myocardial ischemia.

IDEAL PERFUSION TRACER PROPERTIES

The most important (necessary) properties for a tracer to be used for relative MPI with SPECT or PET are listed in **Table 1**. High-quality (contrast, resolution, noise) images should be obtained regardless of patient size and shape. Interpretation should be highly reliable and related to the underlying disease processes of CAD and myocardial ischemia to direct appropriate therapy and improve patient outcomes.

Additional properties (desirable) for a tracer to be used for absolute quantification of MBF (mL/min/g) as well as relative MPI are listed in **Table 2**. MBF quantification offers incremental diagnostic and prognostic information, but should not compromise the necessary properties for MPI listed above. A tracer with high first-pass extraction fraction is ideally suited for accurate MBF quantification with high precision and test-retest repeatability. The use of PET imaging with simple and accurate attenuation correction reduces artifacts that may otherwise be interpreted as false-positive MPI or MBF defects, but at the expense of increased capital equipment and operating costs currently.

MBF quantification requires data acquisition starting from the time of tracer injection, and reconstruction of a dynamic image series measuring the time-dependent distribution of the tracer from arterial blood into the myocardial tissue. Dynamic imaging is not compatible with treadmill exercise stress and therefore requires the use of pharmacologic stress, typically with coronary vasodilators. The use of short-lived PET tracers such as ^{82}Rb, ^{13}N-ammonia, or ^{15}O-water enables rapid single-session acquisition of combined MBF and MPI at rest and stress. Similar throughput may be possible with longer-lived ^{18}F- or ^{99m}Tc-labeled tracers, but requires subtraction of residual rest activity from the subsequent stress scan to maintain accuracy. The supply cost of the PET tracers is currently a limiting

Table 1
Necessary tracer properties for myocardial perfusion imaging

Property	Clinical Benefit
High heart-to-background contrast (low lung, liver, stomach, gut uptake)	Reduced spillover of activity from adjacent organs
High retention; slow washout from the heart (stable over time)	Effective myocardial perfusion visualization
High normal-to-disease contrast	Identification of defects reflecting stenosis
High stress-to-rest contrast	Identification of reversibility reflecting ischemia
Compatible with exercise and pharmacological-stress	Effective ECG interpretation
Measures electrocardiogram (ECG)-gated left ventricle function	Determination of contractile reserve
High diagnostic accuracy	Identification of CAD and ischemia
High prognostic value	Risk stratification
High patient outcome benefit	Direct effective therapy
Good availability	Cost-effective

Table 2
Desirable tracer properties for absolute myocardial blood flow and relative myocardial perfusion imaging

Property	Clinical Benefit
High physiologic extraction and high retention	High sensitivity
Low rate of false-positive artifacts	High specificity
Low test-retest variability	High precision
High diagnostic confidence	Direct effective therapy
Low radiation dose	Maximize benefit-to-risk ratio
Available supply and low operating costs	Minimize expenses
Low overhead and fixed costs (scanners, staffing)	Effective resource utilization
Fast imaging times	Maximize throughput and patient convenience

factor for widespread adoption. The availability of small dedicated cyclotrons may help to reduce the cost of ^{15}O-water and ^{13}N-ammonia, and the fixed costs of ^{82}Rb generators can be offset at sites with high cardiac patient volumes.

List-mode imaging with PET (**Fig. 1**) provides the capability for routine MBF quantification in addition to MPI without the need for additional tracer administration or imaging time, because images are typically acquired immediately following tracer injection at rest or using pharmacologic stress agents. Similar methods are also under development for MBF quantification using dynamic SPECT imaging.[8–11]

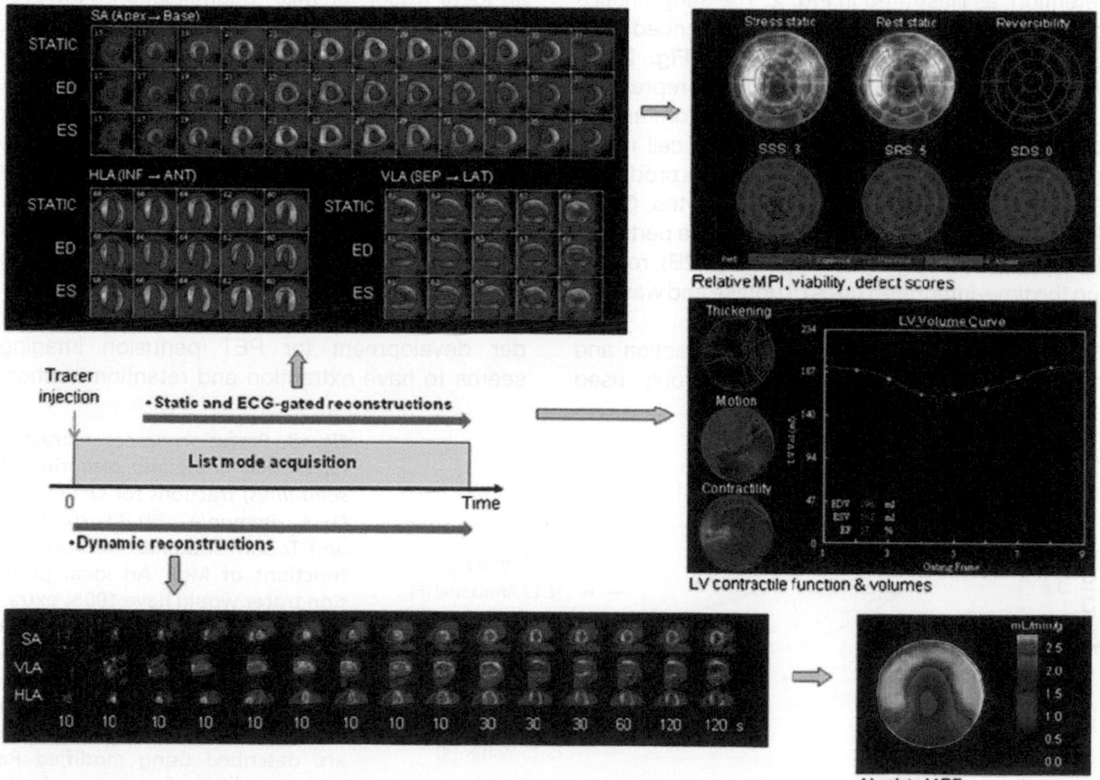

Fig. 1. List-mode acquisition for PET and SPECT perfusion imaging is used to store all recorded counts in a single scan-file starting at the time of tracer injection. The list-mode files can be used to reconstruct separate series of electrocardiogram-gated, respiratory-gated (not shown), ungated (*static*), and dynamic images. LV, left ventricle. (*From* Renaud JM, Beanlands RSB, deKemp RA. PET instrumentation. In: Heller GV, Hendel RC, editors. Handbook of nuclear cardiology: cardiac PET and SPECT. London: Springer; 2013. p. 131; with permission.)

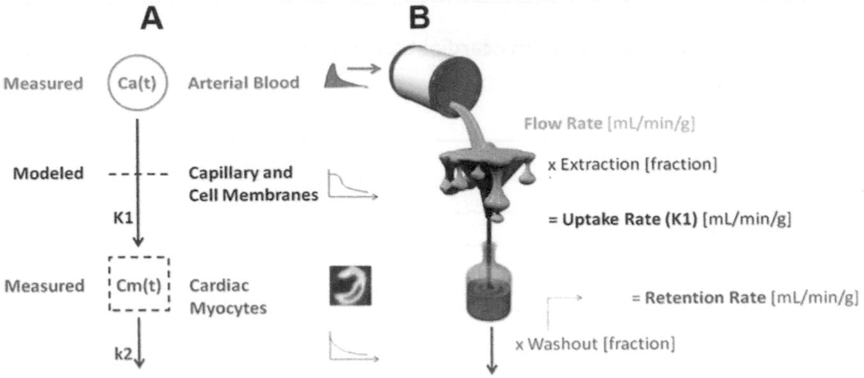

Fig. 2. Perfusion tracer kinetics described using a one-tissue-compartment model in (*A*). Tracer concentration is measured in arterial blood Ca(t) and in the target tissues Cm(t). K1 is the rate of uptake from blood to tissue, which is equal to MBF (Flow) times the tracer extraction fraction ($1 - e^{-PS/Flow}$); PS is the capillary (and cell) membrane permeability × surface-area product (mL/min/g). k2 is the rate of washout from the target tissues. The concepts of tracer extraction and retention are illustrated in (*B*). Tracer extraction fraction is the uptake rate ÷ flow rate, whereas tracer retention fraction is the retention rate ÷ flow rate (including the effect of tracer washout = e^{-k2t}). The units of measurement are shown in square brackets.

Among the criteria listed above for relative MPI and MBF quantification, it is important to emphasize the distinction between tracer extraction and retention, as illustrated in **Fig. 2**. The early kinetics of most perfusion tracers can be described by a one-tissue-compartment model (see **Fig. 2**A).[12] The tracer uptake rate, K1 (mL/min/g), represents the unidirectional transport (or influx) from arterial blood, Ca(t), across the capillary and cell membranes (with Permeability × Surface-area product = PS [mL/min/g]) into the cardiac myocytes, Cm(t). For MPI, tracer retention is measured at a particular time point following injection (see **Fig. 2**B), reflecting the time-integrated rates of uptake and washout (efflux), denoted as k2 (fraction/min).

Fig. 3 shows the differences in extraction and retention fractions for several commonly used PET and SPECT perfusion tracers. ^{15}O-water has close to 100% extraction over a wide range of flow values and is therefore often referred to as an ideal tracer for MBF quantification. However, the washout rate of water is also very high (and proportional to flow); therefore, this tracer is not retained in the myocardium and is not suitable for standard MPI, including assessment of cardiac function: ejection fraction, wall motion, and thickening. ^{13}N-ammonia extraction also remains close to 100% at rest and stress, and therefore, is an excellent MBF tracer. It also has the highest retention of all the conventional perfusion tracers, remaining higher than 50% over the full range of rest and stress flows. ^{18}F-flurpiridaz, which is under development for PET perfusion imaging, seems to have extraction and retention fractions

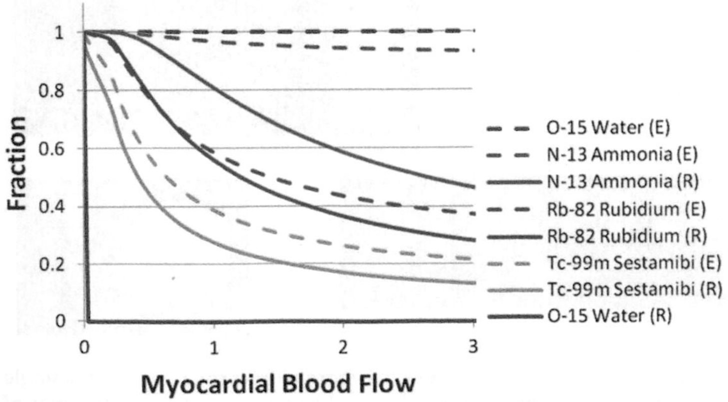

Fig. 3. Perfusion tracer extraction (E; *dashed lines*) and retention (R; *solid lines*) fractions for O-15 water, N-13 ammonia, Rb-82 rubidium, and Tc-99m sestamibi, as nonlinear functions of MBF. An ideal perfusion tracer would have 100% extraction and 100% retention (no washout). Current tracers all have retention less than extraction due to some degree of tracer washout. The extraction and retention curves are described using modified Renkin-Crone[14,15] functions of the form $1 - e^{-PS/MBF}$. (*Data from* Renkin EM. Transport of potassium-42 from blood to tissue in isolated mammalian skeletal muscles. Am J Physiol 1959;197:1205–10; and Crone C. Permeability of capillaries in various organs as determined by use of the indicator diffusion method. Acta Physiol Scand 1963;58:292–305.)

Table 3
Common perfusion tracer properties (in order of decreasing extraction)

Tracer	Half-life (Production)	Extraction (Stress-Rest)	Retention (Stress-Rest)	Dose (mSv/GBq)	MPI	MBF	Strength	Weakness
O-15 water	2 min (cyclotron)	1.00	0.0	1.1	−−	++	MBF standard	MPI not feasible
N-13 ammonia	10 min (cyclotron)	0.95–0.99	0.50–0.90	2.0	++	++	MPI and MBF	Lung, liver uptake
Tl-201 thallium	73 h (cyclotron)	0.45–0.70	0.35–0.70	220	+	−	MPI and viability	High dose
Rb-82 rubidium	1.25 min (generator)	0.40–0.70	0.30–0.70	0.8	++	+	Fast MPI and MBF	High cost
Tc-99m sestamibi	6 h (generator)	0.20–0.50	0.15–0.45	9.0	+	−	MPI standard	MBF not available
Tc-99m tetrofosmin	6 h (generator)	0.15–0.40	0.10–0.35	7.6	+	−	MPI standard	MBF not available

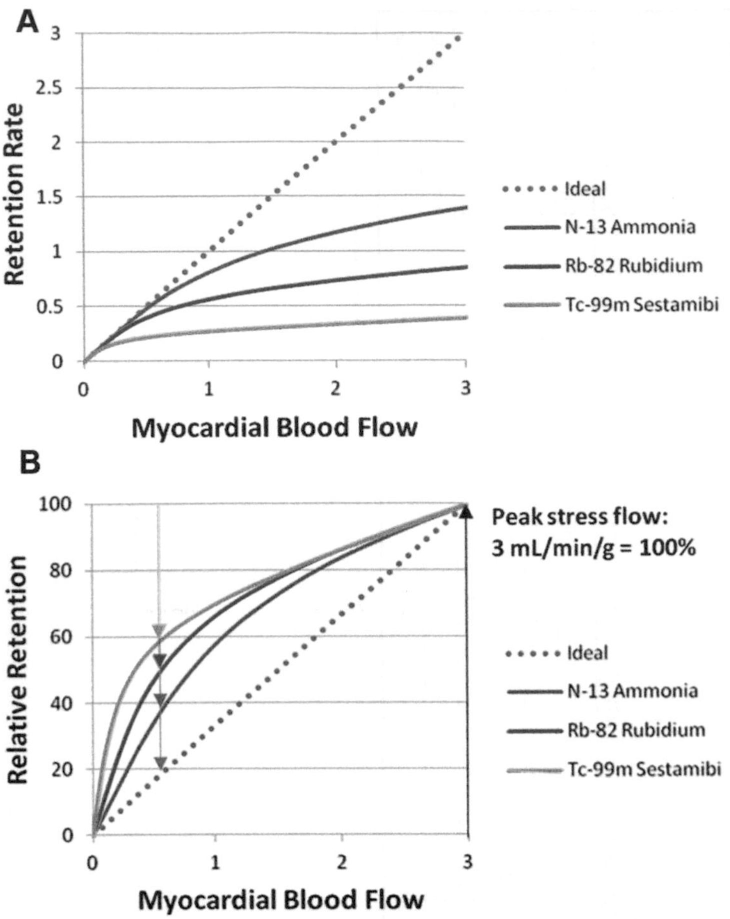

Fig. 4. Tracer retention rate (MBF × Retention fraction) as functions of MBF for 3 commonly used perfusion tracers (*A*). Retention increases more linearly with MBF above resting flow values ~1 mL/min/g. For MPI, relative tracer retention is interpreted visually on a scale from 0% to 100% of maximum (*B*). An ideal perfusion tracer would change linearly with MBF. Note that typical tracer uptake continues to increase with MBF, even for the Tc-99m sestamibi curve, which appears to plateau in (*A*), that is, there is no roll-off or decrease in tracer uptake with increasing MBF. The differences in tracer relative retention (and defect severity) are most apparent in regions of low flow ~0.5 mL/min/g, as shown by the colored arrows. A defect region with 20% of peak stress flow has relative tracer retention of ~40%, 50%, or 60% using ammonia, rubidium, or sestamibi, respectively, thereby underestimating the severity of the true underlying disease.

similar to or higher than ^{13}N-ammonia.[13] ^{82}Rb-rubidium has lower extraction (40%–70%) compared with ammonia and water, but the washout rate is slow; therefore, most of the tracer uptake is also retained, resulting in good MPI quality. ^{201}Tl-thallium has similar properties to ^{82}Rb-rubidium, because both are potassium analogues. The ^{99m}Tc SPECT tracers, sestamibi and tetrofosmin, have extraction and retention fractions that are slightly lower than ^{82}Rb-rubidium.[11] Tracer extraction and retention fractions, radiation dosimetry, relative strengths, and weaknesses are listed for the most common perfusion tracers in **Table 3**.

STANDARD MYOCARDIAL PERFUSION IMAGING

For standard MPI, high tracer retention is required in addition to the initial extraction, as described above. With perfusion tracers, retention is always lower than the initial extraction, because of the added effects of washout. Ideally, tracer retention should be stable over time, with minimal leakage or washout over the period used clinically for relative perfusion imaging (**Fig. 4**).

A clinical example illustrating the effect of tracer retention on perfusion defect contrast is shown in **Fig. 5**. This patient underwent dipyridamole ^{82}Rb-rubidium PET and treadmill exercise ^{99m}Tc-tetrofosmin SPECT 3 months following revascularization by PCI. SPECT MPI shows mild residual ischemia in the left anterior descending (LAD) artery territory, suggesting some residual flow-limiting disease. The ^{82}Rb PET scan confirmed similar extent of disease in the LAD, but much higher severity of ischemia compared with SPECT. Assuming that the degree of hyperemia was similar using dipyridamole and exercise stress, the difference in defect contrast can be explained by the lower tracer retention of tetrofosmin versus rubidium at stress. The increase in tetrofosmin retention at stress was not sufficient to unmask the true flow limitation in the diseased vessel compared with imaging at rest, a limitation that was overcome by the higher retention of ^{82}Rb.

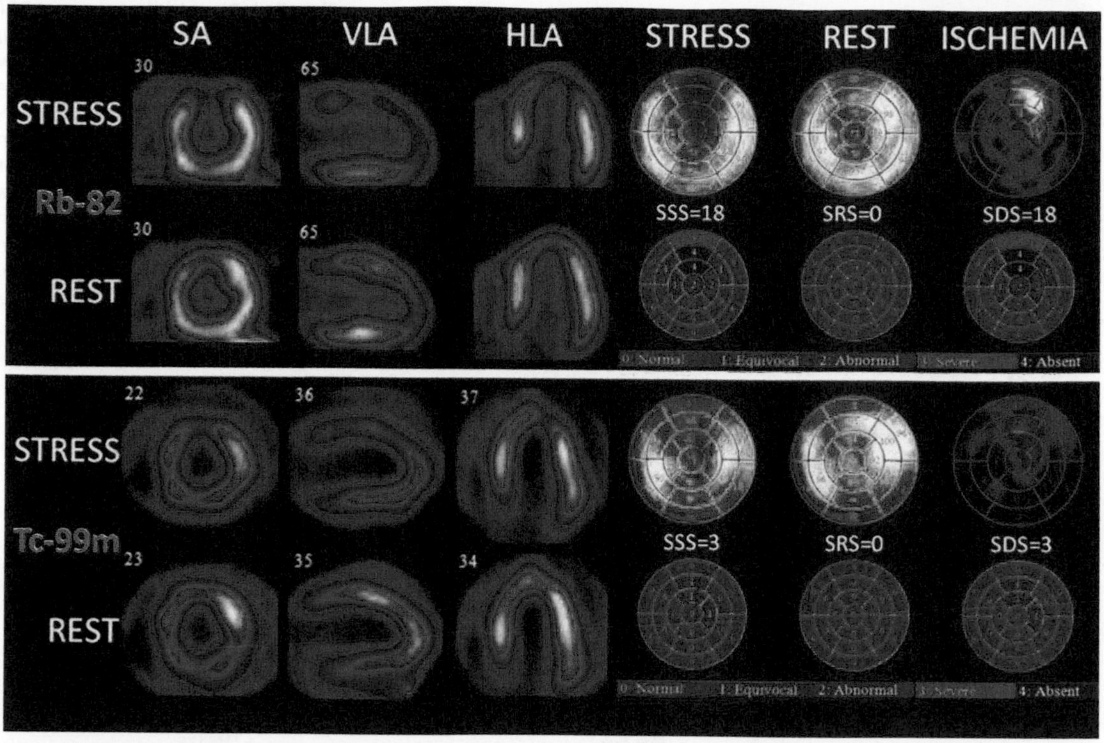

Fig. 5. ^{82}Rb PET-CT (A) and ^{99m}Tc SPECT-cadmium zinc telluride images in a 52-year-old man 3 months post-PCI of the proximal LAD coronary artery. Dipyridamole stress-rest ^{82}Rb PET images demonstrate residual severe ischemia in the entire LAD territory (summed stress score [SSS] = summed difference score [SDS] = 18) equivalent to 26% of the left ventricle myocardium. Exercise ^{99m}Tc SPECT images show only mild ischemia (SSS = SDS = 3) corresponding to 4.4% of the left ventricle. SA, short axis; VLA, vertical long axis; HLA, horizontal long axis; SRS, summed rest score.

QUANTITATIVE MYOCARDIAL BLOOD FLOW IMAGING

The tracer extraction fraction ($1 - e^{-PS/MBF}$) determines the rate of uptake (K1) into the target cells; therefore, if the extraction is high (close to 1.0), then K1 can provide a direct estimate of flow (MBF), for example, using ^{15}O-water or ^{13}N-ammonia, as shown in **Fig. 6**. For tracers with extraction substantially less than 1.0, a correction function (=1/extraction fraction) must be used to obtain estimates of MBF from the K1 values; note that the correction factors are larger at stress compared with rest because the tracer extraction fraction decreases more as MBF increases.

The stress polar-maps of ^{82}Rb uptake, K1, and MBF are shown in **Fig. 7** for the same patient as

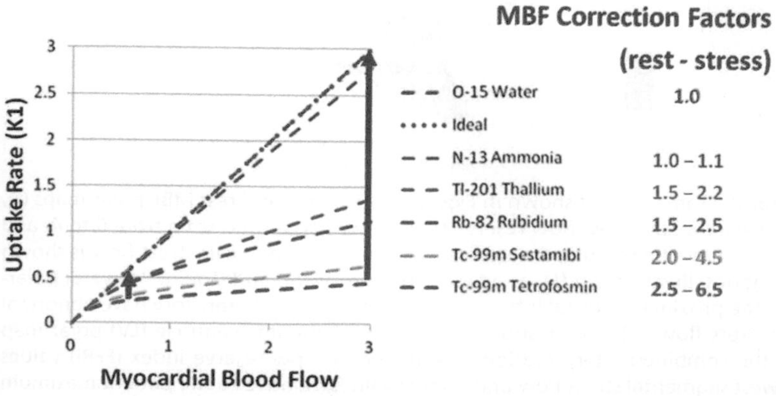

Fig. 6. Tracer uptake rate (K1) is the extraction fraction × MBF. Therefore, to estimate MBF, the tracer uptake rate must be multiplied by a correction factor (=1/extraction fraction), as illustrated by the red arrows. N-13-ammonia correction factors are close to unity (extraction >95%) over the whole range of rest and stress flows. Tc-99m-sestamibi correction factors are close to 5 (extraction ~20%) at peak stress flow of 3 mL/min/g.

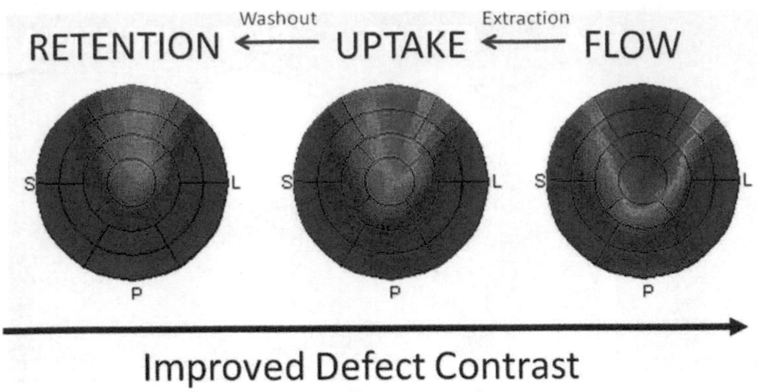

Fig. 7. ^{82}Rb-rubidium stress PET polar-maps of tracer retention, uptake rate (K1), and blood flow (MBF) for the same patient shown in **Fig. 5**. Defect contrast is determined by the tracer extraction and retention properties. For ^{82}Rb, the tracer extraction has a larger effect on defect contrast than tracer washout, reflected in the difference between the uptake and flow polar-maps.L, lateral; P, posterior; S, septum.

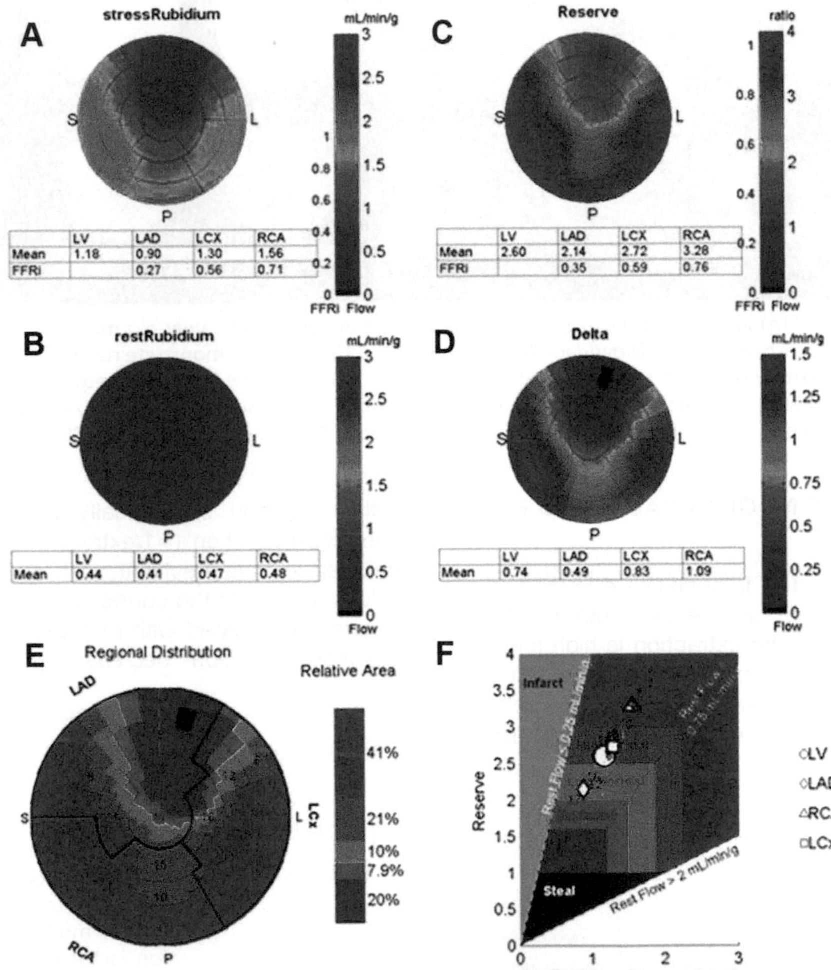

Fig. 8. Flow quantification report for the same patient shown in **Figs. 5** and **7**. Stress and rest MBF polar-maps (*A*, *B*) are shown on a scale of 0 to 3 mL/min/g. Stress/rest flow reserve (*C*) is shown on a ratio scale from 0 to 4, and stress–rest delta (*D*) from 0 to 1.5 mL/min/g. The combined classification of flow reserve AND stress flow is shown in (*E*), according to the clinical categories illustrated in (*F*), as adapted from Johnson and Gould.[16] Several polar-map segments (numbers 1, 7, 13) in the proximal-to-distal left anterior descending (LAD) territory have abnormal flow reserve (<1.6) AND abnormal stress flow (<1.2) corresponding to 20% of the left ventricle (LV) polar map shown in dark blue, according to the combined interpretation. The fractional flow reserve index (FFRi) values in (*A*) and (*C*) correspond to the lowest segmental stress flow and reserve values, relative to the patient maximum normal values. L, lateral; P, posterior; S, septum; LCx, left circumflex; RCA, right coronary artery.

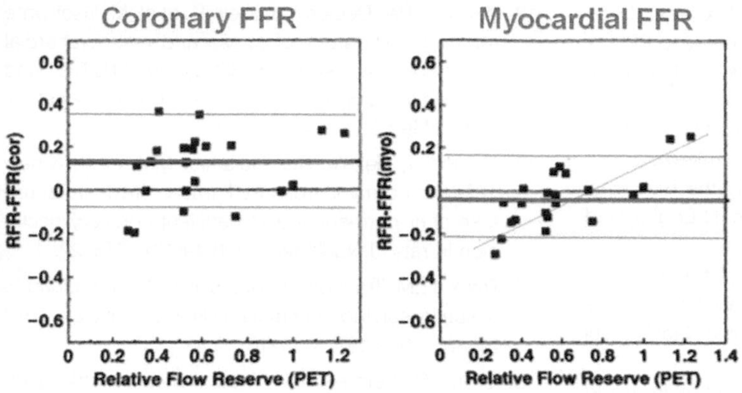

Fig. 9. PET relative flow reserve (RFR) used as the original validation gold standard for invasive pressure measurements of FFR in the coronary arteries (FFR(cor)) and myocardial perfusion bed (FFR(myo)). Coronary FFR measurements are ~10% higher than PET measurements of relative MFR. Myocardial FFR measurements are accurate on average, but show a trend toward overestimation at higher flow reserve values. (*Adapted from* De Bruyne B, Baudhuin T, Melin JA, et al. Coronary flow reserve calculated from pressure measurements in humans. Validation with positron emission tomography. Circulation 1994;89(3):1017–18; with permission.)

in **Fig. 5**. The MBF polar-map reflects the true underlying perfusion defect contrast at peak stress. The contrast is reduced on the uptake (K1) map due to the limited tracer extraction of ~40% at peak stress in this case (see **Fig. 3**). Defect contrast on the retention polar-map is further reduced due to the incremental effects of tracer washout, reflecting somewhat lower retention of ~30% compared with the initial extraction.

MBF quantification at rest and stress in this patient is shown in the flow reserve report of **Fig. 8**. Peak stress flow (~2.0 mL/min/g) and stress/rest reserve (4.0) in the lateral wall confirm that an adequate hyperemic response was achieved using the dipyridamole protocol. The lowest stress flow in the LAD territory is below the reported ischemic threshold of ~1.0 mL/min/g[16]; stress/rest reserve is absent (~1.0), and stress–rest delta is close to zero, indicating that the proximal LAD territory was not able to increase flow in response to coronary vasodilatation.

O-15-water measurements of relative PET flow reserve were used originally to validate invasive measurements of FFR,[17] as shown in **Fig. 9**. Assessment of abnormal FFR less than 0.80 is now used widely in Europe to guide PCI revascularization of intermediate coronary artery lesions (50%–70% stenosis), based largely on the results of the FAME trial[18] and subsequent class 1A recommendations of the European Society of Cardiology.[19] With the current routine availability of noninvasive quantification of MFR using Rb-82, N-13-ammonia, and O-15-water tracers, PET MFR imaging is being used increasingly to direct revascularization decisions as proposed recently by Gould and colleagues.[20] The incremental prognostic value of PET flow reserve (physiology) in addition to angiographic CAD (anatomy) has been confirmed recently[21] and should continue to see increasing application in the management of patients with CAD.

SUMMARY

MPI is performed most commonly using Tc-99m-sestamibi or tetrofosmin SPECT as well as Rb-82-rubidium or N-13-ammonia PET. Diseased-to-normal tissue contrast is determined by the tracer retention fraction, which decreases nonlinearly with flow. Reduced tissue perfusion results in reduced tracer retention, but the severity of perfusion defects is typically underestimated by 20% to 40%. Retention of the PET tracers is more linearly related to flow, and therefore, the perfusion defects are measured more accurately using N-13-ammonia or Rb-82.

O-15-water is an ideal tracer for MBF imaging due to the very high extraction fraction, but it is not suitable for MPI because it washes out quickly and is not retained in the myocardial tissues. Quantitative MBF imaging is performed most commonly using Rb-82 or N-13-ammonia dynamic PET. Tracer extraction corrections at peak stress vary from factors as low as 1.1 for N-13-ammonia to values around 2.5 for Rb-82 or Tl-201-thallium, or as high as 5 for Tc-99m-sestamibi or tetrofosmin. With accurate corrections for tracer extraction and washout, MBF imaging can restore the true diseased-to-normal contrast compared with conventional MPI.

REFERENCES

1. Renaud JM, Mylonas I, McArdle B, et al. Clinical interpretation standards and quality assurance for the multicenter PET/CT trial: 82Rb as an alternative radiopharmaceutical for myocardial imaging. J Nucl Med 2014;55:1–7.

2. McArdle BA, Dowsley TF, deKemp RA, et al. Does rubidium-82 PET have superior accuracy to SPECT perfusion imaging for the diagnosis of obstructive coronary disease?: a systematic review and meta-analysis. J Am Coll Cardiol 2012;60(18):1828–37.
3. Pijls NH, De Bruyne B, Peels K, et al. Measurement of fractional flow reserve to assess the functional severity of coronary-artery stenoses. N Engl J Med 1996;334(26):1703–8.
4. Parkash R, deKemp RA, Ruddy TD, et al. Potential utility of rubidium-82 PET quantification in patients with 3-vessel coronary artery disease. J Nucl Cardiol 2004;11(4):440–9.
5. Ziadi MC, deKemp RA, Williams KA, et al. Impaired myocardial flow reserve on rubidium-82 positron emission tomography imaging predicts adverse outcomes in patients assessed for myocardial ischemia. J Am Coll Cardiol 2011;58(7):740–8.
6. Murthy VL, Naya M, Foster CR, et al. Improved cardiac risk assessment with noninvasive measures of coronary flow reserve. Circulation 2011;124(20):2215–24.
7. Danad I, Uusitalo V, Kero T, et al. Quantitative assessment of myocardial perfusion in the detection of significant coronary artery disease: cutoff values and diagnostic accuracy of quantitative [(15)O] H2O PET imaging. J Am Coll Cardiol 2014;64(14):1464–75.
8. Ben-Haim S, Murthy VL, Breault C, et al. Quantification of myocardial perfusion Reserve using dynamic SPECT imaging in humans: a feasibility study. J Nucl Med 2013;54(6):873–9.
9. Hsu B, Chen FC, Wu TC, et al. Quantitation of myocardial blood flow and myocardial flow reserve with 99mTc-sestamibi dynamic SPECT/CT to enhance detection of coronary artery disease. Eur J Nucl Med Mol Imaging 2014;41(12):2294–306.
10. Klein R, Hung G-U, Wu T-C, et al. Feasibility and operator variability of myocardial blood flow and reserve measurements with 99m Tc-sestamibi quantitative dynamic SPECT/CT imaging. J Nucl Cardiol 2014;21(6):1075–88.
11. Wells RG, Timmins R, Klein R, et al. Dynamic SPECT measurement of absolute myocardial blood flow in a porcine model. J Nucl Med 2014;55(10):1685–91.
12. deKemp RA, Declerck J, Klein R, et al. Multisoftware reproducibility study of stress and rest myocardial blood flow assessed with 3D dynamic PET/CT and a 1-tissue-compartment model of 82Rb kinetics. J Nucl Med 2013;54(4):571–7.
13. Higuchi T, Nekolla SG, Huisman MM, et al. A new 18F-labeled myocardial PET tracer: myocardial uptake after permanent and transient coronary occlusion in rats. J Nucl Med 2008;49(10):1715–22.
14. Renkin EM. Transport of potassium-42 from blood to tissue in isolated mammalian skeletal muscles. Am J Physiol 1959;197:1205–10.
15. Crone C. Permeability of capillaries in various organs as determined by use of the indicator diffusion method. Acta Physiol Scand 1963;58:292–305.
16. Johnson NP, Gould KL. Physiological basis for angina and ST-segment change PET-verified thresholds of quantitative stress myocardial perfusion and coronary flow reserve. JACC Cardiovasc Imaging 2011;4(9):990–8.
17. De Bruyne B, Baudhuin T, Melin JA, et al. Coronary flow reserve calculated from pressure measurements in humans. Validation with positron emission tomography. Circulation 1994;89(3):1013–22.
18. Tonino PA, De Bruyne B, Pijls NH, et al, FAME Study Investigators. Fractional flow reserve versus angiography for guiding percutaneous coronary intervention. N Engl J Med 2009;360(3):213–24.
19. Wijns W, Kolh P, Danchin N, et al. Guidelines on myocardial revascularization. Eur Heart J 2010;31:2501–55.
20. Gould KL, Johnson NP, Bateman TM, et al. Anatomic versus physiologic assessment of coronary artery disease. Role of coronary flow reserve, fractional flow reserve, and positron emission tomography imaging in revascularization decision-making. J Am Coll Cardiol 2013;62(18):1639–53.
21. Taqueti VR, Hachamovitch R, Murthy VL, et al. Global coronary flow reserve is associated with adverse cardiovascular events independently of luminal angiographic severity and modifies the effect of early revascularization. Circulation 2015;131(1):19–27.

Automated Quantitative Nuclear Cardiology Methods

Manish Motwani, PhD[a], Daniel S. Berman, MD[a,b], Guido Germano, PhD[a,b], Piotr Slomka, PhD[a,b,*]

KEYWORDS

• SPECT • PET • Automated quantitation • Myocardial function • Left ventricular ejection fraction • Myocardial perfusion • Total perfusion deficit • Ischemia

KEY POINTS

- One of the main advantages of nuclear techniques over other imaging modalities is the development of standardized methods for automated quantitation.
- Current software can automatically segment the left ventricle, quantify left ventricular ejection fraction, establish myocardial perfusion maps, and estimate global and local measures of stress/rest perfusion, all with minimal user input.
- Quantitative analysis of myocardial perfusion imaging has shown better reproducibility, and at least similar diagnostic accuracy as qualitative visual analysis by expert readers.
- The accuracy of the quantitative perfusion analysis can be compromised by imaging artifacts, because they may mimic true abnormalities.
- Recent advances, such as automated contour checking and application of machine learning, bring us closer to *fully* automated analysis with strong diagnostic and prognostic impact.

INTRODUCTION

Radionuclide myocardial perfusion imaging (MPI) with single-photon emission computed tomography (SPECT) or PET is the most widely used technique for detecting coronary artery disease (CAD) in clinical practice.[1] Currently, one of the main advantages of nuclear techniques over other modalities, such as stress echocardiography or cardiac MRI, is the development of standardized methods for automated quantitation. Automated analysis of 3-dimensional SPECT and PET images is now routine for both clinical and research purposes. Current software can automatically segment the left ventricle (LV), quantify left ventricular ejection fraction (LVEF), establish myocardial perfusion maps, and estimate global and local measures of stress/rest perfusion, all with minimal user input. These methods have demonstrated better reproducibility, and at least similar diagnostic accuracy to qualitative visual analysis by expert readers.

Furthermore, automated quantitation continues to be an active field of research, with several recent developments. For example, new software that checks automated LV contours for potential errors has been shown to further reduce the level of human supervision required.[2] Another promising development has been the use of machine learning

Conflicts of Interest: This research was supported in part by grants R01HL089765 from the National Heart, Lung, and Blood Institute/National Institutes of Health (NHLBI/NIH). Cedars-Sinai Medical Center receives royalties for the quantitative assessment of function, perfusion, and viability, a minority portion of which is distributed to some of the authors of this manuscript (DB, GG, PS).
[a] Departments of Imaging and Medicine, Cedars-Sinai Medical Center, 8700 Beverly Boulevard, Los Angeles, CA 90048, USA; [b] David Geffen School of Medicine at UCLA, Los Angeles, CA, USA
* Corresponding author.
E-mail address: piotr.slomka@cshs.org

Cardiol Clin 34 (2016) 47–57
http://dx.doi.org/10.1016/j.ccl.2015.08.003
0733-8651/16/$ – see front matter

to integrate a combination of automated imaging parameters with clinical data for greater diagnostic accuracy, and prediction of prognostic outcomes on a personalized basis.[3,4] In this article, we briefly review the principles, strengths, and limitations of current automated quantitation methods, and discuss some of these latest developments.

OVERVIEW OF QUANTITATIVE METHODS

Gated MPI with SPECT or PET generates information on reversible perfusion defects, fixed perfusion defects, LV function, LV volumes, regional wall motion, and thickening. Although visual interpretation for all these parameters is feasible, it is more time-consuming, less reproducible, and ultimately more dependent on the observer's expertise than using automated methods. It has been demonstrated that computer-based quantitation provides an important means of improving consistency of interpretation.[5] A number of validated software packages are available for automated quantification (QPS-QGS (Cedar Sinai Medical Center, Los Angeles, CA, USA), Emory Toolbox (Emory University, Atlanta, GA, USA), 4D-MSPECT (Invia Medical Imaging Solutions, Ann Arbor, MI, USA), and Wackers-Liu CQ (Eclipse Systems, Branford, CT, USA))[6–9] and are distributed by the main vendors of nuclear medicine imaging equipment. The basic principles are similar for each of these software packages: after segmentation of the LV, normalized relative radiotracer uptake in reconstructed slices is quantitatively compared against normal data files.

Left Ventricular Segmentation

The first step in quantification of perfusion and function is segmentation of the LV from both gated and static reconstructed data. Segmentation of the myocardium may sometimes be challenging due to possible large perfusion defects, extracardiac activity, and image noise. Typically, the most common sources of incorrect automated contours are gut activity and incorrect definition of the valve plane (**Fig. 1**). Nonetheless, current software tools allow accurate automatic definition of LV contours in up to 90% of cases.[2] Incorrect segmentation in the minority of cases can result in spurious defects mimicking perfusion abnormalities, and therefore, some supervision by an experienced observer is still required during this step. However, this can be accomplished by an experienced technologist before scan interpretation. Furthermore, recent software developments, which are discussed in this review, can be used to check automated LV contours, allowing readers to target manual adjustment only to those studies flagged by the algorithm for potential errors.

Left Ventricular Function

Using the endocardial surfaces from LV segmentation, a volume curve spanning the cardiac cycle can be generated. From the volume curve data, LV end-diastolic volume (EDV), LV end-systolic volume (ESV), LVEF, cardiac output, myocardial mass, and diastolic function parameters (peak and time to peak filling and ejection rates) can then be calculated. Several studies confirm strong agreement between gated MPI and reference standard measurements of quantitative LVEF and LV volumes.[7,10–15] This relationship is relatively independent of the isotope, protocol, standard, and algorithm used. Reproducibility and repeatability for LVEF and LV volumes have also been shown to be high.[16,17] With regard to cross-algorithm reproducibility, a number of studies confirm strong correlation between different approaches, but systematic differences in the measurements do exist, and therefore normal limits for the specific imaging approach are required.[15,18–20] Prognostic thresholds for LVEF, EDV, and ESV have also been reported for quantitative software.[21,22]

Myocardial Perfusion

Polar maps

Evaluating myocardial perfusion involves the detection of significant differences between stress and rest images. For the visual observer, this is only a subjective analysis and can be particularly challenging if the differences are subtle or if there are differences in stress and rest alignment. By contrast, automated software offers several objective quantitative measures of myocardial perfusion. After LV segmentation, the standard processing sequence for automated analysis involves extraction of myocardial count densities to polar map coordinates (typically the maximal values for a given polar map pixel), and subsequent comparison of polar map samples to normal limits (**Fig. 2**).[5,11,23] Site-specific or protocol-specific normal limits are derived from a small number of visually normal studies from low-likelihood patients (20–40 is usually sufficient) in the local population.[23,24] For any given myocardial location, the image count can be used to grade the *severity* of hypoperfusion, based on the number of SDs below the lower limit of normal. Polar maps can then be plotted with severity mapped to a color scale, or as so-called "blackout maps" where all pixels below normal limits are blacked-out (**Fig. 3**). Another advantage of this quantitative approach is that the use of common polar map coordinates for all subjects allows

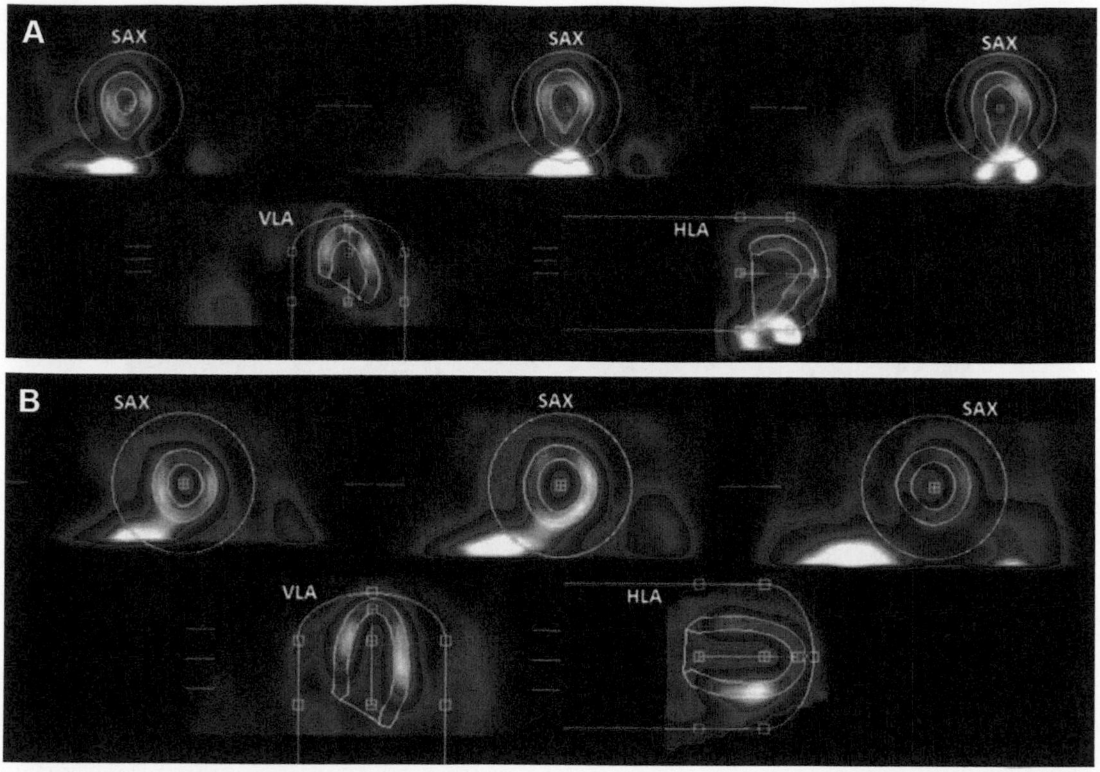

Fig. 1. LV segmentation errors. In each panel, top images are in short-axis orientation (SAX), and bottom images are in horizontal and vertical (long)-axis orientation (HLA, VLA). Yellow circles show initial masks, and LV contours are shown in white. Panel (*A*) shows an example of mask-failure due to extracardiac activity. Panel (*B*) shows an example of valve-plane overshooting. (*Adapted from* Xu Y, Kavanagh P, Fish M, et al. Automated quality control for segmentation of myocardial perfusion SPECT. J Nucl Med 2009;50:1420–1; with permission.)

objective intersubject comparison of relative count intensities, as the image counts in each study are normalized to a common level.

Quantitative parameters of perfusion

Various quantitative parameters can be derived from myocardial perfusion scans, and reported at a regional (per vascular territory) or global (per ventricle) level. These parameters are most commonly obtained by comparison with normal limits. For example, the *extent* of a perfusion defect can be expressed as the percentage of pixels in the polar map for which severity is greater than a predefined statistical threshold

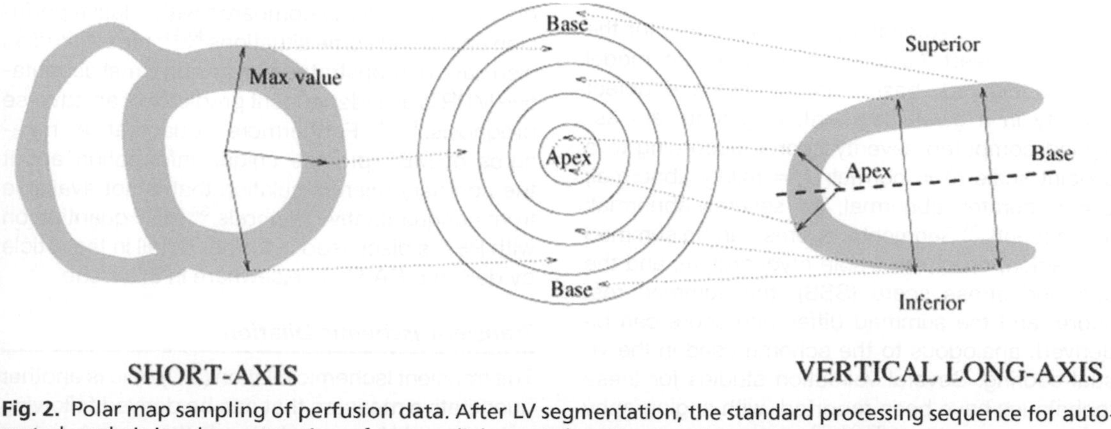

Fig. 2. Polar map sampling of perfusion data. After LV segmentation, the standard processing sequence for automated analysis involves extraction of myocardial count densities to polar map coordinates.

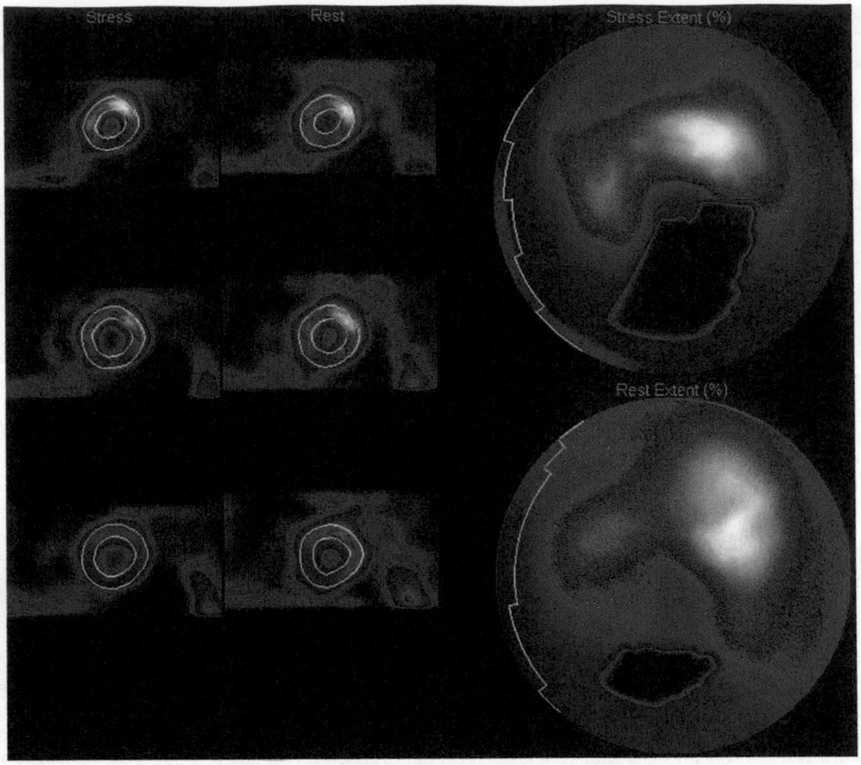

Fig. 3. Blackout maps are derived by the quantitative software obtained by masking the polar maps pixels below normal limits. Corresponding short-axis stress (*top right*) and rest images (*bottom right*) are shown.

(eg, 2.0–2.5 SD below normal limits). This measure reflects the size of the perfusion defect and it has been validated against delayed enhancement MRI for infarct imaging.[25]

Most commonly, a single parameter combining both pixel-based *severity and extent* is used to quantify the overall magnitude of hypoperfusion; for example, the total perfusion deficit (TPD), as used by the Cedars-Sinai QPS module.[23] The difference in TPD at stress and rest (ie, ischemic TPD) can be used to quantify ischemia. A similar concept to TPD is used by other quantification packages.

In addition, segmental perfusion scores for the American Heart Association 17-segment model can be derived, based on the average defect severity in a given segment. Segments are assigned computed severity scores according to a 5-point scale (0 = normal; 1 = mildly abnormal; 2 = moderately abnormal; 3 = severely abnormal; 4 = absent).[26] Segmental scores can be summed per region, or for the whole myocardium, and the summed stress score (SSS), the summed rest score, and the summed difference score can be derived, analogous to the scheme used in the visual scoring. Several validation studies for these techniques have been reported, with angiography as the gold standard.[23,27–29]

Standard tools with the previously discussed general functionality for both SPECT and PET (but with some differences in the computational analysis methods) are available in all the main software packages available commercially.

Myocardial Blood Flow

PET can additionally be used to quantify absolute myocardial blood flow (MBF) and myocardial perfusion reserve (MPR), and it is currently the noninvasive reference standard for these measures. Such analysis has been shown to improve diagnostic accuracy compared with relative perfusion analysis in some situations[30,31]; recent studies also have demonstrated that an abnormal quantitative MPR is an independent predictor of an adverse prognosis.[32,33] Furthermore, quantitative measures of MBF provide unique information about the coronary microcirculation that is not available from nonquantitative methods.[34] MBF quantitation with PET is discussed in further detail in the article by deKemp RA et al., elsewhere in this issue.

Transient Ischemic Dilation

The transient ischemic dilation (TID) ratio is another quantitative measure that can be derived following automated LV segmentation.[35] It is calculated as the ratio of ungated poststress LV cavity volume to that at rest. Abnormally high values of the TID ratio are associated with severe and extensive CAD.[36] It is debated as to whether an increased TID ratio reflects true stress-induced stunning of the LV, or extensive subendocardial ischemia, or indeed a combination. TID ratio can be effective in avoiding the problem of underestimating disease extent, which is inherent in the assessment of relative perfusion defects, particularly with subjective visual analysis. For example, in one study, the sensitivity for detecting severe disease improved significantly (from 64% to 71%; $P<.05$) when TID was combined with TPD.[37]

QUANTITATIVE ANALYSIS OF MYOCARDIAL PERFUSION IMAGING IN PRACTICE

Diagnostic Accuracy

A recent study confirmed that diagnostic accuracy in terms of area under the curve (AUC) for detecting CAD, by using the latest automated quantitative MPI methods, is at least similar or marginally superior to that achieved by expert visual readers.[38] The latter was true for both attenuation-corrected and not corrected data and even when additional information such as patient age and symptom history (not used by the computer software) was revealed to the reader (**Fig. 4**).

Prognostic Accuracy

Previously, a number of studies demonstrated the prognostic value of standard visual scoring of MPI, but this also has been shown to be valid for automated quantitative parameters.[39–41] Cox models based on automated stress TPD have been shown to have similar prognostic performance for predicting cardiac death as those based on expert visual analysis incorporating clinical information (AUC: 0.72 vs 0.71).[42]

Ischemic Change

A particularly useful application for quantitative analysis is the estimation of subtle changes in ischemic burden during longitudinal follow-up of

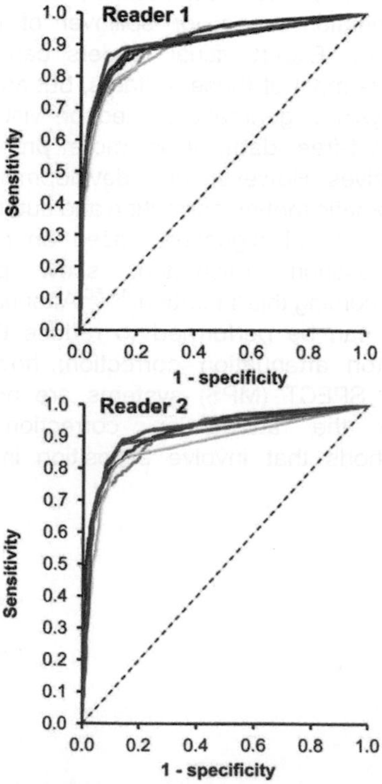

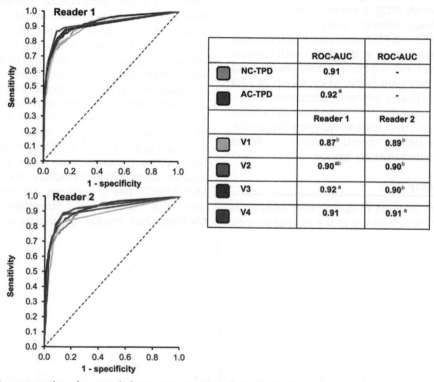

		ROC-AUC	ROC-AUC
	NC-TPD	0.91	-
	AC-TPD	0.92[a]	-
		Reader 1	Reader 2
	V1	0.87[b]	0.89[b]
	V2	0.90[ab]	0.90[b]
	V3	0.92[a]	0.90[b]
	V4	0.91	0.91[a]

Fig. 4. Receiver operating characteristic curves: automated versus visual analysis. A recent study confirmed that diagnostic accuracy for detecting CAD (≥70% stenosis) on a per-patient basis using automated methods is at least similar or marginally superior to that achieved by 2 expert visual readers. Comparisons were made for both AC and non-AC (NC) data, and using variable amounts of imaging and clinical data available to the reader (V1-V4). V1, NC only; V2, NC + AC; V3, NC + AC + computer analysis results; V4, NC + AC + computer analysis results + clinical information. [a] Comparison with previous step $P<.01$. [b] Fully automated TPD versus visual analysis $P<.01$ (red *b* indicates fully automated TPD analysis was superior to visual). (*From* Arsanjani R, Xu Y, Hayes SW, et al. Comparison of fully automated computer analysis and visual scoring for detection of coronary artery disease from myocardial perfusion SPECT in a large population. J Nucl Med 2013;54:224; with permission.)

the same patient. This can provide a reliable objective measure of a patient's response to therapy. Although this can also be performed with visual assessment, small but clinically important improvements can be underinterpreted due to the subjective scoring of different readers. The most common approach using quantitative analysis is to report the difference in the overall quantitative parameter between repeat scans such as TPD, and this has shown good reproducibility and repeatability.[43,44]

Newer automated software can further refine longitudinal follow-up by analyzing serial stress/rest studies together in pairs, thereby eliminating errors associated with multiple comparisons to normal limits and variations in contour placements.[45,46] This approach also has the advantage that it does not require normal limits.

In the nuclear substudy of the Clinical Outcomes Utilizing Revascularization and Aggressive Drug Evaluation (COURAGE) trial, quantitative analysis of perfusion was compared before and after 2 different treatment strategies (percutaneous coronary intervention [PCI] + medical therapy versus medical therapy alone).[41] Greater reduction of ischemia (TPD: −2.7%) was shown in the group with PCI therapy than in the group with medical therapy alone (TPD: −0.5%; *P*<.0001). Such small group differences are harder to demonstrate with visual scoring due to greater interobserver and intraobserver variability.[47,48] Consequently, clinical trials based on visual analysis may require considerably larger patient cohorts to show significant differences between study groups.

Reproducibility

An important strength of quantitative analysis is the inherent reproducibility of the measurements. Lower variability directly translates to improved detection of true differences in hypoperfusion. The reproducibility of quantitative perfusion analysis has been compared with visual analysis for a stress and rest SPECT scan, repeated on the same day.[43] Quantitative measures of stress, rest, and ischemic (stress-rest) defects were significantly more reproducible than visual scores, with smaller repeatability coefficients (stress: 3.3% vs 4.8%; rest: 1.8% vs 3.8%; ischemic: 3.2% vs 4.3%; all *P*<.002). Bland-Altman plots for repeated measures of visual stress and automated stress perfusion size are shown in **Fig. 5**. These comparisons clearly demonstrate the advantages of the quantitative perfusion analysis over visual expert analysis.

Limitations of Myocardial Perfusion Imaging Quantification

Accuracy of quantitative perfusion analysis can be reduced by imaging artifacts, which can mimic true defects. Artifacts can be caused by patient motion, photon attenuation, misalignment of attenuation maps, or spillover of extracardiac activity. Expert visual readers can detect and ignore most of these artifacts, but as quantitative analysis is generally trained on visually normal, artifact-free data, it is more prone to false-positives. However, new developments, such as automatic motion correction and automatic recognition of misalignment based on myocardium-mediastinum mismatch, show potential in overcoming this limitation.[49,50] Attenuation correction can be performed to reduce the effect of photon attenuation correction; however, most MPI SPECT (MPS) systems are not equipped with the attenuation correction hardware. Methods that involve 2-position imaging have

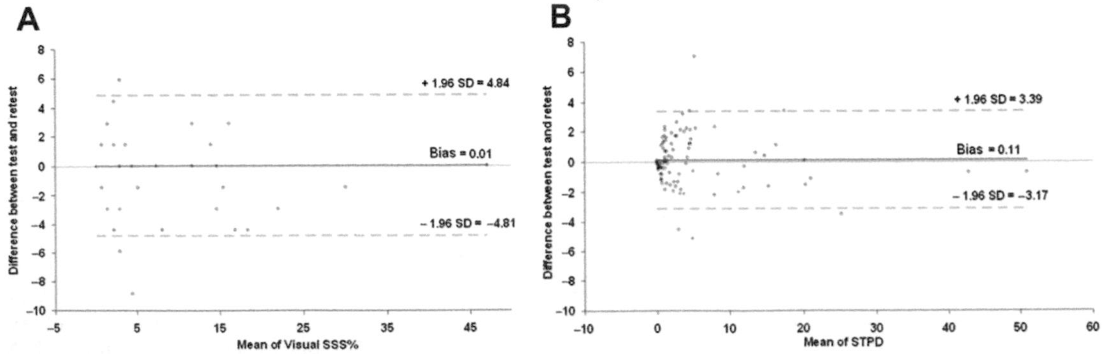

Fig. 5. Reproducibility: automated versus visual analysis Bland-Altman plots for visual (*A*) and automatic (*B*) repeated measurements of myocardial perfusion at stress are shown. The plot for automated stress total perfusion defect (STPD) shows better reproducibility with narrower limits of agreement compared with the plot for visual summed stress score as % of total myocardium (SSS%). (*From* Xu Y, Hayes S, Ali I, et al. Automatic and visual reproducibility of perfusion and function measures for myocardial perfusion SPECT. J Nucl Cardiol 2010;17:1054; with permission.)

been proposed for mitigation of attenuation-correction artifacts if attenuation correction is not available.[51] These methods are of particular use on newer dedicated cardiac SPECT scanners that often are not equipped with attenuation correction (AC) but can perform fast imaging, making 2-position imaging practical clinically.[52,53] Novel fast-MPS protocols have been adopted with 2 sequential scans in 2 patient positions (supine/upright or supine/prone, depending on the scanner), allowing differentiation of true perfusion defects from artifacts, if AC is not available[53,54]; however, they make visual reading more complex. The 2-position approach also may allow for detection of position-related artifacts, which may occur with limited field-of-view gantry of the new scanners.[55]

Another acknowledged limitation of the quantitative approach is the need for normal perfusion databases, specific to the scanner, tracer, acquisition algorithm, and patient demographic, to establish valid normal limits for quantitative parameters. Such factors can all result in differing myocardial count distributions, resolution, photon attenuation, and scatter.

RECENT ADVANCES AND FUTURE DIRECTIONS

Quality Control Flags: Toward Full Automation

The only element of human interaction required in quantitative MPI analysis is the potential adjustment of computer-generated contours during LV segmentation in a minority of cases. This manual interaction introduces user variability in an otherwise fully automated workflow. Therefore, in efforts to reduce the requirement for this step, a quality control (QC) algorithm for automatic identification of potentially incorrect contours has recently been developed.[2] This automated contour check algorithm derives 2 parameters to categorize segmentation failure: the "shape flag" to detect mask-failure cases, and the "valve-plane flag" to detect mitral valve-plane overshooting or undershooting. This method has been shown to be very accurate for detecting both types of error (AUC: 1.00 and 0.96, respectively), compared with expert readers.[2] A follow-up study using this technique in 995 rest/stress 99mTc-sestamibi MPI studies has shown it to be reliable in directing the attention of technologists to those contours that need manual correction; and in this way, with some refinement, we are one step closer to *fully* unsupervised automated perfusion scoring without sacrificing accuracy.[38] Furthermore, enhanced automation of quantitative analysis enabled by such algorithms may allow accelerated QC for clinical trials on a large scale.

Motion-Frozen Quantification of Perfusion

Cardiac motion can lead to blurring, and therefore, most MPI protocols now use cardiac gating during acquisition. It has been suggested that analysis of only the end-diastolic images can improve the detection of CAD, particularly in smaller hearts.[56] However, using end-diastolic images in isolation is not suitable for reliable computer quantification, because they only contain counts from a limited portion of the cardiac cycle. Therefore, quantification of perfusion has most commonly been performed on summed (added) image frames from all cardiac gates, without consideration for cardiac motion.

A novel "motion-frozen" display and quantification technique, using all gated frames and taking cardiac motion into account, has therefore been developed to address this issue.[57] This technique eliminates image blurring due to cardiac motion, with noticeable improvement in image quality. "Motion-freezing" of perfusion data is accomplished by detection and subsequent motion tracking of the LV endocardial and epicardial borders, with an established LV myocardial contour extraction algorithm such as QGS. Subsequently, 3-dimensional (3D) nonlinear image warping is applied to all phases of the gated data, deforming each image phase to match the position of the end-diastolic phase (**Fig. 6**). The warped images can be summed, forming "motion-frozen" perfusion images. Such "motion-frozen" perfusion images have a visual appearance similar to the end-diastolic frames but are less noisy because they contain counts from all or most cardiac cycles.

Image quantification algorithms can use the motion information in polar map coordinates to derive cardiac motion–corrected polar maps. Therefore, "motion-frozen" quantification can be performed by using polar maps that are created from individual polar map samples for each portion of the cardiac cycle, as defined by the gated 3D contours. Such "motion-frozen" perfusion quantification has been demonstrated to improve the diagnostic performance in obese patients and the improvement in image quality is likely to be most useful for resolving borderline findings in patients with high ejection fractions, in which cardiac motion significantly reduces the image resolution.[58] Furthermore, as image resolution increases, cardiac motion becomes the dominant degrading effect; therefore, this novel technique may be of greater

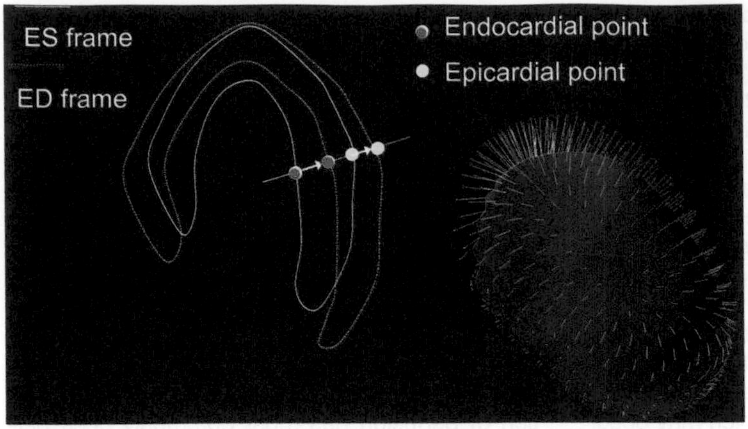

Fig. 6. The principle of motion-frozen technique. Three-dimensional LV contours are identified on images from different cardiac phases. End-systolic (ES, *white*) and end-diastolic (ED, *red*) frames are shown on the left. The 3D phase-to-phase motion vectors are derived by sampling epicardial and endocardial surfaces. The 3D motion vectors are shown on the right, superimposed on epicardial surface of the LV ventricle. A nonlinear image warping is then applied to warp all image phases to fit the ED phase. (*Adapted from* Slomka PJ, Nishina H, Berman DS, et al. "Motion-frozen" display and quantification of myocardial perfusion. J Nucl Med 2004;45:1129; with permission.)

importance for PET or future high-resolution SPECT imaging.

Machine Learning

Machine learning is a form of artificial intelligence that has proven to be highly effective for prediction and decision-making in a multitude of disciplines, including Internet search engines, natural language processing, and finance trending. Increasingly it is finding applications in medicine, particularly in genomics, but more recently in risk assessment for various disease processes.[59–61] Fundamentally, it differs from traditional risk assessment methods by making no priori assumptions about causative factors, thus allowing for an unbiased exploration of all available data for patterns that predict a patient's individual risk.[61]

Quantitative parameters from automated analysis of MPI provide a rich source of objective reproducible cardiac data that can be mined with machine-learning algorithms for highly accurate diagnostics and prognostic risk assessment. Recent studies applying machine learning to automated MPI analysis have confirmed this postulation. For example, Arsanjani and colleagues[62] integrated various parameters from automated analysis (TPD, ischemic changes, and ejection fraction changes between stress and rest) with a support vector machines algorithm to generate a diagnostic score for significant CAD that was significantly superior to any single parameter in isolation. Moreover, further studies showed it is also possible to combine quantitative parameters with clinical parameters, akin to the integrative clinical scan analysis performed by physicians for both diagnostic and prognostic risk assessments.[3,4] A LogitBoost ensemble machine learning method trained in a 10-fold cross-validation experiment was compared with TPD and visual scores in a large study (n = 1181) with correlating invasive angiography. When clinical and imaging information was provided to LogitBoost, it achieved a significantly higher diagnostic accuracy for detection of significant CAD (87%) than one of the expert readers (82%) or TPD (83%; P<.01), and a higher AUC (0.94 ± 0.01) than TPD (0.88 ± 0.01) or 2 visual readers (0.89, 0.85; P<.001) (**Fig. 7**).[3] A similar method was

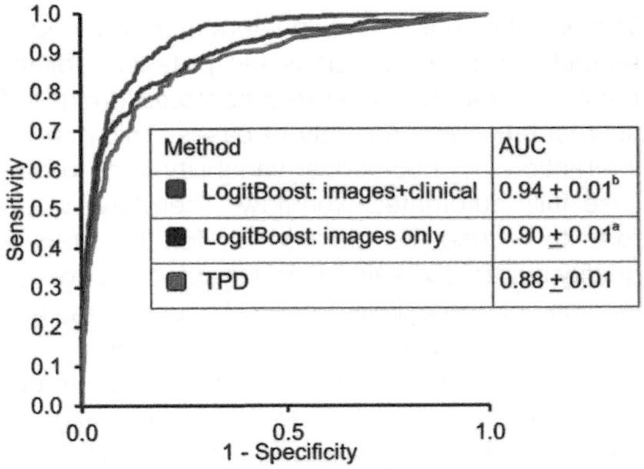

Fig. 7. Application of machine learning to automated quantitation. When clinical and imaging information was provided to the LogitBoost machine-learning technique in a large study (n = 1181), it achieved a significantly higher diagnostic accuracy for detection of significant CAD (87%) than one of the expert readers (82%) or TPD (83%; P<.01); and a higher AUC (0.94 ± 0.01) than TPD (0.88 ± 0.01) or 2 visual readers (0.89, 0.85; P<.001). [a] Better than TPD (P<.001). [b] Better than image-only LogitBoost (P<.0001). (*From* Arsanjani R, Xu Y, Dey D, et al. Improved accuracy of myocardial perfusion SPECT for detection of coronary artery disease by machine learning in a large population. J Nucl Cardiol 2013;20:558; with permission.)

used to combine quantitative perfusion and function parameters with clinical parameters to predict early revascularization from MPI.[4]

These recent efforts using machine learning methods dismiss the myth that the integrative characteristics of visual reading cannot be emulated with automated software.

SUMMARY

Current tools for automated quantitative analysis are now readily available and in widespread use. These methods have been proven to be clinically robust with superior reproducibility and at least comparable diagnostic and prognostic performance compared with visual scoring, even by experts. Nonetheless, some challenges remain in the pursuit of a fully unsupervised quantitative approach. For example, LV segmentation still needs to be verified by a skilled operator, and multiple quantitative parameters may need to be reconciled by the thought processes of an expert reader for the final interpretation. However, recent developments in software and machine learning show that even these challenges can be overcome by the latest technology.

REFERENCES

1. Salerno M, Beller GA. Noninvasive assessment of myocardial perfusion. Circ Cardiovasc Imaging 2009;2:412–24.
2. Xu Y, Kavanagh P, Fish M, et al. Automated quality control for segmentation of myocardial perfusion SPECT. J Nucl Med 2009;50:1418–26.
3. Arsanjani R, Xu Y, Dey D, et al. Improved accuracy of myocardial perfusion SPECT for detection of coronary artery disease by machine learning in a large population. J Nucl Cardiol 2013;20:553–62.
4. Arsanjani R, Dey D, Khachatryan T, et al. Prediction of revascularization after myocardial perfusion SPECT by machine learning in a large population. J Nucl Cardiol 2014;1–8.
5. Slomka P, Xu Y, Berman D, et al. Quantitative analysis of perfusion studies: strengths and pitfalls. J Nucl Cardiol 2012;19:338–46.
6. Ficaro EP, Lee BC, Kritzman JN, et al. Corridor4DM: the Michigan method for quantitative nuclear cardiology. J Nucl Cardiol 2007;14:455–65.
7. Garcia EV, Faber TL, Cooke CD, et al. The increasing role of quantification in clinical nuclear cardiology: the Emory approach. J Nucl Cardiol 2007;14:420–32.
8. Germano G, Kavanagh PB, Slomka PJ, et al. Quantitation in gated perfusion SPECT imaging: the Cedars-Sinai approach. J Nucl Cardiol 2007;14:433–54.
9. Liu Y-H. Quantification of nuclear cardiac images: the Yale approach. J Nucl Cardiol 2007;14:483–91.
10. Germano G, Kiat H, Kavanagh PB, et al. Automatic quantification of ejection fraction from gated myocardial perfusion SPECT. J Nucl Med 1995;36:2138.
11. Faber TL, Cooke CD, Folks RD, et al. Left ventricular function and perfusion from gated SPECT perfusion images: an integrated method. J Nucl Med 1999;40:650–9.
12. Kumita S, Cho K, Nakajo H, et al. Assessment of left ventricular diastolic function with electrocardiography-gated myocardial perfusion SPECT: comparison with multigated equilibrium radionuclide angiography. J Nucl Cardiol 2001;8:568–74.
13. Bax JJ, Lamb H, Dibbets P, et al. Comparison of gated single-photon emission computed tomography with magnetic resonance imaging for evaluation of left ventricular function in ischemic cardiomyopathy. Am J Cardiol 2000;86:1299–305.
14. Chua T, Yin LC, Thiang TH, et al. Accuracy of the automated assessment of left ventricular function with gated perfusion SPECT in the presence of perfusion defects and left ventricular dysfunction: correlation with equilibrium radionuclide ventriculography and echocardiography. J Nucl Cardiol 2000;7:301–11.
15. Faber TL, Vansant JP, Pettigrew RI, et al. Evaluation of left ventricular endocardial volumes and ejection fractions computed from gated perfusion SPECT with magnetic resonance imaging: comparison of two methods. J Nucl Cardiol 2001;8:645–51.
16. Nakajima K, Nishimura T. Inter-institution preference-based variability of ejection fraction and volumes using quantitative gated SPECT with 99mTc-tetrofosmin: a multicentre study involving 106 hospitals. Eur J Nucl Med Mol Imaging 2006;33:127–33.
17. Hyun IY, Kwan J, Park KS, et al. Reproducibility of Tl-201 and Tc-99m sestamibi gated myocardial perfusion SPECT measurement of myocardial function. J Nucl Cardiol 2001;8:182–7.
18. Nichols K, Santana CA, Folks R, et al. Comparison between ECTb and QGS for assessment of left ventricular function from gated myocardial perfusion SPECT. J Nucl Cardiol 2002;9:285–93.
19. Nakajima K, Higuchi T, Taki J, et al. Accuracy of ventricular volume and ejection fraction measured by gated myocardial SPECT: comparison of 4 software programs. J Nucl Med 2001;42:1571–8.
20. Véra P, Koning R, Cribier A, et al. Comparison of two three-dimensional gated SPECT methods with thallium in patients with large myocardial infarction. J Nucl Cardiol 2000;7:312–9.
21. Sharir T, Germano G, Kavanagh PB, et al. Incremental prognostic value of post-stress left ventricular ejection fraction and volume by gated myocardial perfusion single photon emission computed tomography. Circulation 1999;100:1035–42.

22. Sharir T, Kang X, Germano G, et al. Prognostic value of poststress left ventricular volume and ejection fraction by gated myocardial perfusion SPECT in women and men: gender-related differences in normal limits and outcomes. J Nucl Cardiol 2006; 13:495–506.
23. Slomka PJ, Nishina H, Berman DS, et al. Automated quantification of myocardial perfusion SPECT using simplified normal limits. J Nucl Cardiol 2005;12:66–77.
24. Van Train KF, Areeda J, Garcia EV, et al. Quantitative same-day rest-stress technetium-99m-Sestamibi SPECT: definition and validation of stress normal limits and criteria for abnormality. J Nucl Med 1993;34:1494–502.
25. Slomka PJ, Fieno D, Thomson L, et al. Automatic detection and size quantification of infarcts by myocardial perfusion SPECT: clinical validation by delayed-enhancement MRI. J Nucl Med 2005;46: 728–35.
26. Tilkemeier PL, Cooke CD, Ficaro EP, et al. American Society of Nuclear Cardiology information statement: standardized reporting matrix for radionuclide myocardial perfusion imaging. J Nucl Cardiol 2006; 13:e157–71.
27. Ficaro EP, Fessler JA, Shreve PD, et al. Simultaneous transmission/emission myocardial perfusion tomography diagnostic accuracy of attenuation-corrected 99mTc-Sestamibi single-photon emission computed tomography. Circulation 1996;93:463–73.
28. Wolak A, Slomka PJ, Fish MB, et al. Quantitative myocardial-perfusion SPECT: comparison of three state-of-the-art software packages. J Nucl Cardiol 2008;15:27–34.
29. Xu Y, Fish M, Gerlach J, et al. Combined quantitative analysis of attenuation corrected and non-corrected myocardial perfusion SPECT: method development and clinical validation. J Nucl Cardiol 2010;17:591–9.
30. Ziadi MC, Williams K, Guo A, et al. Does quantification of myocardial flow reserve using rubidium-82 positron emission tomography facilitate detection of multivessel coronary artery disease? J Nucl Cardiol 2012;19:670–80.
31. Fiechter M, Ghadri JR, Gebhard C, et al. Diagnostic value of 13N-ammonia myocardial perfusion PET: added value of myocardial flow reserve. J Nucl Med 2012;53:1230–4.
32. Kajander SA, Joutsiniemi E, Saraste M, et al. Clinical value of absolute quantification of myocardial perfusion with 15O-water in coronary artery disease. Circ Cardiovasc Imaging 2011;4:678–84.
33. Herzog BA, Husmann L, Valenta I, et al. Long-term prognostic value of 13n-ammonia myocardial perfusion positron emission tomography added value of coronary flow reserve. J Am Coll Cardiol 2009;54: 150–6.
34. Camici PG, Crea F. Coronary microvascular dysfunction. N Engl J Med 2007;356:830–40.
35. Mazzanti M, Germano G, Kiat H, et al. Identification of severe and extensive coronary artery disease by automatic measurement of transient ischemic dilation of the left ventricle in dual-isotope myocardial perfusion SPECT. J Am Coll Cardiol 1996;27: 1612–20.
36. Weiss AT, Berman DS, Lew AS, et al. Transient ischemic dilation of the left ventricle on stress thallium-201 scintigraphy: a marker of severe and extensive coronary artery disease. J Am Coll Cardiol 1987;9:752–9.
37. Xu Y, Arsanjani R, Clond M, et al. Transient ischemic dilation for coronary artery disease in quantitative analysis of same-day sestamibi myocardial perfusion SPECT. J Nucl Cardiol 2012;19:465–73.
38. Arsanjani R, Xu Y, Hayes SW, et al. Comparison of fully automated computer analysis and visual scoring for detection of coronary artery disease from myocardial perfusion SPECT in a large population. J Nucl Med 2013;54:221–8.
39. Pazhenkottil AP, Ghadri J-R, Nkoulou RN, et al. Improved outcome prediction by SPECT myocardial perfusion imaging after CT attenuation correction. J Nucl Med 2011;52:196–200.
40. Leslie WD, Tully SA, Yogendran MS, et al. Prognostic value of automated quantification of 99mTc-sestamibi myocardial perfusion imaging. J Nucl Med 2005;46:204–11.
41. Shaw LJ, Berman DS, Maron DJ, et al. Optimal medical therapy with or without percutaneous coronary intervention to reduce ischemic burden: results from the Clinical Outcomes Utilizing Revascularization and Aggressive Drug Evaluation (COURAGE) trial nuclear substudy. Circulation 2008;117:1283–91.
42. Xu Y, Nakazato R, Hayes S, et al. Prognostic value of automated vs visual analysis for adenosine stress myocardial perfusion SPECT in patients without prior coronary artery disease: a case-control study. J Nucl Cardiol 2011;18:1003–9.
43. Xu Y, Hayes S, Ali I, et al. Automatic and visual reproducibility of perfusion and function measures for myocardial perfusion SPECT. J Nucl Cardiol 2010;17:1050–7.
44. Berman DS, Kang X, Gransar H, et al. Quantitative assessment of myocardial perfusion abnormality on SPECT myocardial perfusion imaging is more reproducible than expert visual analysis. J Nucl Cardiol 2009;16:45–53.
45. Prasad M, Slomka PJ, Fish M, et al. Improved quantification and normal limits for myocardial perfusion stress–rest change. J Nucl Med 2010;51:204–9.
46. Slomka PJ, Nishina H, Berman DS, et al. Automatic quantification of myocardial perfusion stress–rest change: a new measure of ischemia. J Nucl Med 2004;45:183–91.
47. Mahmarian JJ, Cerqueira MD, Iskandrian AE, et al. Regadenoson induces comparable left ventricular

perfusion defects as adenosine: a quantitative analysis from the ADVANCE MPI 2 trial. JACC Cardiovasc Imaging 2009;2:959–68.
48. Cerqueira MD, Nguyen P, Staehr P, et al. Effects of age, gender, obesity, and diabetes on the efficacy and safety of the selective A2A agonist regadenoson versus adenosine in myocardial perfusion imaging: integrated ADVANCE-MPI trial results. JACC Cardiovasc Imaging 2008;1:307–16.
49. Matsumoto N, Berman DS, Kavanagh PB, et al. Quantitative assessment of motion artifacts and validation of a new motion-correction program for myocardial perfusion SPECT. J Nucl Med 2001;42:687–94.
50. Chen J, Caputlu-Wilson SF, Shi H, et al. Automated quality control of emission-transmission misalignment for attenuation correction in myocardial perfusion imaging with SPECT-CT systems. J Nucl Cardiol 2006;13:43–9.
51. Nishina H, Slomka PJ, Abidov A, et al. Combined supine and prone quantitative myocardial perfusion SPECT: method development and clinical validation in patients with no known coronary artery disease. J Nucl Med 2006;47:51–8.
52. Nakazato R, Slomka PJ, Fish M, et al. Quantitative high-efficiency cadmium-zinc-telluride SPECT with dedicated parallel-hole collimation system in obese patients: results of a multi-center study. J Nucl Cardiol 2014;22:266–75.
53. Nakazato R, Tamarappoo BK, Kang X, et al. Quantitative upright–supine high-speed SPECT myocardial perfusion imaging for detection of coronary artery disease: correlation with invasive coronary angiography. J Nucl Med 2010;51:1724–31.
54. Duvall WL, Sweeny JM, Croft LB, et al. Comparison of high efficiency CZT SPECT MPI to coronary angiography. J Nucl Cardiol 2011;18:595–604.
55. Fiechter M, Gebhard C, Fuchs TA, et al. Cadmium-zinc-telluride myocardial perfusion imaging in obese patients. J Nucl Med 2012;53:1401–6.
56. Taillefer R, DePuey EG, Udelson JE, et al. Comparison between the end-diastolic images and the summed images of gated 99mTc-sestamibi SPECT perfusion study in detection of coronary artery disease in women. J Nucl Cardiol 1999;6:169–76.
57. Slomka PJ, Nishina H, Berman DS, et al. "Motion-frozen" display and quantification of myocardial perfusion. J Nucl Med 2004;45:1128–34.
58. Suzuki Y, Slomka PJ, Wolak A, et al. Motion-frozen myocardial perfusion SPECT improves detection of coronary artery disease in obese patients. J Nucl Med 2008;49:1075–9.
59. Singal AG, Mukherjee A, Joseph Elmunzer B, et al. Machine learning algorithms outperform conventional regression models in predicting development of hepatocellular carcinoma. Am J Gastroenterol 2013;108:1723–30.
60. Xiong HY, Alipanahi B, Lee LJ, et al. The human splicing code reveals new insights into the genetic determinants of disease. Science 2015;347(6218):1254806.
61. Waljee AK, Higgins PDR. Machine learning in medicine: a primer for physicians. Am J Gastroenterol 2010;105:1224–6.
62. Arsanjani R, Xu Y, Dey D, et al. Improved accuracy of myocardial perfusion SPECT for the detection of coronary artery disease using a support vector machine algorithm. J Nucl Med 2013;54:549–55.

Stress-first Myocardial Perfusion Imaging

Nasir Hussain, MD[a], Matthew W. Parker, MD[a], Milena J. Henzlova, MD[b], William Lane Duvall, MD[a,*]

KEYWORDS

- Myocardial perfusion imaging • Stress only • Stress first • Radiation reduction • Stress protocols • SPECT

KEY POINTS

- Normal stress-only myocardial perfusion imaging (MPI) studies have the same prognosis as full rest-stress MPI studies.
- Stress-only MPI studies decrease test time by 38% compared with conventional rest-stress protocols.
- Stress-only MPI studies decrease radiation exposure to patients by 27% to 76% compared with conventional rest-stress protocols.
- Successful stress-first protocols require attenuation correction for maximal effectiveness.

INTRODUCTION

Myocardial perfusion imaging (MPI) is traditionally conceptualized as 2 images. First, an image of radiotracer distribution under stress conditions is reviewed for any areas of decreased activity. The reader then compares these areas with a resting scan to determine whether the defect is reversible (ischemia) or fixed (infarction). However, when stress MPI is normal, the rest image becomes superfluous.

As far back as 1992,[1] nuclear cardiologists suggested reviewing stress MPI before deciding on the need to image the patient at rest. This stress-first strategy provides high-quality perfusion data equivalent to a full rest-stress study, saves time in the imaging laboratory, and reduces radiation exposure in appropriately selected patients. However, only a minority of nuclear cardiology laboratories use a stress-first protocol, perhaps reflecting challenges such as the need for attenuation correction, feasibility of real-time review of stress images, and concerns about reimbursement.[2,3]

In current clinical practice, most appropriately indicated diagnostic stress MPI studies are found to be normal, especially in patients with no prior history of coronary artery disease (CAD). In a study by Rozanski and colleagues[4] of 39,515 patients with no history of CAD who underwent diagnostic stress MPI from 1991 to 2009, the prevalence of normal MPI studies had increased among all subgroups from a prevalence rate of 59.1% in 1991, to 91.3% in 2009. The prevalence rate of normal studies reached as high as 97.1% among exercising patients without typical angina. In a recent multicenter study of 108,654 patients undergoing clinically indicated stress MPI studies, an overall increase in the prevalence of normal studies was seen from 1996 to 2012 in all patients (46.2%–68.2%), patients without CAD (67.8%–82%), and patients with CAD (25.3%–39.2%).[5] With the increasing prevalence of normal MPI studies, it is imperative that more cost-effective strategies be developed for the initial evaluation of patients who are presently at low risk for abnormal findings during stress MPI studies, and stress-first protocols represent and attractive option.

[a] Division of Cardiology, Hartford Hospital, 80 Seymour Street, Hartford, CT 06102, USA; [b] Mount Sinai Heart, Mount Hospital, One Gustave L Levy Place, New York, NY 10029, USA
* Corresponding author.
E-mail address: lane.duvall@hhchealth.org

Cardiol Clin 34 (2016) 59–67
http://dx.doi.org/10.1016/j.ccl.2015.06.006
0733-8651/16/$ – see front matter

DIAGNOSIS/PROGNOSIS

The diagnostic accuracy of single-photon emission computed tomography (SPECT) MPI for detecting flow-limiting CAD is well established, such that patients are unlikely to undergo diagnostic angiography after a normal SPECT MPI result and they have a benign 1-year prognosis.[6–8] This is a relevant issue for clinicians when interpreting stress-only SPECT MPI; that is, given normal stress-only SPECT MPI, are the expected rates of cardiac events in the coming year similar to those suggested by a full rest-stress MPI study?

A recent review cited 10 studies that all showed annualized cardiac event rates less than 1% following a normal stress-only MPI.[9] The pooled patient experience from the 4 studies directly comparing the prognosis of rest-stress and stress-only imaging suggests that the cardiac event rate is marginally lower following a normal stress-only MPI than following a normal rest-stress MPI (**Fig. 1**).[10–13] Low all-cause mortality and cardiac event rates following normal stress-only MPI suggest that rest imaging can be omitted without any reduction in the prognostic value of the test.

PATIENT SELECTION

At present, there are no published guidelines for the determination of which patients are suitable candidates for stress-first MPI protocols. The first step in the appropriate selection of patients for any imaging protocol is to ensure that the study is appropriately indicated.[14,15] Once MPI is deemed appropriate, selecting patients for a stress-first protocol requires some initial evaluation of the patient in order to customize the patient's experience in the nuclear laboratory. In general, patients with low to intermediate pretest probability for CAD (based on age, gender, risk factors, symptoms, and rest electrocardiogram [ECG]) are suitable candidates for a stress-first or stress-only MPI protocol. Another suitable group is patients with a high body mass index (>35 kg/m^2) or weight more than 115 kg (250 pounds); patients with recent (<3 years) negative noninvasive or invasive tests for the presence of obstructive CAD also seem to be suitable candidates.

A clinical scoring system has been proposed as a prediction model for determining which patients will undergo a successful stress-first technetium-99m (Tc-99m) MPI study and not require rest images.[16] Eight clinical variables with their assigned scores are listed in **Table 1** (a higher score correlates with an unsuccessful stress-first MPI study). Using this prediction model, patients were stratified into low-risk (−2 to <5), intermediate-risk (≥5 and <10), and high-risk (≥10) score groups. The low-risk cohort had a success rate of 92% for not requiring rest images, whereas the intermediate-risk and high-risk cohorts had 27% and 65% of patients requiring rest images, respectively.

In order to simplify the triage of patients to a stress-first protocol, we reevaluated the predictive accuracy of this model in a new population and analyzed CAD status alone as the determination of imaging protocol.[17] A history of CAD was defined as a previous myocardial infarction, a history of percutaneous coronary intervention, or previous coronary artery bypass grafting. Simply assigning all patients with no history of CAD to a stress-first protocol resulted in an 88% success rate for not needing subsequent rest images. Note that 54% of patients with known CAD did not require rest images as well. A simplified approach with a high success rate may therefore be to triage all patients without known CAD to a stress-first MPI protocol, with most patients with

Meta Analysis of Studies Comparing Prognosis of Normal Stress-only to Normal Stress-Rest MPI

	Study name	Statistics for each study			
Rate ratio		Lower limit	Upper limit	Z-value	*P*-value
1.139	Chang 2010	1.047	1.239	3.018	0.003
1.337	Duvall 2010	0.951	1.879	1.673	0.094
0.886	Ueyama 2012	0.512	1.534	−0.431	0.667
2.431	Edenbrandt 2013	1.816	3.255	5.964	0.000
1.206		1.116	1.304	4.708	0.000

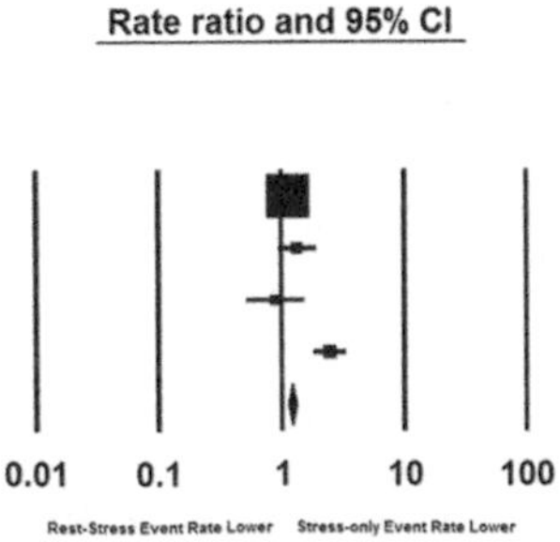

Fig. 1. Meta-analysis of studies investigating the prognosis of normal stress-only MPI studies. CI, confidence interval.

Table 1
Clinical and demographic variables with associated previously defined score

Variable	Score
Emergency department location	−2
Age>65 y	1
Diabetes mellitus	2
Typical chest pain	2
Congestive heart failure	3
Abnormal resting ECG	4
Male gender	4
Documented CAD	5

Data from Duvall WL, Baber U, Levine EJ, et al. A model for the prediction of a successful stress-first Tc-99m SPECT MPI. J Nucl Cardiol 2012;19:1124–34.

known CAD undergoing a standard rest-stress protocol.

A protocol that uses a provisional dose of radiotracer and perfusion imaging in patients undergoing exercise stress only when needed is an extension of the logic behind stress-first imaging that would further shorten test duration, decrease radiation exposure, and reduce health care costs. In this protocol, patients would not have the isotope administered if 10 or more Metabolic Equivalents (METs) of exercise were achieved without symptoms or ECG changes. The most obvious application of a provisional protocol in routine clinical practice would be to downgrade negative high-level exercise MPI studies to an Exercise Treadmill Test (ETT), thereby avoiding unnecessary injections of isotope and saving time and resources. Another use would be to facilitate the efficient diagnosis of patients and encourage adherence to the current guidelines encouraging the use of ETT.[14,15] In this case, by upgrading the study by adding imaging to an ETT when abnormal, a patient's evaluation can be completed efficiently in a single session as opposed to having the patient return for another stress and imaging session. This approach is similar to that used in the What is the Optimal Method for Ischemia Evaluation in Women (WOMEN) trial, only more efficient.[18] Preliminary work on this novel protocol has found that few of these patients (5.9%) had abnormal perfusion images and all had a benign prognosis at 5 years (1.1% all-cause mortality).[19] A recent prospective evaluation of this protocol in patients referred for stress testing as part of their emergency department evaluation showed that provisional injection of radioisotope saved time, reduced radiation exposure and health care costs compared with standard imaging protocols, but also conferred a very low mortality and fewer follow-up diagnostic tests.[20]

ADVANTAGES OF STRESS-FIRST MYOCARDIAL PERFUSION IMAGING

Radiation Reduction

Stress-first imaging results in substantial reductions in radiation exposure to patients and laboratory staff when stress images are normal and no rest images are performed. The rest-stress protocol recommended by the American Society of Nuclear Cardiology (ASNC), with a 10-mCi rest dose followed by a 30-mCi stress dose of Tc-99m sestamibi, results in total radiation exposure of 12.1 mSv.[21] Administering a high dose (30 mCi Tc-99m sestamibi) at stress and canceling the rest scan decreases total effective dose to 8.8 mSv, a 27% reduction in radiation. If the stress-first image is performed with the lower (10 mCi) dose, effective dose is only 2.9 mSv, 76% less than the standard rest-stress protocol. This reduced effective dose to patients is especially important in younger patients and women when it comes to the lifetime risk of developing cancer.[22] Further dose reduction can be achieved with the half-dose protocols made possible by new high-efficiency SPECT cameras as well as with PET imaging (**Fig. 2**). Rest-stress protocols of 5 mCi/15 mCi and the resultant 5-mCi low-dose stress-first approach have recently been made possible by high-efficiency SPECT cameras.[23,24] Although stress-first PET imaging is feasible,[25] the short half-life and imaging time of Rb-82 make it an impractical protocol. The longer half-life of N-13 or future F-18 labeled tracers would lend themselves better to a stress-first approach.

In 2010, an ASNC Information Statement on recommendations for reducing radiation exposure suggested that, by 2014, on average a total radiation exposure of less than or equal to 9 mSv could be achieved in 50% of MPI studies.[26] Recent articles investigating the temporal trends of abnormal or ischemic MPI study results in large clinical cohorts have consistently shown high proportions of normal studies.[4,5] If only half of the patients who undergo a stress-first protocol are normal and do not undergo rest imaging, this ASNC goal could be met solely by converting a laboratory to a stress-first approach instead of the standard rest-stress structure of most nuclear laboratories.

The radiation reduction seen with stress-first protocols can also be realized by laboratory staff. In a study of the effects of the introduction of a stress-first protocol and high-efficiency SPECT technology, there was approximately a 40% reduction in radiation exposure to laboratory

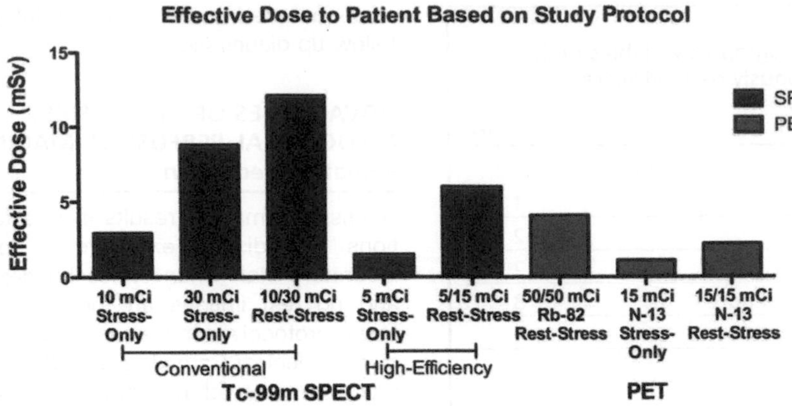

Fig. 2. Effective dose (mSv) to the patient based on imaging modality (conventional SPECT, high-efficiency SPECT, or PET) and study protocol (rest-stress or stress only). Radiation dosimetry calculations from International Commission on Radiological Protection Publication 120,[21] conventional SPECT doses based on current guidelines,[42] high-efficiency doses based on published literature,[23] and PET doses based on current guidelines.[43]

nurses and technologists based on badge dosimetry.[27] Although the effects of the two interventions were not separated, the contribution of stress-only protocols was likely substantial.

Time Savings

A stress-first protocol that becomes a stress-only protocol also results in time savings for patients and for the laboratory. We calculated the time it took to complete a SPECT MPI study from the time a patient checks into the laboratory at the reception desk to the time the study is interpreted based on guideline-specified waiting times, measured preparation and performance times in our laboratory, average exercise stress times, and standard imaging times with a conventional Na-I SPECT camera.[28] A standard rest-stress SPECT MPI study took 203 minutes to perform, whereas a stress-only study took 126 minutes, resulting in a time saving of 77 minutes or a 38% time reduction compared with the standard protocol. This time saving is immediately beneficial to patients who have other, shorter diagnostic modalities, such as cardiac computed tomographic angiography (CTA) and stress echocardiography, to choose from. It is also beneficial to laboratories, potentially allowing the performance of additional MPI studies in the same work day, or allowing a shorter work day, which may limit overtime expenditures.

Although a stress-first protocol has the potential to save time if rest images are not needed, concern has been raised regarding the risk of shine-through with low-dose stress images followed by high-dose rest images, resulting in an underestimation of defect reversibility. This possible scenario involves stress-induced ischemia in which the stress images are abnormal and the rest images are normal, but the rest/stress count density is not great enough to minimize the contribution (shine-through) of the underlying stress defect.[29] Controversy remains as to whether the shine-through phenomenon is clinically significant[29] or merely theoretic.[30] Current practice varies from as low as a 1:2 ratio between the low and high doses to as high as a 1:4 ratio. Also, the minimum recommended time to rest imaging after the stress dose varies considerably, from a few minutes to several hours. More studies or modeling are needed to clarify and codify these issues with modern SPECT cameras and software.

Thallium-201

Thallium is intrinsically stress first given the nature of its stress-redistribution protocol. Thallium studies can be reviewed after the stress images are obtained and the redistribution images forgone if the stress is normal. The prognosis of these normal stress-only thallium perfusion studies is the same as for normal stress-only Tc-99m and rest-stress Tc-99m studies.[31] Stress-only thallium studies do not result in any radiation reduction to patients but they do considerably shorten the study duration for patients and laboratories.

CHALLENGES IN IMPLEMENTING STRESS-FIRST MYOCARDIAL PERFUSION IMAGING

Need for Attenuation Correction

Stress MPI studies have emerged as a mainstay for the diagnosis and prognosis of CAD; however, the presence of soft tissue attenuation often poses challenges for the correct interpretation of the images. With the use of stress and rest ECG-gated wall motion assessment,[32] position-dependent imaging,[33] and advancement in attenuation correction software and hardware technology,[34] the diagnostic accuracy of stress MPI studies has improved. The success of stress-first MPI protocol depends on accurate interpretation of the perfusion images, which is highly dependent on attenuation correction to remove soft tissue artifacts because there are no rest images for comparison (**Fig. 3**). Current attenuation correction

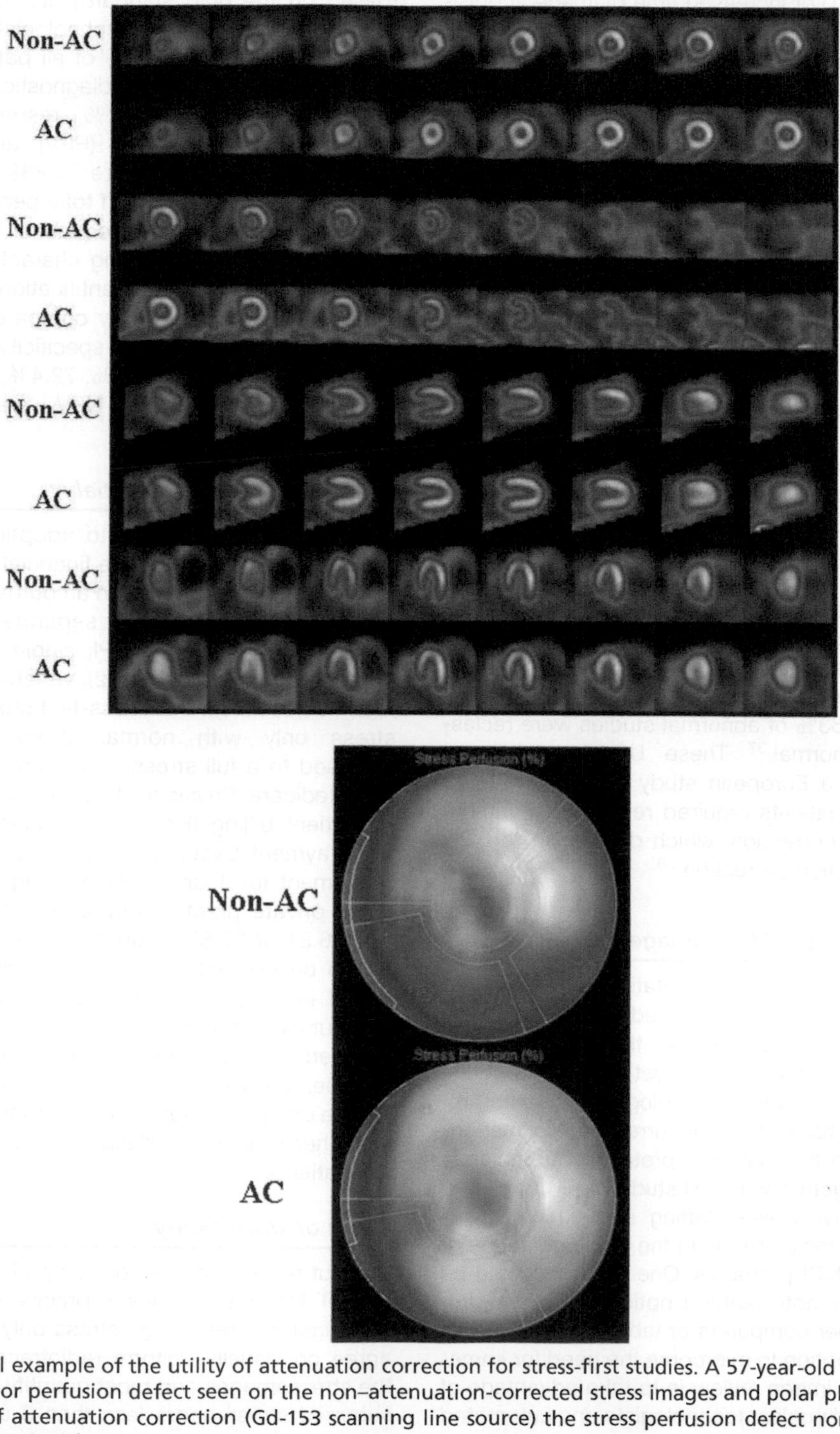

Fig. 3. Clinical example of the utility of attenuation correction for stress-first studies. A 57-year-old man with an obvious inferior perfusion defect seen on the non–attenuation-corrected stress images and polar plot. After the application of attenuation correction (Gd-153 scanning line source) the stress perfusion defect normalizes. AC, attenuation corrected.

options include supine and prone imaging, scanning Gd-153 line sources, and computed tomography (CT).[35]

One of the major drawbacks of a stress-first MPI protocol is the need for some form of attenuation correction with its associated cost (Gd-153 line source or CT) or increased time of image acquisition (supine and prone images). Additional information obtained with ECG gating has little added value for stress-first MPI studies because a given perfusion defect with normal wall motion may still represent ischemia versus residual attenuation and thus a need for rest imaging. Heller and colleagues[36] assessed the impact of the use of ECG gating and attenuation correction on the perceived need for rest imaging and on the level of confidence of interpreting the results of stress-only MPI studies. The application of ECG gating had little influence on the perceived need for rest imaging (77% without ECG gating vs 76% with) and on interpretation (37% vs 42%). However, the application of attenuation correction resulted in a statistically significant decrease in the perceived need for rest imaging (43% vs 77%; *P*-value <.005), and improved definitive interpretation (84% vs 37%; *P*-value <.005) without compromising the diagnostic accuracy of the test. In another study of the clinical importance of attenuation correction, 58% of stress-only images were classified as abnormal without attenuation correction; however, after the application of attenuation correction, 83% of abnormal studies were reclassified as normal.[37] These US findings were mirrored in a European study in which 49% of stress-first patients required rest images without attenuation correction, which decreased to 32% with attenuation correction.[38]

Need to Review Stress Images

For the successful implementation of a stress-first MPI protocol, an experienced reader must be available to timely interpret the stress images and determine the need for rest images. In routine clinical practice, most cardiologists who interpret MPI studies have other concurrent clinical responsibilities and the daily interpretation of studies is grouped together when all studies are completed for efficiency. These staffing and timing issues represent a major hurdle in the implementation of stress-first MPI protocols. One solution would be off-site or remote reading options to review images on other computers or tablets.

Another option to overcome the need for immediate stress image review is to take advantage of experienced nuclear technologists and automated computer quantification to assess the need for rest images. To test this idea, we assessed the ability of nuclear technologists and automated computer quantification to determine the need for rest images compared with the physician gold standard in 250 consecutive attenuation–corrected stress-first studies.[39] Overall, 83.2% of patients (based on the gold standard) did not need any rest images and nuclear technologists were able to correctly classify 91.6% of all patients with a sensitivity, specificity, and diagnostic accuracy of 66.7%, 96.2%, and 91.2%, respectively. The positive predictive value (PPV) and negative predictive value (NPV) were 77.8% and 93.5%, respectively. Using a cut off total perfusion deficit score of greater than or equal to 1.2%, cutoff based on receiver operating characteristic curve analysis, computer quantification classified 71.6% of patients correctly compared with gold standard. The sensitivity, specificity, and diagnostic accuracy were 73.2%, 72.4%, and 72.5%, respectively. The PPV and NPV were 35.3% and 92.9%, respectively.

Reimbursement Differential

One significant deterrent to adopting a stress-first work flow has been the financial disincentive that can occur, especially in an outpatient private practice setting. Because separate CPT billing codes exist for SPECT MPI, single (78451), and SPECT MPI, multiple (78452), variable reimbursement is possible if the stress-first study becomes stress only with normal stress images as opposed to a full stress-rest study. When using the Medicare Physician Fee Schedule, hospital outpatient billing (Hospital Outpatient Prospective Payment System) provides the same reimbursement for 1 or 2 sets of images. However, using private practice outpatient rates, there is a $136.21 or 27.8% reduction in reimbursement based on the 2015 fee schedule when a single set of images is obtained versus 2 sets. With reimbursement already having been substantially reduced for MPI procedures over the past decade, many physicians are unable to contemplate a change in their practices that would result in further reductions, despite the advantages to the patients.

Areas of Uncertainty

Without resting images for comparison, a normal SPECT MPI result requires precise definition. All investigators reporting stress-only techniques agree on visually uniform radiotracer uptake on the stress images and most quantify this as either summed stress score less than 3 using the 17-segment model or total perfusion defect less than 5% without attenuation correction or total perfusion defect of 0% with attenuation correction. Most investigators also stipulate normal left ventricular function after stress as a requirement of a normal stress-only study. The largest study, by Chang and colleagues,[10] specifically stated that electrocardiographic findings during treadmill exercise were not incorporated into the decision for rest imaging and post-hoc analysis, suggested that prognosis was similar for patients with both low-risk and intermediate-risk Duke Treadmill Scores in that cohort. The 2013 study by Edenbrandt and colleagues[13] defined normal perfusion solely by visual inspection and did not find any differences in prognosis when left ventricular ejection fraction and ventricular volumes were abnormal in patients with normal perfusion findings. All of these criteria assume good image quality; when artifacts such as hot spots, patient motion, or low count density are present, rest imaging or repeat acquisition of the stress images is required.

When stress images are not normal, rest imaging is generally recommended and areas of abnormal stress perfusion can then be compared with the resting perfusion pattern to ascertain reversibility (ischemia)[40]; other differential diagnostic possibilities to explain a perfusion defect present at stress include attenuation artifact and infarction. If attenuation correction is used, attenuation artifact becomes unlikely, and, in patients carefully selected for stress-first imaging (normal resting ECG and no personal history of infarction), infarction should also be rare. Therefore, patients with ischemic symptoms and electrocardiographic changes in combination with a significant perfusion defect at stress may benefit from proceeding directly to invasive coronary angiography and intervention without rest imaging.[9] Electrocardiographic evidence of ischemia and preserved or nearly-normal wall motion on the gated stress images may be important corroborating evidence of ischemia as opposed to artifact or infarction in such cases.

A novel approach would be to investigate less dramatic findings, such as small or mild perfusion defects or defects without associated electrocardiographic changes, with coronary CTA. This combined imaging strategy would essentially result in a hybrid SPECT-CTA specifically in those patients with indeterminate stress MPI findings. Coronary CTA can be performed with an effective dose of 2 to 4 mSv or less, resulting in a hybrid strategy that provides more information for less radiation exposure than a stress-rest MPI strategy.[41]

One additional scenario is that of futile rest images. Abnormal stress images caused by left bundle branch block artifact represent a scenario in which rest images are unlikely to clarify the diagnosis of CAD. A fixed defect may indicate a scar or left bundle branch block artifact, and a reversible defect may represent ischemia or left bundle branch block artifact. In another example, homogeneous perfusion at stress-only but abnormal left ventricular systolic function may not require rest images. Rest imaging is not likely to be helpful given that the differential diagnostic possibilities reduce to ischemic versus nonischemic cardiomyopathy and further perfusion imaging does not provide evidence of ischemia or infarction, especially if patient selection criteria are used to reduce the pretest probability of multivessel CAD.

SUMMARY

Stress-first approaches to MPI provide diagnostically and prognostically accurate perfusion data equivalent to a full rest-stress study, save time in the imaging laboratory, and reduce the radiation exposure to patients and laboratory staff. Converting a nuclear cardiology laboratory from a conventional rest-stress strategy to a stress-first approach involves challenges such as the need for attenuation correction, triage of patients to an appropriate protocol, real-time review of stress images, and consideration of differential reimbursement.

REFERENCES

1. Worsley DF, Fung AY, Coupland DB, et al. Comparison of stress-only vs. stress/rest with technetium-99m methoxyisobutylisonitrile myocardial perfusion imaging. Eur J Nucl Med 1992;19:441–4.
2. Lindner O, Bengel FM, Hacker M, et al. Use of myocardial perfusion imaging and estimation of associated radiation doses in Germany from 2005 to 2012. Eur J Nucl Med Mol Imaging 2014;41:963–71.
3. Einstein AJ, Tilkemeier P, Fazel R, et al. Radiation safety in nuclear cardiology-current knowledge and practice: results from the 2011 American Society of Nuclear Cardiology member survey. JAMA Intern Med 2013;173:1021–3.
4. Rozanski A, Gransar H, Hayes SW, et al. Temporal trends in the frequency of inducible myocardial ischemia during cardiac stress testing: 1991 to 2009. J Am Coll Cardiol 2013;61:1054–65.
5. Duvall WL, Rai M, Ahlberg AW, et al. A multi-center assessment of the temporal trends in myocardial perfusion imaging. J Nucl Cardiol 2015;22:539–51.
6. Fleischmann KE, Hunink MG, Kuntz KM, et al. Exercise echocardiography or exercise SPECT imaging? A meta-analysis of diagnostic test performance. JAMA 1998;280:913–20.

7. Kim C, Kwok YS, Heagerty P, et al. Pharmacologic stress testing for coronary disease diagnosis: a meta-analysis. Am Heart J 2001;142:934–44.
8. Klocke FJ, Baird MG, Lorell BH, et al. ACC/AHA/ASNC guidelines for the clinical use of cardiac radionuclide imaging–executive summary: a report of the American College of Cardiology/American Heart Association Task Force on Practice Guidelines (ACC/AHA/ASNC Committee to Revise the 1995 Guidelines for the Clinical Use of Cardiac Radionuclide Imaging). J Am Coll Cardiol 2003;42:1318–33.
9. Gowd BM, Heller GV, Parker MW. Stress-only SPECT myocardial perfusion imaging: a review. J Nucl Cardiol 2014;21:1200–12.
10. Chang SM, Nabi F, Xu J, et al. Normal stress-only versus standard stress/rest myocardial perfusion imaging: similar patient mortality with reduced radiation exposure. J Am Coll Cardiol 2010;55:221–30.
11. Duvall WL, Wijetunga MN, Klein TM, et al. The prognosis of a normal stress-only Tc-99m myocardial perfusion imaging study. J Nucl Cardiol 2010;17:370–7.
12. Ueyama T, Takehana K, Maeba H, et al. Prognostic value of normal stress-only technetium-99m myocardial perfusion imaging protocol. Comparison with standard stress-rest protocol. Circ J 2012;76:2386–91.
13. Edenbrandt L, Ohlsson M, Tragardh E. Prognosis of patients without perfusion defects with and without rest study in myocardial perfusion scintigraphy. EJNMMI Res 2013;3:58.
14. Hendel RC, Berman DS, Di Carli MF, et al. ACCF/ASNC/ACR/AHA/ASE/SCCT/SCMR/SNM 2009 Appropriate Use Criteria for Cardiac Radionuclide Imaging: a report of the American College of Cardiology Foundation Appropriate Use Criteria Task Force, the American Society of Nuclear Cardiology, the American College of Radiology, the American Heart Association, the American Society of Echocardiography, the Society of Cardiovascular Computed Tomography, the Society for Cardiovascular Magnetic Resonance, and the Society of Nuclear Medicine. J Am Coll Cardiol 2009;53:2201–29.
15. Wolk MJ, Bailey SR, Doherty JU, et al. ACCF/AHA/ASE/ASNC/HFSA/HRS/SCAI/SCCT/SCMR/STS 2013 multimodality appropriate use criteria for the detection and risk assessment of stable ischemic heart disease: a report of the American College of Cardiology Foundation Appropriate Use Criteria Task Force, American Heart Association, American Society of Echocardiography, American Society of Nuclear Cardiology, Heart Failure Society of America, Heart Rhythm Society, Society for Cardiovascular Angiography and Interventions, Society of Cardiovascular Computed Tomography, Society for Cardiovascular Magnetic Resonance, and Society of Thoracic Surgeons. J Am Coll Cardiol 2014;63:380–406.
16. Duvall WL, Baber U, Levine EJ, et al. A model for the prediction of a successful stress-first Tc-99m SPECT MPI. J Nucl Cardiol 2012;19:1124–34.
17. Chaudhry W, Ahlberg AW, Mujtaba M, et al. Prediction of successful stress-first SPECT MPI using a clinical pre-rest scoring model. J Nucl Cardiol 2014;21:778.
18. Shaw LJ, Mieres JH, Hendel RH, et al. Comparative effectiveness of exercise electrocardiography with or without myocardial perfusion single photon emission computed tomography in women with suspected coronary artery disease: results from the What is the Optimal Method for Ischemia Evaluation in Women (WOMEN) trial. Circulation 2011;124:1239–49.
19. Duvall WL, Levine EJ, Moonthungal S, et al. A hypothetical protocol for the provisional use of perfusion imaging with exercise stress testing. J Nucl Cardiol 2013;20:739–47.
20. Duvall WL, Savino JA, Levine EJ, et al. Prospective evaluation of a new protocol for the provisional use of perfusion imaging with exercise stress testing. Eur J Nucl Med Mol Imaging 2015;42:305–16.
21. Cousins C, Miller DL, Bernardi G, et al. ICRP PUBLICATION 120: radiological protection in cardiology. Ann ICRP 2013;42:1–125.
22. Berrington de Gonzalez A, Kim KP, Smith-Bindman R, et al. Myocardial perfusion scans: projected population cancer risks from current levels of use in the United States. Circulation 2010;122:2403–10.
23. Duvall WL, Croft LB, Ginsberg ES, et al. Reduced isotope dose and imaging time with a high-efficiency CZT SPECT camera. J Nucl Cardiol 2011;18:847–57.
24. Sharir T, Pinskiy M, Pardes A, et al. Comparison of the diagnostic accuracy of very low stress-dose to standard-dose myocardial perfusion imaging: automated quantification of one-day, stress-first SPECT using a CZT camera. J Nucl Cardiol 2015. [Epub ahead of print].
25. McMahon SR, Kikut J, Pinckney RG, et al. Feasibility of stress only rubidium-82 PET myocardial perfusion imaging. J Nucl Cardiol 2013;20:1069–75.
26. Cerqueira MD, Allman KC, Ficaro EP, et al. Recommendations for reducing radiation exposure in myocardial perfusion imaging. J Nucl Cardiol 2010;17:709–18.
27. Duvall WL, Guma KA, Kamen J, et al. Reduction in occupational and patient radiation exposure from myocardial perfusion imaging: impact of stress-only imaging and high-efficiency SPECT camera technology. J Nucl Med 2013;54:1251–7.
28. Duvall WL, Naib T, Greco G, et al. Cost savings associated with the use of selective stress-only and CZT SPECT myocardial perfusion imaging. J Nucl Cardiol 2013;20:S57.

29. DePuey EG, Ata P, Wray R, et al. Very low-activity stress/high-activity rest, single-day myocardial perfusion SPECT with a conventional sodium iodide camera and wide beam reconstruction processing. J Nucl Cardiol 2012;19:931–44.
30. Herzog BA, Buechel RR, Katz R, et al. Nuclear myocardial perfusion imaging with a cadmium-zinc-telluride detector technique: optimized protocol for scan time reduction. J Nucl Med 2010;51:46–51.
31. Duvall WL, Hiensch RJ, Levine EJ, et al. The prognosis of a normal Tl-201 stress-only SPECT MPI study. J Nucl Cardiol 2012;19:914–21.
32. Taillefer R, DePuey EG, Udelson JE, et al. Comparative diagnostic accuracy of Tl-201 and Tc-99m sestamibi SPECT imaging (perfusion and ECG-gated SPECT) in detecting coronary artery disease in women. J Am Coll Cardiol 1997;29:69–77.
33. Berman DS, Kang X, Nishina H, et al. Diagnostic accuracy of gated Tc-99m sestamibi stress myocardial perfusion SPECT with combined supine and prone acquisitions to detect coronary artery disease in obese and nonobese patients. J Nucl Cardiol 2006;13:191–201.
34. Kluge R, Sattler B, Seese A, et al. Attenuation correction by simultaneous emission-transmission myocardial single-photon emission tomography using a technetium-99m-labelled radiotracer: impact on diagnostic accuracy. Eur J Nucl Med 1997;24:1107–14.
35. Bateman TM, Cullom SJ. Attenuation correction single-photon emission computed tomography myocardial perfusion imaging. Semin Nucl Med 2005;35:37–51.
36. Heller GV, Bateman TM, Johnson LL, et al. Clinical value of attenuation correction in stress-only Tc-99m sestamibi SPECT imaging. J Nucl Cardiol 2004;11:273–81.
37. Mathur S, Heller GV, Bateman TM, et al. Clinical value of stress-only Tc-99m SPECT imaging: importance of attenuation correction. J Nucl Cardiol 2013;20:27–37.
38. Tragardh E, Valind S, Edenbrandt L. Adding attenuation corrected images in myocardial perfusion imaging reduces the need for a rest study. BMC Med Imaging 2013;13:14.
39. Chaudhry W, Ahlberg AW, Duvall WL. The ability of nuclear technologist to determine the need for rest imaging in a stress-first MPI protocol. J Nucl Cardiol 2014;21:772–3.
40. Iskandrian AE. Stress-only myocardial perfusion imaging a new paradigm. J Am Coll Cardiol 2010;55:231–3.
41. Fink C, Krissak R, Henzler T, et al. Radiation dose at coronary CT angiography: second-generation dual-source CT versus single-source 64-MDCT and first-generation dual-source CT. AJR Am J Roentgenol 2011;196:W550–7.
42. Henzlova MJ, Cerqueira MD, Mahmarian JJ, et al. Stress protocols and tracers. J Nucl Cardiol 2006;13:e80–90.
43. Dilsizian V, Bacharach SL, Beanlands R, et al. PET myocardial perfusion and metabolism clinical imaging. American Society of Nuclear Cardiology Web site. 2009. Available at: www.asnc.org/imageuploads/ImagingGuidelinesPETJuly2009.pdf. Accessed April 22, 2015.

Clinical PET Myocardial Perfusion Imaging and Flow Quantification

Daniel Juneau, MD, FRCPC[a,1], Fernanda Erthal, MD[a,1],
Hiroshi Ohira, MD, PhD[a,b], Brian Mc Ardle, MD[a],
Renée Hessian, MD, FRCPC[a],
Robert A. deKemp, PhD, PEng, PPhys[a],
Rob S.B. Beanlands, MD, FRCPC[a,*]

KEYWORDS

• PET • Myocardial perfusion imaging • Rubidium-82 • N-13-ammonia • Myocardial blood flow • Myocardial flow reserve • Flow quantification

KEY POINTS

- Cardiac PET has inherent advantages over single photon emission computed tomography (SPECT) myocardial perfusion imaging (MPI), including better imaging characteristics and the ability to quantify blood flow routinely.
- PET MPI has better sensitivity, specificity and accuracy than SPECT MPI in the detection of obstructive coronary artery disease.
- Myocardial flow reserve assessment can overcome the pitfall of balanced ischemia otherwise observed using conventional MPI in some patients with multivessel disease.
- PET MPI and flow quantification provide independent and incremental prognostic information for risk stratification.

INTRODUCTION

PET has evolved tremendously over the last 40 years. From humble beginnings in brain imaging, limited at first to a few research centers in the 1960s and 1970s,[1,2] PET has now grown to be a widely used modality in many disease areas. The development of numerous tracers imaging a wide range of biological pathways has lead to an ever-increasing reliance on PET in multiple clinical and research fields. The technology itself has seen many advances in recent years, including a 3-dimensional (3D)-mode acquisition, iterative reconstruction, hybrid systems (PET–computed tomography [CT] and PET–MR), and the (re)introduction of time-of-flight capabilities.

Although cardiac applications were first described in the 1970s, it was only once PET gained widespread use in oncologic imaging, with fluorodeoxyglucose (18-FDG), that the

Disclosures: R.A. deKemp is a consultant for and has received grant funding from Jubilant DraxImage. R.A. deKemp receives revenues from rubidium-82 generator technology licensed to Jubilant DraxImage, and from sales of FlowQuant software. R.S.B. Beanlands is or has been a consultant for and receives grant funding from GE Healthcare, Lantheus Medical Imaging, and Jubilant DraxImage.
R.S.B. Beanlands is a career investigator supported by the Heart and Stroke Foundation of Ontario (CI7431), Tier 1 Research Chair supported by the University of Ottawa, and University of Ottawa Heart Institute Vered Chair in Cardiology.
[a] Division of Cardiology, Department of Medicine, National Cardiac PET Centre, University of Ottawa Heart Institute, 40 Ruskin Street, Ottawa, Ontario K1Y 4W7, Canada; [b] First Department of Medicine, Hokkaido University Graduate School of Medicine, Kita 15 Nishi 7, Kita-Ku, Sapporo, Hokkaido 060-8638, Japan
[1] Co-first authors of this work.
* Corresponding author.
E-mail address: rbeanlands@ottawaheart.ca

Cardiol Clin 34 (2016) 69–85
http://dx.doi.org/10.1016/j.ccl.2015.07.013
0733-8651/16/$ – see front matter

availability of PET systems really increased. This has lead to increased availability of PET in other fields, including cardiology. Furthermore, the approval of rubidium-82 generators for clinical use has opened the way for centers without an on-site cyclotron to consider routine PET myocardial perfusion imaging (MPI). Nitrogen-13-ammonia ($^{13}NH_3$) and O-15-water are also used for perfusion and flow measurements in some jurisdictions. A longer lived F-18–labeled radiopharmaceutical is presently undergoing phase III trials to obtain approval in North America and Europe.

This article focuses on the role of PET imaging in patients with known or suspected coronary artery disease (CAD). We start with an overview of the available radiotracers and imaging protocols, discuss their accuracy compared with single photon emission computed tomography (SPECT) MPI, and review the prognostic value and impact on clinical decision making. We will also discuss myocardial blood flow (MBF) quantification, including its role in the diagnosis of CAD and its prognostic value.

PET TRACERS FOR MYOCARDIAL PERFUSION IMAGING AND FLOW QUANTIFICATION

Both PET and SPECT rely on the same general principle: a radiolabeled perfusion tracer with known characteristics is administered to the patient, and external detectors are then used to count photons being emitted from the patient. In SPECT, the tracers emit gamma rays with or without characteristic x-rays, whereas in PET, the tracers emit positrons that, after traveling a short distance in the surrounding tissue, interact with an electron, leading to an annihilation event. This results in two 511-keV annihilation photons being emitted simultaneously at approximately 180° apart, which are then detected in coincidence by several rings of detectors positioned around the patient. PET has several advantages over SPECT, including greater sensitivity and count rate (because it uses electronic coincidence collimation instead of geometric physical collimation), better spatial resolution, and robust attenuation correction, which enables the quantification of regional tracer activity accurately and in absolute units (Bq/cc).[3] PET also allows the dynamic acquisition of activity versus time data, permitting MBF quantification in mL/min/g among other quantifiable biologic parameters. Most current commercial PET cameras are hybrid PET-CT machines, thus allowing fast, reliable, and accurate attenuation correction, with optional coronary artery calcium and/or angiography assessment.

The 4 main tracers used for PET MPI are rubidium-82-chloride (^{82}Rb), $^{13}NH_3$, oxygen-15-water, and fluorine-18-flurpiridaz; their main advantages, disadvantages, and characteristics are listed in **Table 1**. Only ^{82}Rb and $^{13}NH_3$ are currently in routine clinical use in North America; oxygen-15-water is also used in Europe and Japan. An ideal tracer for PET MPI should have a short positron range (better spatial resolution), high uptake within the myocardium and low washout (better myocardium/blood pool contrast), and a linear relationship between tracer uptake and MBF (increased ability to detect milder stenosis and ability to perform accurate MBF measurement).[4] Short and long half-life tracers both have advantages: shorter half-life results in less radiation exposure for the patient and the ability to perform rapid repeat testing, but longer half-life obviates the need for an on-site cyclotron, and also enables exercise stress imaging protocols.

Rubidium-82-Chloride

^{82}Rb is a short-lived radionuclide, with a half-life of only 76 seconds, and is a potassium analog. It enters the myocardium by passive diffusion and active transport, via the adenosine triphosphate–dependent sodium–potassium cotransporter. Because of this active transport, the uptake in the myocardium has a nonlinear relationship with MBF, which may decrease the sensitivity of conventional MPI for mild stenosis. ^{82}Rb also has the drawback of having the longest positron range among the commonly used PET tracers (root mean square of positron range of 2.6 mm for ^{82}Rb vs 0.23 mm for ^{18}F and 0.57 mm for ^{13}N). This can lead to decreased spatial resolution when compared with other tracers; the effects are nonlinear and apparent mainly in high-resolution images. Compared with conventional $^{13}NH_3$ images with ~10 mm reconstructed resolution, the higher ^{82}Rb positron range degrades the resolution by ~15%.

The short half-life has the advantage of enabling very fast imaging protocols while maintaining high count rates and a low effective radiation dose for the patient. A complete rest plus stress examination using weight-based dosing for 3D PET, including a low-dose CT for attenuation correction, can be less than 1.5 to 2 mSv.[5,6] The short half-life also permits repeat imaging within a few minutes should it be required for clinical research studies. On the downside, exercise stress testing is not generally performed. Although exercise PET MPI has been done with ^{82}Rb, the challenges of the short half-life generally preclude this application.[7]

Table 1
Characteristics of cardiac PET radiotracers for myocardial perfusion imaging and flow quantification

Characteristic	^{82}Rb-Chloride	^{13}N-Ammonia	^{18}F-Flurpiridaz	^{15}O-Water
Production method	^{82}Sr/^{82}Rb generator	Onsite cyclotron	Offsite "regional" cyclotron	Onsite cyclotron
Half-life	76 s	9.97 min	110 min	112 s
Positron range (root mean square), mm	2.6	0.57	0.23	1.02
Extraction (stress-rest), %	40–70	94–98	≥90	95–100
Retention (stress-rest), %	30–55	60–90	60–90	No retention
Advantages	Commercially available generator Approved for clinical use Fast scan time Low radiation dose Short half-life permits quick testing	Excellent contrast resolution Approved for clinical use Low radiation dose	Excellent contrast resolution and spatial resolution Exercise stress possible No need for onsite cyclotron or investment in generator system	Low radiation dose Short half-life permits quick testing Ideal kinetics for quantification (free diffusion) Excellent extraction at high flow rates
Disadvantages	Lowest spatial resolution (still superior to SPECT) Lowest retention at high flow Exercise stress almost impossible	Requires onsite cyclotron Lung and liver uptake Lateral wall relative hypocaptation Exercise stress impractical Moderate retention at high flow rates	Highest radiation dose (still less than routine ^{201}Tl or ^{99m}Tc agents protocols) Not yet approved for clinical use Moderate retention at high flow rates	Exercise stress impossible Requires onsite cyclotron Low contrast resolution Low spatial resolution

Adapted from Mc Ardle B, Renaud J, DeKemp R, et al. Role of PET in diagnosis and risk assessment in patients with known or suspected CAD. In: Iskandrian A, Garcia E, editors. Nuclear cardiac imaging. 5th edition. Oxford University Press; 2015; with permission.

^{82}Rb is produced from strontium-82/rubidium-82 generators (^{82}Sr/Rb), which are approved for clinical use by the US Food and Drug Administration (FDA; CardioGen) and Health Canada (Ruby-Fill) currently. ^{82}Rb is eluted from the generator using physiologic saline, and because it has such a short half-life, full activity can be eluted from the generator every 5 to 10 minutes.[8] Because ^{82}Sr has a half-life of 25.5 days, a single generator can be used for 4 to 8 weeks depending on the manufacturer and the dose administered for 2-dimensional or 3D PET. This obviates the need for an on-site cyclotron, and is among the main reasons why ^{82}Rb is currently the most widely used tracer for PET MPI in clinical practice. Finally, the ability of ^{82}Rb dynamic PET imaging to accurately and reproducibly quantify absolute MBF is now well-established.[9,10]

N-13-Ammonia

$^{13}NH_3$ was the first radiotracer used for PET MPI,[1] and with ^{82}Rb, is 1 of only 2 tracers approved for clinical use in the US. It has a relatively short half-life of 10 minutes. This means it must be produced by an onsite cyclotron for immediate use. $^{13}NH_3$ enters the myocardium both by free diffusion and via the ammonium transporter. Once it has entered the myocardium, retention is predominantly via the conversion of $^{13}NH_3$ and glutamic acid to ^{13}N-glutamine, which is mediated by glutamine synthetase. This is an adenosine triphosphate–dependent process.

$^{13}NH_3$ has first-pass extraction of greater than 90% from the blood, even at high flow rates. This extraction results in a near linear relationship between the myocardial uptake rate and blood flow. Despite a relatively fast initial clearance rate, it still has superior retention when compared with ^{82}Rb, as well as a shorter positron range. Its longer half-life also permits longer acquisition time, with better count statistics. These advantages all contribute to better image quality with better contrast resolution and better spatial resolution. It is also possible to perform exercise stress imaging, but this remains impractical in most settings owing to the difficultly in timing with tracer production.[11]

Liver uptake is part of the normal biodistribution of $^{13}NH_3$. Diffuse lung uptake is also frequently seen in smokers and in patients with congestive heart failure. This can in turn lead to CT used for attenuation correction (CTAC) misalignment artifacts and diminished image quality. Last, lateral wall defects are often present, which can be difficult to distinguish from a true perfusion defect.[12] The exact cause and mechanism of this "normal variant" are still unknown.

F-18-Flurpiridaz

^{18}F-flurpiridaz Is a recently introduced PET tracer developed specifically for PET MPI. The results from recently completed phase III(a) studies have been presented at the International Congress for Nuclear Cardiology and CT.[13] Final phase III(b) studies are being planned to further support the FDA investigational new drug and application for approval. Flurpiridaz is a pyridaben analog, a mitochondrial complex 1 inhibitor, a protein predominantly found in viable myocardium. The toxicity of F-18–labeled flurpiridaz has been investigated and the results show that, with a maximum clinical dose of less than 0.07 μg/kg, flurpiridaz has an ample safety margin for clinical cardiac imaging.[14]

Flurpiridaz has excellent first-pass extraction and good retention, similar to $^{13}NH_3$. It does not seem to suffer from the lateral wall "normal variant" defect or the lung uptake seen with $^{13}NH_3$, although it is metabolized predominantly by the liver. Its greatest advantage, however, is the longer ^{18}F half-life of 110 minutes, which enables delivery from a regional cyclotron, obviating the need for on-site tracer production. This is an even greater advantage when one considers that smaller centers, with smaller throughput, might thus be able to purchase a few doses per week, as needed, without investing in a cyclotron or $^{82}Sr/Rb$ generator. The longer half-life also easily permits exercise stress testing. It does, however, lead to a greater effective radiation dose for the patient when compared with ^{82}Rb and $^{13}NH_3$. Although the longer half-life complicates same-day rest–stress flow quantification, it has been demonstrated that flurpiridaz dynamic studies can accurately and reproducibly quantify absolute MBF using appropriate corrections for the residual rest activity.[15]

O-15-Water

O-15-water, unlike the other tracers discussed, is not retained within the myocardium. It diffuses freely across capillary and myocardial cell membranes. It has a first-pass extraction fraction of close to 100%, and the relationship between tracer clearance and MBF is linear, making it an ideal tracer for absolute measurement of MBF.

The lack of retention in the myocardium means that relative perfusion imaging cannot be performed without the use of additional parametric imaging software, because there is no contrast in tracer uptake between the myocardium and the blood pool. Although some centers in Europe use it clinically, $H_2{}^{15}O$ use is mainly limited to the research setting in Canada and US.

PET IMAGING PROTOCOLS FOR MYOCARDIAL PERFUSION IMAGING AND MYOCARDIAL BLOOD FLOW QUANTIFICATION

Patient Preparation and Image Acquisition

Patient preparation is similar to SPECT imaging, whether proceeding to pharmacologic or exercise stress. The use of PET instead of SPECT does not entail any modification of the stress protocol itself. Patient positioning is the same as with SPECT. In the case of the shortest lived tracers, ^{82}Rb and $H_2{}^{15}O$, the patient generally remains in the scanner throughout the rest–stress imaging protocol. Because their half-lives are so short, there is no need to wait for radioactive decay between rest and stress imaging.

A typical ^{82}Rb protocol using a modern 3D PET-CT system is described as follows: a CT scout and a transmission CT for attenuation correction are acquired. A rapid infusion, over about 10 to 30 seconds, follows the CT scan, while the patient is at rest. The dose (750–1500 MBq) is calculated based on body weight (eg, 10–15 MBq/kg; **Fig. 1**).[16] Acquisition in list mode starts immediately, and lasts 6 to 8 minutes. Pharmacologic stress testing is then performed, without the need for any delay, while the patient remains in the scanner. ^{82}Rb is again injected while the patient is at peak stress and image acquisition is repeated. The whole acquisition is generally electrocardiography (ECG) and respiration gated, and can be completed in less than 30 minutes. The

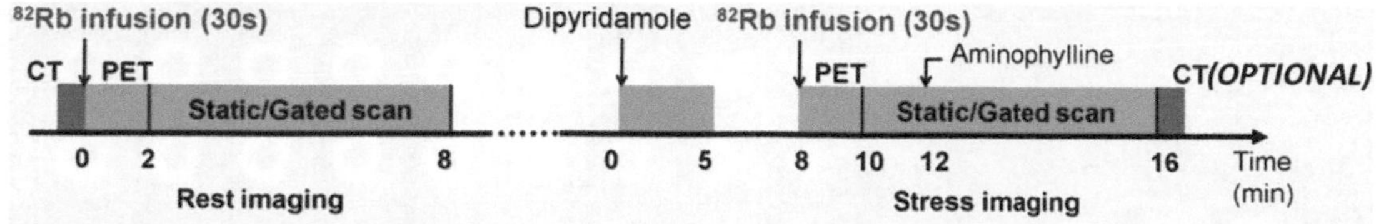

Fig. 1. Example of typical rubidium-82-chloride (^{82}Rb) PET myocardial perfusion imaging protocol. Rest CT includes a scout to localize the heart and a low-dose end-expiration CT for attenuation correction. (*Adapted from* Renaud JM, Mylonas I, McArdle B, et al. Clinical interpretation standards and quality assurance for the multicenter PET/CT trial rubidium-ARMI. J Nucl Med 2014;55(1):61; with permission.)

use of list-mode acquisition (where every single coincidence count is saved individually) allows multiple series, including dynamic images, ECG-gated images, respiratory-gated images, and ungated uptake images to be reconstructed from a single acquisition or dataset. An $H_2{}^{15}O$ protocol would be similar; the only significant change being the activity injected (350–1100 MBq). For $^{13}NH_3$, acquisition time is longer (10–20 minutes), and a 30- to 40-minute delay between the rest study and stress testing is typically required to allow for isotope decay. Less activity is injected (350–750 MBq) to minimize radiation dose.[17] Optimal protocols for ^{18}F-flurpiridaz imaging are still being established.

The CTAC should generally be a low-dose (0.2–0.4 mSv), ungated, helical scan performed either during shallow breathing or end-tidal expiration. Some centers routinely perform a second CTAC after stress testing imaging, whereas other centers, including ours, have reported excellent results using only 1 CTAC scan.[18] A second CTAC should always be considered in cases where the patient experienced significant discomfort or other side effects during stress testing and if any kind of mobilization was required, because patient positioning might not be identical, and the attenuation map might thus be inaccurate if using only 1 CTAC. If calculation of a coronary artery calcium score is desired, the CTAC scan can be changed to an ECG-gated protocol, thus allowing end-diastolic acquisition. This addition may, however, lead to a slightly higher radiation dose, although initial experience suggests that a single low-dose CT–coronary artery calcium scan may also be used for attenuation correction in most cases.[18]

Image Reconstruction, Quality Assurance, and Artifacts

Modern PET-CT systems use iterative reconstruction, thus eliminating artifacts associated with filtered back-projection. Recent PET detector hardware advances have also seen the addition of time-of-flight technology that, by measuring the miniscule time difference between the arrival of the annihilation photons, can better position the event along the line of response between detector pairs. This method has the benefit of reducing background image noise, particularly in larger patients.

The most common source of artifact in PET MPI is incorrect attenuation correction. A misaligned attenuation map can, instead of helping to correct for attenuation artifacts, create new artifacts in the images or even mask real perfusion defects. It is, therefore, vital to verify visually the correct alignment of the CT and PET images, and apply manual correction if needed.[19] Visual alignment of the PET and CTAC images can be challenging in cases with lung uptake, for example, ^{13}N-ammonia scans in smokers; lung uptake shifted medially toward the left ventricular (LV) lateral wall can give the false impression of cardiac hypertrophy or relative increased uptake compared with the rest of the LV, on the attenuation corrected PET images. Automated image alignment software is being developed, which could lead to more reliable and less operator-dependent correction.[20] The images should also be inspected visually to rule out patient motion (including respiratory motion), another important source of image artifact.[21]

Image Interpretation

PET MPI images are generally reconstructed and displayed similarly to SPECT MPI images, using orthogonal slices along the 3 anatomic axes of the heart (**Fig. 2**). Semiquantitative interpretation is based on the standardized 17-segments model, using the same severity and extent criteria as SPECT.[22,23] ECG-gated images are also evaluated for the presence of any wall motion abnormality, and to quantify LV ejection fraction. The presence of induced wall motion abnormality on poststress images has a different meaning with PET versus SPECT. With PET MPI using $^{13}NH_3$ or ^{82}Rb, it represents ischemia during peak stress, whereas with Tc-99m–based SPECT imaging, it represents poststress stunning (ie, postischemic dysfunction). This difference is explained by the delay

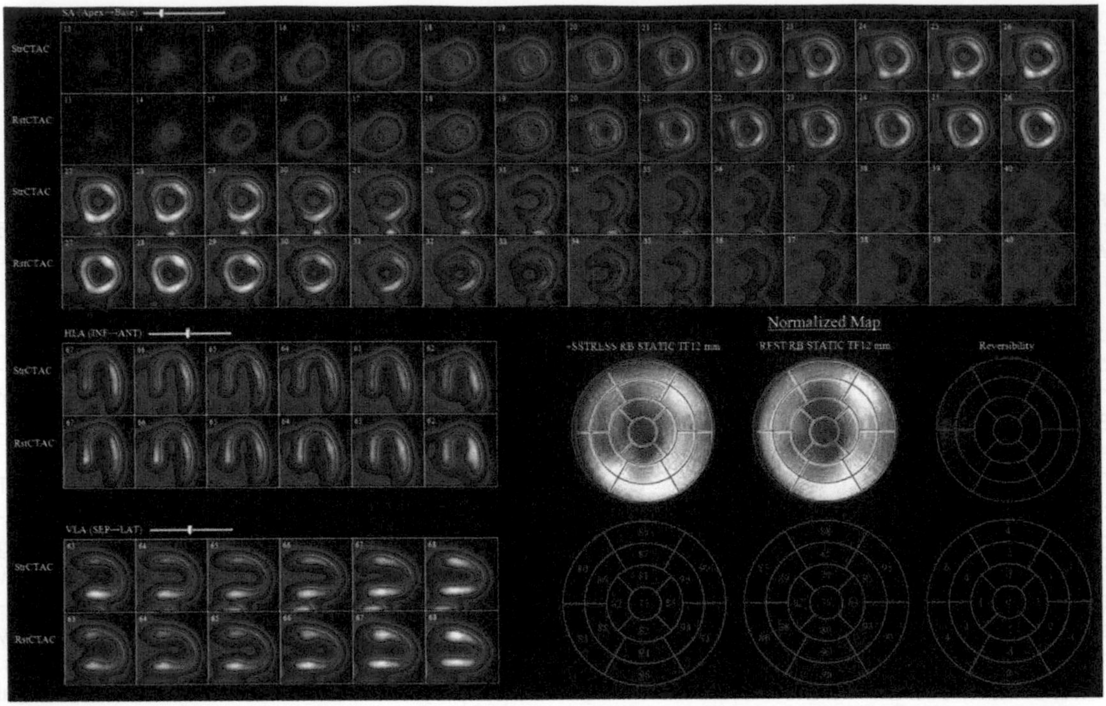

Fig. 2. PET myocardial perfusion imaging in a 48-year-old obese man with a history of atypical chest pain. Both rest and poststress images, along all 3 axes, show normal left ventricular perfusion. (*From* Mc Ardle B, Renaud J, DeKemp R, et al. Role of PET in diagnosis and risk assessment in patients with known or suspected CAD. In: Iskandrian A, Garcia E, editors. Nuclear cardiac imaging. 5th edition. Oxford University Press; 2015; with permission.)

between injection and imaging in SPECT, whereas patients are imaged during or immediately after maximum stress when using ^{82}Rb or $^{13}NH_3$.

Most high-risk imaging features (**Box 1**) are similar to those used for the interpretation of SPECT. Similar to SPECT, it has been demonstrated that there is an inverse relationship between the summed stress score and event-free survival using ^{82}Rb PET MPI.[24] A recent multicenter study[25] showed that increasing percentage of abnormal (ischemic or scarred) myocardium on PET MPI with ^{82}Rb, was a significant univariable predictor of cardiac death and all-cause death.

Box 1
High-risk imaging features

Perfusion defect size/severity: inverse relationship between Summed Stress Score and event-free survival[24,25,34]

Transient ischemic dilation: ratio stress/rest greater than 1,15[26]

Reduced stress LVEF: increased annual mortality proportional to decrease in LVEF[27,28]

Severely impaired myocardial flow reserve on quantification[47,51,52]

Right ventricle uptake increased with stress[29]

Abbreviation: LVEF, left ventricular ejection fraction.

Adapted from Mc Ardle B, Renaud J, DeKemp R, et al. Role of PET in diagnosis and risk assessment in patients with known or suspected CAD. In: Iskandrian A, Garcia E, editors. Nuclear Cardiac Imaging. 5th edition. Oxford University Press; 2015; with permission.

Transient ischemic dilation after stress testing is indicative of more severe ischemia (**Fig. 3**). As in SPECT MPI, the exact threshold used varies between centers and is the subject of some debate. At least 1 group has demonstrated that a total ionizing dose cutoff of 1.15 using ^{82}Rb had a high sensitivity for single and multiple vessel CAD (100% and 93%, respectively).[26]

As with SPECT, decreasing the LV ejection fraction (LVEF) on ECG-gated PET MPI is associated with increased mortality.[27] Patients with an LVEF of less than 40% had annual mortality rates of 9.2% versus 2.4% for patients with an LVEF of greater than 50%. Patients who had diminished LVEF after stress testing when compared with rest LVEF also had a worse outcome, with increased rates of adverse cardiac event and death.[28]

Increased RV uptake with stress has also been described as a high-risk feature. This phenomena is likely owing to the relative decrease of maximal perfusion in the LV compared with the RV and may reflect multivessel disease.[29]

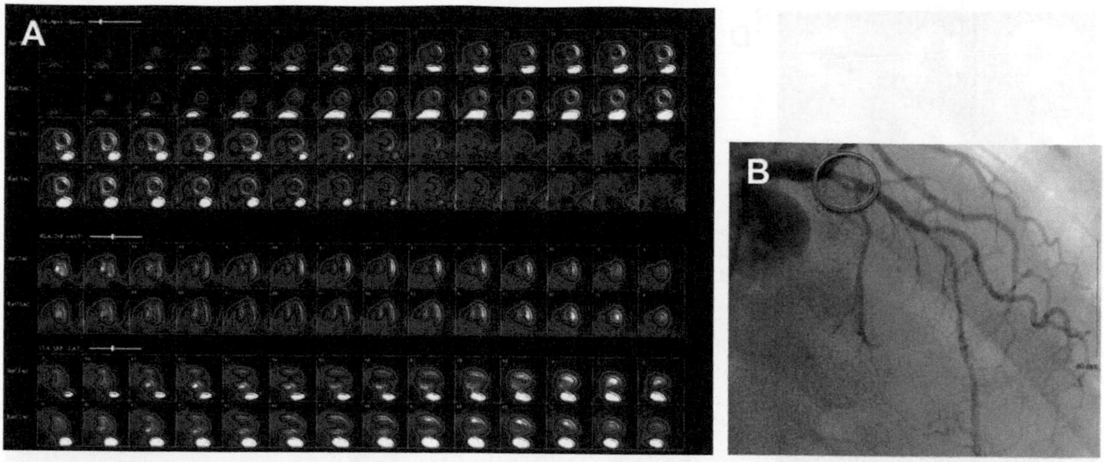

Fig. 3. Rubidium-82-chloride (^{82}Rb) PET myocardial perfusion imaging of a 68-year-old diabetic male patient with history of atypical chest pain. (*A*) Postdipyridamole images showed severe reduction in tracer uptake along the distal anterior and anteroseptal wall as well as the apex; rest images are normal. There was transient ischemic dilation of the LV on poststress images (ratio 1.34) and ST segment depression during dipyridamole stress. (*B*) Coronary angiography revealed serial stenosis of the mid (*circle*) and distal left anterior descending coronary artery. (*From* Mc Ardle B, Renaud J, DeKemp R, et al. Role of PET in diagnosis and risk assessment in patients with known or suspected CAD. In: Iskandrian A, Garcia E, editors. Nuclear cardiac imaging. 5th edition. Oxford University Press; 2015; with permission.)

DIAGNOSTIC ACCURACY

Many studies have shown that PET MPI is highly sensitive and specific for the detection of obstructive coronary disease.[30–33] Although many of those studies had important limitations (most were small series, retrospective, used older 2-dimensional PET systems, and most did not use MBF quantification), more recent data, using modern 3D PET-CT systems, support the same conclusions (**Fig. 4**). This includes 2 recent studies by Kaster and colleagues[30] and Nakazato and colleagues,[31] both using modern 3D PET-CT systems and ^{82}Rb, both aiming to evaluate the accuracy of PET MPI. Nakazato and colleagues used MBF quantification whereas Kaster and colleagues used only MPI. Nakazato reported a sensitivity/specificity of 86%/86% for stenosis of 50% or greater and 93%/77% for stenosis of 70% or greater, whereas Kaster reported a sensitivity of nearly 100% for the detection of CAD and a specificity of 87% (**Fig. 5**).

Two recent metaanalyses demonstrated that PET MPI is superior to SPECT MPI. Mc Ardle and colleagues[32] compared ^{82}Rb PET MPI and contemporary ^{99m}Tc-based SPECT imaging. They only included SPECT studies that used ECG-gated and attenuation corrected images, because this method best reflects contemporary practice. In the final analysis, PET and SPECT had sensitivities of 90% and 85%, respectively, and specificities of 88% and 85% (**Fig. 6**). Parker and colleagues,[33] in another metaanalysis, also demonstrated the superior accuracy of PET. They reported sensitivities of 93% and 88% for PET and SPECT, respectively, and specificities of 81% and 76%. They included studies that used ^{82}Rb, $H_2{}^{15}O$, and $^{13}NH_3$ for PET versus ^{99m}Tc-based agents and ^{201}Tl for SPECT.

RISK STRATIFICATION AND PROGNOSIS

The prognostic value of PET MPI, mainly with ^{82}Rb but also with $^{13}NH_3$, has been well-established in multiple studies.[34] Although these studies vary greatly in design, including the type of patients and type of events included, all agreed that a normal PET MPI was indicative of low risk (annual cardiac event rate of <1%), whereas abnormal scans were associated with greater risk, proportionate to the severity of findings.[24,25] The incremental prognostic value of rest LVEF, stress LVEF, and LVEF reserve have also all been clearly established with ^{82}Rb.[27,28]

Results from a recently completed multicenter registry have been published.[25] These results supported previously published data from smaller, single-center, observational studies.[35] The data showed increasing risk of cardiac events and cardiac death in patients with abnormal scans, with the risk-adjusted hazard of such events being proportional to the severity of findings on stress images (**Fig. 7**). Furthermore, 2 substudies from this registry demonstrated that the prognostic value of PET MPI was the same in men and women, and was preserved in overweight and

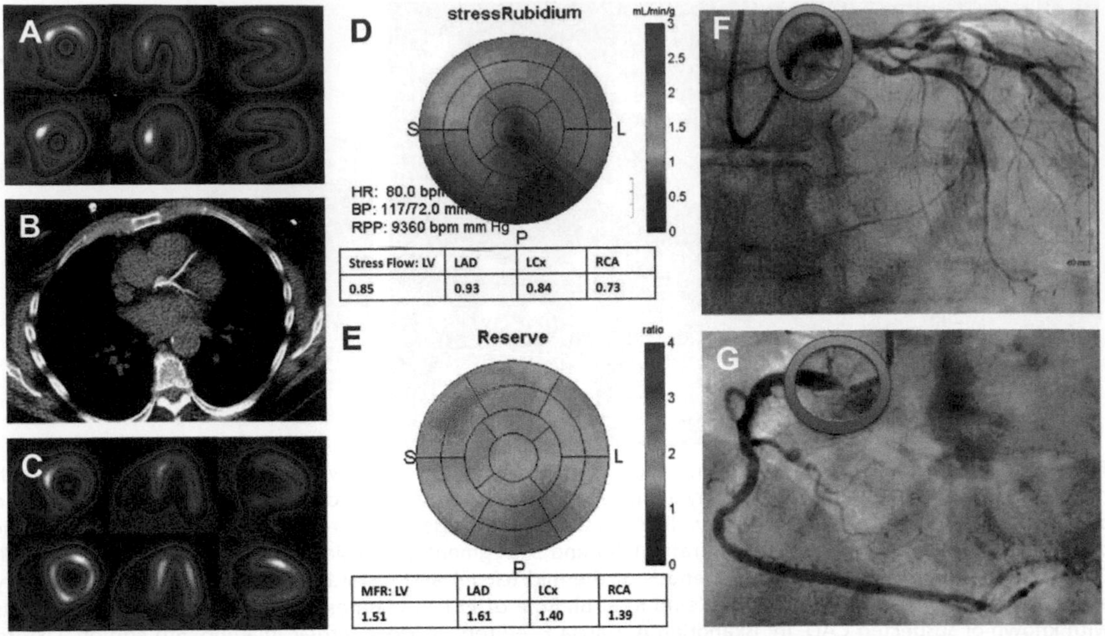

Fig. 4. A 64-year-old man presented after 1 episode of resting chest pain, with negative cardiac enzymes. (*A*) ^{99m}Tc-tetrofosmin single photon emission CT myocardial perfusion imaging (MPI) was normal, but ST segment depression was observed during dypiridamole stress testing. Further testing was recommended and patient underwent rubidium-82-chloride (^{82}Rb) PET MPI. (*B*) Severe calcification was present on CT used for attenuation correction (CTAC) images. (*C*) PET MPI images showed mild inferolateral ischemia. (*D*) Absolute stress myocardial blood flow was decreased globally in the left ventricle (LV; <1.5 mL/min/g), as seen on polar map, with most severe decrease in the inferior wall. (*E*) LV myocardial flow reserve (MFR) was also reduced globally (<2.0), as seen on polar map, particularly in the inferior and lateral wall. (*F, G*) Coronary angiogram revealed severe left main (circled, F) and ostial right coronary artery (RCA) disease (circled, G). BP, blood pressure; HR, heart rate; LAD, left anterior descending; LCx, left circumflex; RCA, right coronary artery; RPP, right perfusion pressure. (*From* Mc Ardle B, Renaud J, DeKemp R, et al. Role of PET in diagnosis and risk assessment in patients with known or suspected CAD. In: Iskandrian A, Garcia E, editors. Nuclear cardiac imaging. 5th edition. Oxford University Press; 2015; with permission.)

obese patients.[36,37] This finding is of particular interest because these are specific patient subgroups in which the accuracy and prognostic value of other modalities, including SPECT, is known to be reduced.

PET MYOCARDIAL PERFUSIONS IMAGING IMPACT ON CLINICAL DECISION MAKING

Ultimately, the role of diagnostic imaging is to guide the clinician in making the best possible clinical decision, and thus to improve patient outcome. Many studies have evaluated the use of radionuclide MPI to guide patient management and to assess response to therapy.[38,39] However, most of the data is based on SPECT, and there is a lack of prospective data regarding PET. The results of the International Study of Comparative Health Effectiveness with Medical and Invasive Approaches (ISCHEMIA, https://ischemiatrial.org/), a large, ongoing, international, multicenter trial, will possibly help to remedy part of the problem if a sufficient number who undergo PET MPI are enrolled, hopefully shedding light on whether or not the identification of myocardial ischemia on PET MPI can guide patient management and lead to improved outcomes.

In the meantime, PET MPI is still incorporated in the current American College of Cardiology/American Heart Association appropriate use documents guiding coronary angiography and coronary revascularization.[40,41] These recommendations are based on expert opinion, SPECT data, and PET data from observational studies. They deem coronary angiography appropriate based on diagnostic imaging findings in patients with high risk features, such as high-risk MPI (≥10% LV ischemic myocardium), transient ischemic dilation (TID) or poststress LV dysfunction, or in patients with intermediate-risk findings on PET MPI but who are symptomatic. As for coronary revascularization, it was deemed appropriate in patients

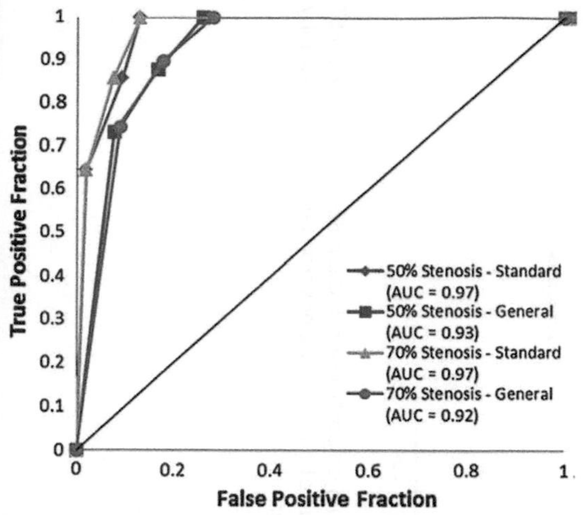

Fig. 5. Receiver operator characteristics curves for detection of coronary artery disease at 50% and 70% stenosis. AUC, area under the curve. (*From* Kaster T, Mylonas I, Renaud JM, et al. Accuracy of low-dose rubidium-82 myocardial perfusion imaging for detection of coronary artery disease using 3D PET and normal database interpretation. J Nucl Cardiol 2012;19(6):1141; with permission.)

with high-risk findings on PET-MPI who have significant symptoms (Canadian Cardiovascular Society class 3 or 4 angina). On the contrary, coronary angiography and coronary revascularization were deemed inappropriate in patients with normal PET MPI, who have been shown to have an excellent prognosis.

QUANTIFICATION OF MYOCARDIAL BLOOD FLOW

Over the past 3 decades, PET has evolved into the modality of choice to evaluate MBF noninvasively.[42] The quantification is performed by analyzing the dynamic data acquired immediately after injection of the PET tracer. A tracer kinetic model is used to describe the shape of the myocardial time-versus-activity curve based on an image-derived arterial blood input function and the first-pass extraction fraction of the tracer by the myocardium. This leads to values of absolute MBF measured in mL/min/g at rest and stress. From this the myocardial flow reserve (MFR), the ratio of stress/rest MBF, can be calculated. The accuracy and reproducibility of these measurements have been demonstrated using ^{82}Rb, $^{13}NH_3$, $H_2{}^{15}O$, and ^{18}F-flurpiridaz.[9,15,42]

MBF and MFR as determined using PET are not the same as invasive measurement of epicardial coronary flow reserve or fractional flow reserve, although they are closely linked.[1,43] Fractional flow reserve evaluates the pressure decrease across a stenosis to define its hemodynamic impact on the downstream myocardium, but this is not able to consider the effect of the microcirculation or collateral flow. Conversely, MFR evaluates the combined effects of the stenosis and the microcirculation, but cannot differentiate the effect of one and the other independently. It is thus possible to have discordant MFR and fractional flow reserve values in the case of a dominant focal lesion with minimal microcirculatory disease, or in the case of diffuse epicardial

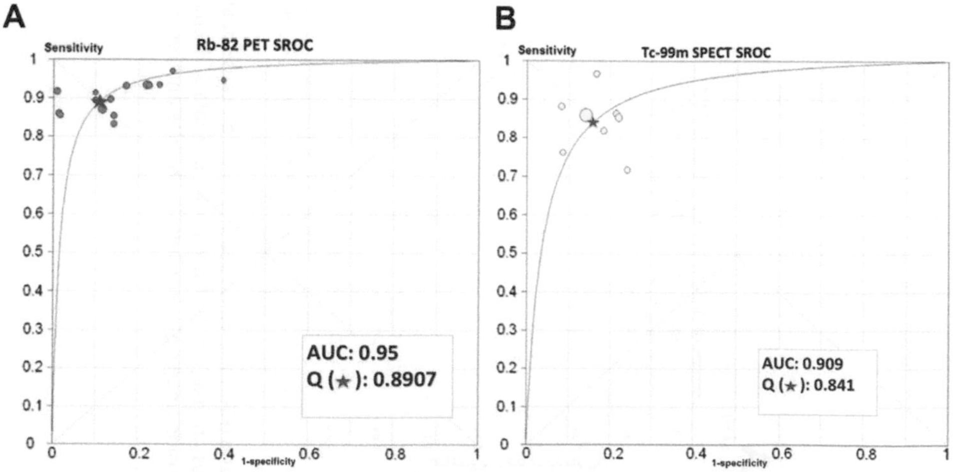

Fig. 6. Area under the curve (AUC) comparing the diagnostic accuracy of (*A*) rubidium-82-chloride (^{82}Rb) PET and (*B*) ^{99m}Tc-based single photon emission CT (SPECT) with electrocardiographic gating and attenuation correction, using epicardial stenosis on invasive coronary angiography as a gold standard. Comparison of the AUC showed superior accuracy for ^{82}Rb PET ($P<.001$). (*From* Mc Ardle BA, Dowsley TF, deKemp RA, et al. Does rubidium-82 PET have superior accuracy to SPECT perfusion imaging for the diagnosis of obstructive coronary disease? A systematic review and meta-analysis. J Am Coll Cardiol 2012;60(18):1833; with permission.)

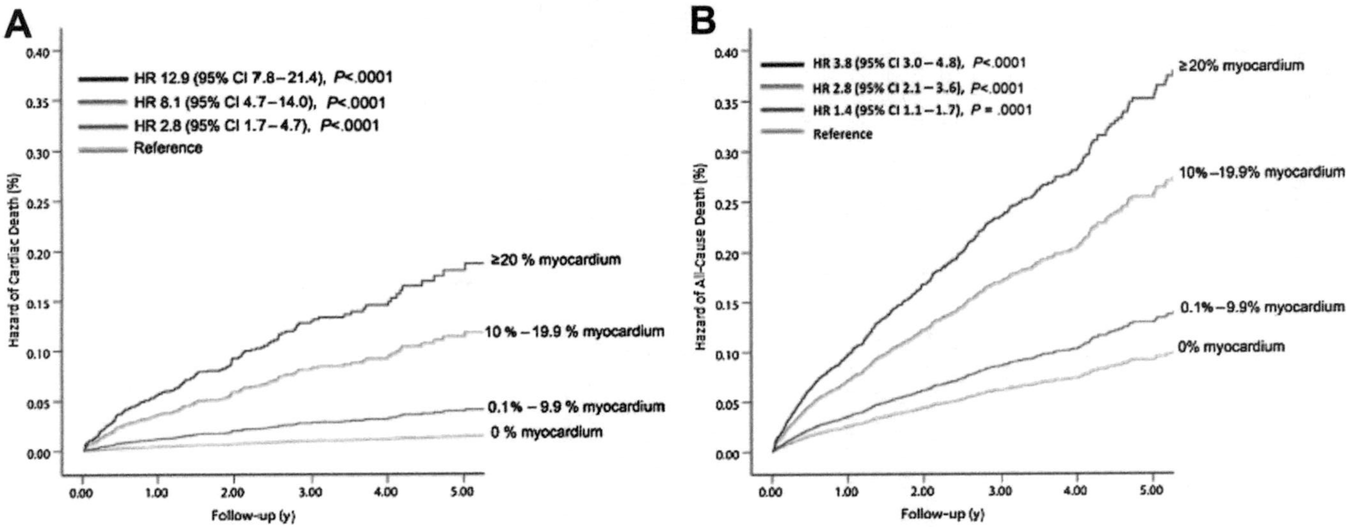

Fig. 7. Hazard ratio (HR) for cardiac death (*A*) and all-cause death (*B*) compared with percentage of abnormal myocardium on poststress rubidium-82-chloride (^{82}Rb) PET myocardial perfusion imaging. (*Adapted from* Dorbala S, Hachamovitch R, Curillova Z, et al. Incremental prognostic value of gated Rb-82 positron emission tomography myocardial perfusion imaging over clinical variables and rest LVEF. JACC Cardiovasc Imaging 2009;2(7):846–54; with permission.)

disease combined with severe microcirculatory disease[43,44] (**Fig. 8**).

The Role of Quantification in the Diagnosis of Coronary Artery Disease

One of the main drawbacks shared by both SPECT and PET MPI is that the evaluation of myocardial perfusion is based on relative tracer distribution. This can lead to misdiagnosis of a so-called balanced ischemia, in which 3-vessel CAD (3VD) causes decreased perfusion in all vascular territories, leading to apparently "normal" relative MPI, with no visually identifiable defects. Although the exact prevalence of balanced ischemia remains uncertain, there is evidence that SPECT MPI is less sensitive in the detection of left-main or 3VD, and some studies report that as many as 40% of patients with 3VD cannot be identified correctly with SPECT MPI.[45] Although PET MPI is more accurate than SPECT MPI, we know that relative PET MPI suffers from the same limitation. Quantification can be particularly useful in these patients because it will demonstrate diminished MBF after stress, with globally decreased MFR (<2.0). Parkash and colleagues[46] demonstrated that quantification with ^{82}Rb correctly Identified diminished perfusion in 92% of patients of patients with 3VD, and in a more recent study by Ziadi and colleagues,[47] diminished MFR using ^{82}Rb detected 88% of patients with 3VD.

Another strength of PET MPI with MBF quantification is its ability to detect ischemia resulting from disease at the level of secondary or even tertiary coronary branches, something previously impossible using SPECT.[43] This feature of PET, combined with its ability to evaluate the physiologic severity of CAD using quantification, could result in a unique new opportunity for individualized management of patients[43,48–50] (**Table 2**).

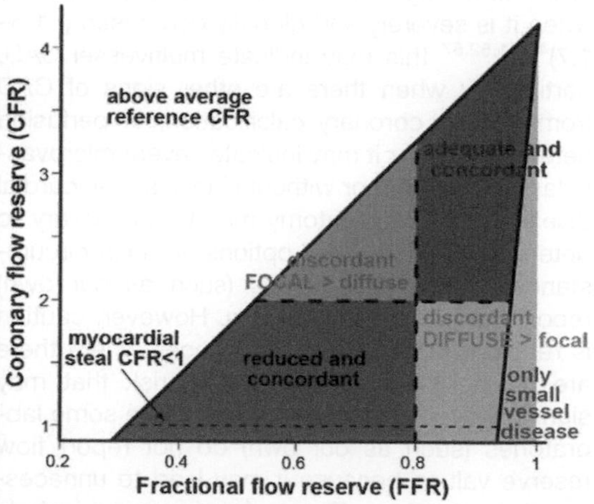

Fig. 8. Conceptual plot of coronary flow reserve (CFR) and fractional flow reserve regions. (*From* Johnson NP, Kirkeeide RL, Gould KL. Is discordance of coronary flow reserve and fractional flow reserve due to methodology or clinically relevant coronary pathophysiology? JACC Cardiovasc Imaging 2012;5(2):199; with permission.)

RISK STRATIFICATION AND PROGNOSIS

Flow quantification has incremental value for risk stratification and prognosis. Multiple studies have demonstrated that abnormally decreased flow with ^{82}Rb is an independent predictor of major cardiac events.[51,52] Murthy and colleagues[52] also showed that the severity of the reduction in MFR was proportionate to worsening clinical outcome (**Fig. 9**). Furthermore, in their study, 50% of patients with intermediate risk study before flow quantification were reclassified as either low- or high-risk patients using flow quantification. These results, and those from similar studies, clearly demonstrate the added value of flow quantification for risk stratification.

Table 2
Potential applications of absolute flow quantification

Application	Description
Early atherosclerosis	Evaluation of microvascular dysfunction in diabetes, hypertension, metabolic syndrome, etc
Advanced atherosclerosis	Improved detection of multivessel disease Evaluation of hemodynamic significance of stenosis
Nonatherosclerotic microvascular disease	Syndrome X Transplant vasculopathy Dilated cardiomyopathy Hypertrophic cardiomyopathy
Defining prognosis	
Evaluation of therapies	

Data from Refs.[43,48–50]

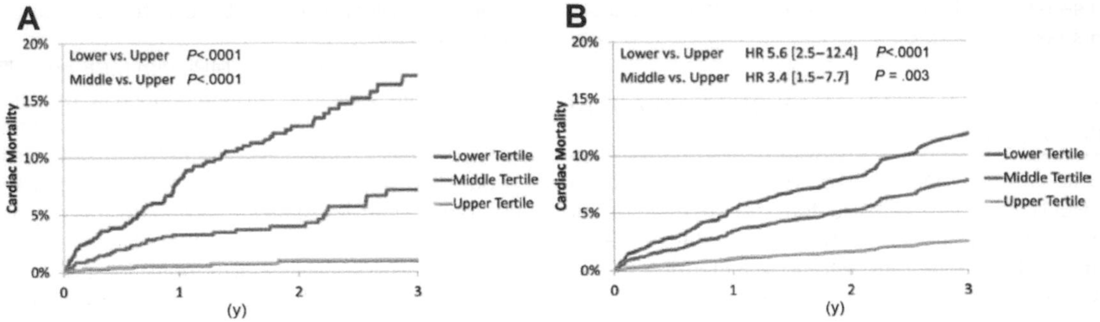

Fig. 9. Cardiac mortality. Cumulative incidence of cardiac mortality for tertiles of cardiac flow reserve (CFR) before (*A*) and after (*B*) adjustment for risk factors (age, sex, body mass index, hypertension, dyslipidemia, diabetes, family history of coronary artery disease [CAD], tobacco use, prior CAD, chest pain, dyspnea, left ventricular ejection fraction [LVEF], LVEF reserve, summed stress score, and early revascularization). Both analyses show significant correlation between CFR and cardiac mortality. (*From* Murthy VL, Naya M, Foster CR, et al. Improved cardiac risk assessment with noninvasive measures of coronary flow reserve. Circulation 2011;124(20):2221; with permission.)

Flow quantification and MFR have also been shown to have prognostic value in patients with nonischemic cardiomyopathy, including those with hypertrophic cardiomyopathy and dilated cardiomyopathy.[53,54]

WHEN TO USE PET MYOCARDIAL PERFUSION IMAGING AND FLOW QUANTIFICATION

Current practice guidelines do not distinguish between SPECT MPI and PET MPI in their recommendations, and although the availability of PET systems has increased tremendously over the last 2 decades, it remains limited in many smaller centers. In these circumstances, it seems to be reasonable to target the patients who have the most to gain from this technology. This includes obese patients, patients with known or suspected 3VD, and patients who have previously undergone other diagnostic imaging tests with equivocal or nondiagnostic findings. Flow quantification can also play an important role in patients with anatomic stenosis where the hemodynamic and functional impact is uncertain, helping to stratify correctly the patient and guiding the need for revascularization. Last, radiation dose to patients are substantially less in PET than SPECT, an argument that can be used for all patients, but particularly in younger patients or those who require serial studies.

Special circumstances may also call for flow quantification, such as the assessment for patients with suspected angina with normal coronary arteries, to rule out true isolated microvascular disease as a cause of angina.[55] Likewise, for patients with cardiac transplantation, flow quantification may be of value to assess for transplant vasculopathy and this may have some prognostic value.[56]

The specific interpretation of flow quantification data is beyond the scope of this review. Suffice it to say that certain patterns do emerge when patients are referred for the assessment of myocardial ischemia. When relative perfusion is normal combined with normal global and regional flow quantification (flow reserve values of >2.0 are generally accepted),[50–52,57–59] this is very reassuring that ischemia is not playing a role in the patient's symptoms and prognosis is excellent. When flow augmentation is reduced, particularly when it is severely and globally decreased (<1.5–1.7)[43,51,52,57] this may indicate multivessel CAD, particularly when there are other signs of CAD from history, coronary calcification, or perfusion heterogeneity; or it may indicate severe microvascular disease with or without significant epicardial disease. Defining anatomy may be necessary to determine management options. In such circumstances, some laboratories (such as our own) report the flow reserve values. However, caution is required in certain circumstances where there are other reasons for increased risk that may significantly impair flow reserve, where some laboratories (such as our own) do not report flow reserve values because it may lead to unnecessary investigations. These circumstances include where diffuse CAD and/or flow reserve reduction may be expected, such as patients with severe renal failure, prior coronary artery bypass grafting, or severe LV dysfunction. In patients with large prior infarction, flow reserve values can be misleading owing to low resting blood flow.

Finally, complete and uniform lack of flow augmentation may indicate a lack of response to vasodilator stress owing to recent caffeine intake or patient-specific characteristics. When this is suspected, we consider the patient for alternative stress agents, such as dobutamine. As can be appreciated, although flow quantification has improved value for diagnosis and prognosis, care, caution, and experience are required to optimize its use in a given clinical laboratory[50,58,59] (**Fig. 10**, **Table 3**).

FUTURE DEVELOPMENTS

Some centers have adopted hybrid approaches to define structure and function in the same setting using CT angiography and PET perfusion and flow imaging.[60] This strategy can increase accuracy, but is at the expense of radiation (although recent CT protocols have lessened radiation considerably). Another disadvantage is the more complex preparation with CTA requiring β-blockade and low heart rate, whereas β-blockers are usually withheld before diagnostic pharmacologic stress imaging. The role of PET-MRI in the setting of assessment of flow and perfusion is still being investigated but may have a role in several cardiomyopathies.

The clinical value of PET perfusion imaging is now well-recognized and its application is increasing. A recent American Society of Nuclear Cardiology PET Summit highlighted some of the steps needed to enable patients and physicians to take greater advantage of the accuracy, radiation dosimetry, convenience, and flow quantification advantages of PET.[58,59] The panel recommended strategies that emphasize quality and add value for patients for PET as well as newer

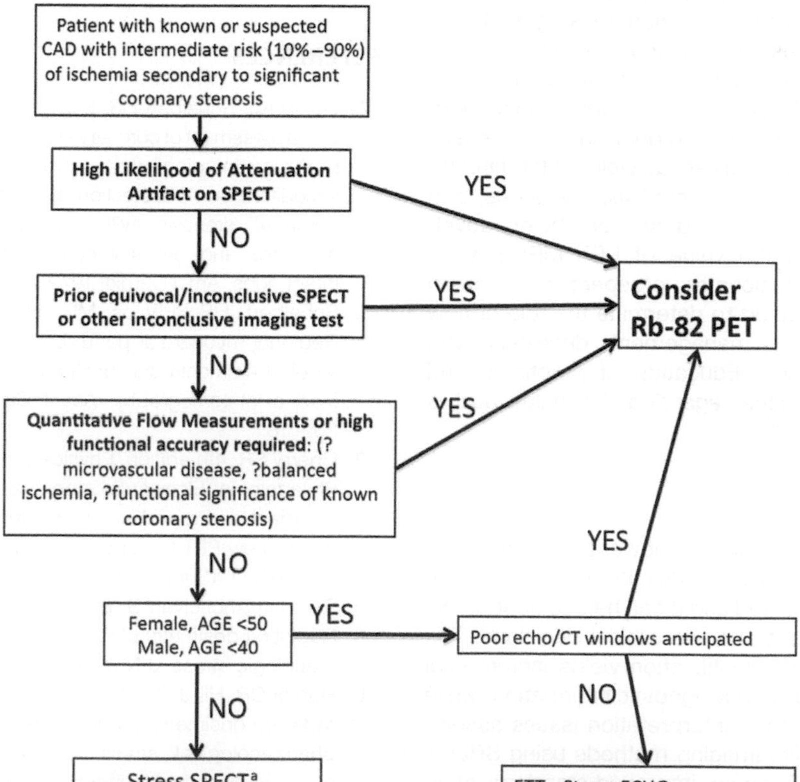

Fig. 10. Proposed clinical algorithm for use of rubidium-82-chloride (Rb-82) PET myocardial perfusion imaging. Based on recommendations from American Society of Nuclear Cardiology. CAD, coronary artery disease; ECHO, echocardiography; ETT, exercise treadmill test; SPECT, single photon emission computed tomography. [a] Where possible and appropriate, stress only and/or low radiation dose imaging should be considered for reduction in patient radiation exposure. (*From* Ohira H, Mc Ardle B, Cocker MS, et al. Current and future clinical applications of cardiac positron emission tomography. Circ J Off J Jpn Circ Soc 2013;77(4):838; with permission.)

Table 3
Reporting MFR in clinical practice

When to Report MFR	When Not to Report MFR
Anytime MFR has added value toward diagnostic and/or stratification: • Normal perfusion - high normal MFR • Abnormal perfusion with more severely of diffusely reduced MFR than expected • Microvascular measurements specifically requested • Assessment of hemodynamic significance of a lesion specifically requested	When MFR provides no diagnostic and/or prognostic value add or when MFR might confuse management or lead to unnecessary tests: • Patient with condition known to impair long-term microvascular function ○ Chronic renal failure ○ Prior CABG ○ Global LV dysfunction (suspected CM) • Accurate MFR measurement not possible or might be misleading ○ Large prior MI

Abbreviations: CABG, coronary artery bypass graft; LV, left ventricular; MFR, myocardial flow reserve; MI, myocardial infarction.

SPECT approaches. The true clinical value of flow quantification needs to be better defined, including its role in defining microvascular disease and how it impacts decision making that can impact outcomes and resource use. We also wait with anticipation to determine whether ^{18}F-flurpiridaz can fulfill the potential to enable routine exercise PET imaging. Updated guidelines, consensus statements for clinical use, as well as standardization of approaches for acquisition, analysis, and interpretation are needed and are being developed. Although the value of PET MPI is well-established, multicenter prospective research studies are required to determine the role of flow quantification in management decisions and patient outcomes. Education of practicing and referring physicians regarding this value add is also required.[58,59]

SUMMARY

Cardiac PET imaging is a powerful and accurate tool for the diagnosis of CAD. Its prognostic value is clearly established and it can help to adequately stratify patients and guide clinical decisions. The addition of flow quantification yields incremental diagnostic value and prognostic information, while solving some of the interpretation issues associated with relative imaging methods using SPECT and PET MPI. Even so, improved standardization is needed and more research is required to determine its full impact on decisions that affect patient outcomes and resource use, and thus enable full use of this valuable tool for diagnosis and risk stratification for our patients. Although the clinical availability remains somewhat limited today, the ever-increasing use of PET technology in cardiology and other fields, combined with advances in radiotracers, is expected to lead to an increasingly important role for cardiac PET imaging in the future.

REFERENCES

1. Gould KL, Schelbert HR, Phelps ME, et al. Noninvasive assessment of coronary stenoses with myocardial perfusion imaging during pharmacologic coronary vasodilatation. V. Detection of 47 percent diameter coronary stenosis with intravenous nitrogen-13 ammonia and emission-computed tomography in intact dogs. Am J Cardiol 1979;43(2):200–8.
2. Schelbert HR, Phelps ME, Hoffman EJ, et al. Regional myocardial perfusion assessed with N-13 labeled ammonia and positron emission computerized axial tomography. Am J Cardiol 1979;43(2):209–18.
3. Cherry SR. 4th edition. Physics in nuclear medicine. Philadelphia: Elsevier/Saunders; 2012.
4. Maddahi J. Properties of an ideal PET perfusion tracer: new PET tracer cases and data. J Nucl Cardiol 2012;19(Suppl 1):S30–7.
5. Senthamizhchelvan S, Bravo PE, Lodge MA, et al. Radiation dosimetry of 82Rb in humans under pharmacologic stress. J Nucl Med 2011;52(3):485–91.
6. Hunter CR, Hill J, Ziadi MC, et al. Biodistribution and radiation dosimetry of 82Rb at rest and during peak pharmacological stress in patients referred for myocardial perfusion imaging. Eur J Nucl Med Mol Imaging 2015;42(7):1032–42.
7. Chow BJ, Ananthasubramaniam K, dekemp RA, et al. Comparison of treadmill exercise versus dipyridamole stress with myocardial perfusion imaging using rubidium-82 positron emission tomography. J Am Coll Cardiol 2005;45(8):1227–34.
8. Klein R, Adler A, Beanlands RS, et al. Precision-controlled elution of a 82Sr/82Rb generator for

cardiac perfusion imaging with positron emission tomography. Phys Med Biol 2007;52(3):659–73.
9. Lortie M, Beanlands RS, Yoshinaga K, et al. Quantification of myocardial blood flow with 82Rb dynamic PET imaging. Eur J Nucl Med Mol Imaging 2007; 34(11):1765–74.
10. Nesterov SV, Deshayes E, Sciagrà R, et al. Quantification of myocardial blood flow in absolute terms using (82)Rb PET imaging: the RUBY-10 Study. JACC Cardiovasc Imaging 2014;7(11):1119–27.
11. Chow BJW, Beanlands RS, Lee A, et al. Treadmill exercise produces larger perfusion defects than dipyridamole stress N-13 ammonia positron emission tomography. J Am Coll Cardiol 2006;47(2):411–6.
12. Beanlands RS, Muzik O, Hutchins GD, et al. Heterogeneity of regional nitrogen 13-labeled ammonia tracer distribution in the normal human heart: comparison with rubidium 82 and copper 62-labeled PTSM. J Nucl Cardiol 1994;1(3):225–35.
13. Maddahi J, Udelson J, Heller G, et al; on behalf of the Flurpiridaz F18 Study 301 Investigators. Flurpiridaz F18 PET MPI: recent clinical trial data; International Congress of Nuclear Cardiology and Cardiac CT 12 [abstract]. Madrid (Spain), May 3–5, 2015. p. 23.
14. Yu M, Nekolla SG, Schwaiger M, et al. The next generation of cardiac positron emission tomography imaging agents: discovery of flurpiridaz F-18 for detection of coronary disease. Semin Nucl Med 2011;41(4):305–13.
15. Packard RR, Huang SC, Dahlbom M, et al. Absolute quantitation of myocardial blood flow in human subjects with or without myocardial ischemia using dynamic flurpiridaz F 18 PET. J Nucl Med 2014;55(9): 1438–44.
16. Renaud JM, Mylonas I, McArdle B, et al. Clinical interpretation standards and quality assurance for the multicenter PET/CT trial rubidium-ARMI. J Nucl Med 2014;55(1):58–64.
17. Dilsizian V, Bacharach SL, Beanlands RS, et al. PET myocardial perfusion and metabolism clinical imaging. J Nucl Cardiol 2009;16(4):651.
18. Kaster TS, Dwivedi G, Susser L, et al. Single low-dose CT scan optimized for rest-stress PET attenuation correction and quantification of coronary artery calcium. J Nucl Cardiol 2015;22(3):419–28.
19. Case JA, Bateman TM. Taking the perfect nuclear image: quality control, acquisition, and processing techniques for cardiac SPECT, PET, and hybrid imaging. J Nucl Cardiol 2013;20(5):891–907.
20. Nakazato R, Dey D, Alexánderson E, et al. Automatic alignment of myocardial perfusion PET and 64-slice coronary CT angiography on hybrid PET/CT. J Nucl Cardiol 2012;19(3):482–91.
21. Wells RG, Ruddy TD, DeKemp RA, et al. Single-phase CT aligned to gated PET for respiratory motion correction in cardiac PET/CT. J Nucl Med 2010;51(8):1182–90.
22. Cerqueira MD, Weissman NJ, Dilsizian V, et al. Standardized myocardial segmentation and nomenclature for tomographic imaging of the heart. A statement for healthcare professionals from the Cardiac Imaging Committee of the Council on Clinical Cardiology of the American Heart Association. Int J Cardiovasc Imaging 2002;18(1):539–42.
23. Mc Ardle B, Renaud J, DeKemp R, et al. Role of PET in diagnosis and risk assessment in patients with known or suspected CAD. In: Iskandrian A, Garcia E, editors. Nuclear cardiac imaging. 5th edition. Oxford University Press, in press.
24. Yoshinaga K, Chow BJ, Williams K, et al. What is the prognostic value of myocardial perfusion imaging using Rubidium-82 positron emission tomography? J Am Coll Cardiol 2006;48(5):1029–39.
25. Dorbala S, Di Carli MF, Beanlands RS, et al. Prognostic value of stress myocardial perfusion positron emission tomography. J Am Coll Cardiol 2013;61(2): 176–84.
26. Shi H, Santana CA, Rivero A, et al. Normal values and prospective validation of transient ischaemic dilation index in 82Rb PET myocardial perfusion imaging. Nucl Med Commun 2007;28(11):859–63.
27. Lertsburapa K, Ahlberg AW, Bateman TM, et al. Independent and incremental prognostic value of left ventricular ejection fraction determined by stress gated rubidium 82 PET imaging in patients with known or suspected coronary artery disease. J Nucl Cardiol 2008;15(6):745–53.
28. Dorbala S, Vangala D, Sampson U, et al. Value of vasodilator left ventricular ejection fraction reserve in evaluating the magnitude of myocardium at risk and the extent of angiographic coronary artery disease: a 82Rb PET/CT study. J Nucl Med 2007; 48(3):349–58.
29. Abraham A, Kass M, Ruddy TD, et al. Right and left ventricular uptake with Rb-82 PET myocardial perfusion imaging: markers of left main or 3 vessel disease. J Nucl Cardiol 2010;17(1):52–60.
30. Kaster T, Mylonas I, Renaud JM, et al. Accuracy of low-dose rubidium-82 myocardial perfusion imaging for detection of coronary artery disease using 3D PET and normal database interpretation. J Nucl Cardiol 2012;19(6):1135–45.
31. Nakazato R, Berman DS, Dey D, et al. Automated quantitative Rb-82 3D PET/CT myocardial perfusion imaging: normal limits and correlation with invasive coronary angiography. J Nucl Cardiol 2012;19(2): 265–76.
32. Mc Ardle BA, Dowsley TF, deKemp RA, et al. Does rubidium-82 PET have superior accuracy to SPECT perfusion imaging for the diagnosis of obstructive coronary disease?: a systematic review and meta-analysis. J Am Coll Cardiol 2012;60(18):1828–37.
33. Parker MW, Iskandar A, Limone B, et al. Diagnostic accuracy of cardiac positron emission tomography

versus single photon emission computed tomography for coronary artery disease: a bivariate meta-analysis. Circ Cardiovasc Imaging 2012;5(6):700–7.
34. Dorbala S, Di Carli MF. Cardiac PET perfusion: prognosis, risk stratification, and clinical management. Semin Nucl Med 2014;44(5):344–57.
35. Dorbala S, Hachamovitch R, Curillova Z, et al. Incremental prognostic value of gated Rb-82 positron emission tomography myocardial perfusion imaging over clinical variables and rest LVEF. JACC Cardiovasc Imaging 2009;2(7):846–54.
36. Kay J, Dorbala S, Goyal A, et al. Influence of sex on risk stratification with stress myocardial perfusion Rb-82 positron emission tomography: results from the PET (Positron Emission Tomography) Prognosis Multicenter Registry. J Am Coll Cardiol 2013; 62(20):1866–76.
37. Chow BJW, Dorbala S, Di Carli MF, et al. Prognostic value of PET myocardial perfusion imaging in obese patients. JACC Cardiovasc Imaging 2014; 7(3):278–87.
38. Hachamovitch R, Hayes SW, Friedman JD, et al. Comparison of the short-term survival benefit associated with revascularization compared with medical therapy in patients with no prior coronary artery disease undergoing stress myocardial perfusion single photon emission computed tomography. Circulation 2003;107(23):2900–7.
39. Hachamovitch R, Rozanski A, Shaw LJ, et al. Impact of ischaemia and scar on the therapeutic benefit derived from myocardial revascularization vs. medical therapy among patients undergoing stress-rest myocardial perfusion scintigraphy. Eur Heart J 2011;32(8):1012–24.
40. Patel MR, Dehmer GJ, Hirshfeld JW, et al. ACCF/SCAI/STS/AATS/AHA/ASNC/HFSA/SCCT 2012 appropriate use criteria for coronary revascularization focused update: a report of the American College of Cardiology Foundation Appropriate Use Criteria Task Force, Society for Cardiovascular Angiography and Interventions, Society of Thoracic Surgeons, American Association for Thoracic Surgery, American Heart Association, American Society of Nuclear Cardiology, and the Society of Cardiovascular Computed Tomography. J Am Coll Cardiol 2012;59(9):857–81.
41. Patel MR, Bailey SR, Bonow RO, et al. ACCF/SCAI/AATS/AHA/ASE/ASNC/HFSA/HRS/SCCM/SCCT/SCMR/STS 2012 appropriate Use criteria for diagnostic Catheterization: a report of the American College of Cardiology Foundation Appropriate Use Criteria Task Force, Society for Cardiovascular Angiography and Interventions, American Association for Thoracic Surgery, American Heart Association, American Society of Echocardiography, American Society of Nuclear Cardiology, Heart Failure Society of America, Heart Rhythm Society, Society of Critical Care Medicine, Society of Cardiovascular Computed Tomography, Society for Cardiovascular Magnetic Resonance, and Society of Thoracic Surgeons. J Am Coll Cardiol 2012;59(22):1995–2027.
42. Kaufmann PA, Camici PG. Myocardial blood flow measurement by PET: technical aspects and clinical applications. J Nucl Med 2005;46(1):75–88.
43. Gould KL, Johnson NP, Bateman TM, et al. Anatomic versus physiologic assessment of coronary artery disease. Role of coronary flow reserve, fractional flow reserve, and positron emission tomography imaging in revascularization decision-making. J Am Coll Cardiol 2013;62(18):1639–53.
44. Johnson NP, Kirkeeide RL, Gould KL. Is discordance of coronary flow reserve and fractional flow reserve due to methodology or clinically relevant coronary pathophysiology? JACC Cardiovasc Imaging 2012; 5(2):193–202.
45. Lima RSL, Watson DD, Goode AR, et al. Incremental value of combined perfusion and function over perfusion alone by gated SPECT myocardial perfusion imaging for detection of severe three-vessel coronary artery disease. J Am Coll Cardiol 2003;42(1):64–70.
46. Parkash R, deKemp RA, Ruddy TD, et al. Potential utility of rubidium 82 PET quantification in patients with 3-vessel coronary artery disease. J Nucl Cardiol 2004;11(4):440–9.
47. Ziadi MC, deKemp RA, Williams K, et al. Does quantification of myocardial flow reserve using rubidium-82 positron emission tomography facilitate detection of multivessel coronary artery disease? J Nucl Cardiol 2012;19(4):670–80.
48. Schelbert HR. Quantification of myocardial blood flow: what is the clinical role? Cardiol Clin 2009; 27(2):277–89 [Table of Contents].
49. Camici PG, Crea F. Coronary microvascular dysfunction. N Engl J Med 2007;356(8):830–40.
50. Ohira H, Dowsley T, Dwivedi G, et al. Quantification of myocardial blood flow using PET to improve the management of patients with stable ischemic coronary artery disease. Future Cardiol 2014;10(5): 611–31.
51. Ziadi MC, Dekemp RA, Williams KA, et al. Impaired myocardial flow reserve on rubidium-82 positron emission tomography imaging predicts adverse outcomes in patients assessed for myocardial ischemia. J Am Coll Cardiol 2011;58(7):740–8.
52. Murthy VL, Naya M, Foster CR, et al. Improved cardiac risk assessment with noninvasive measures of coronary flow reserve. Circulation 2011;124(20): 2215–24.
53. Cecchi F, Olivotto I, Gistri R, et al. Coronary microvascular dysfunction and prognosis in hypertrophic cardiomyopathy. N Engl J Med 2003;349(11):1027–35.
54. Neglia D, Michelassi C, Trivieri MG, et al. Prognostic role of myocardial blood flow impairment in idiopathic left ventricular dysfunction. Circulation 2002; 105(2):186–93.

55. Geltman EM, Henes CG, Senneff MJ, et al. Increased myocardial perfusion at rest and diminished perfusion reserve in patients with angina and angiographically normal coronary arteries. J Am Coll Cardiol 1990;16(3):586–95.
56. Mc Ardle BA, Davies RA, Chen L, et al. Prognostic value of rubidium-82 positron emission tomography in patients after heart transplant. Circ Cardiovasc Imaging 2014;7(6):930–7.
57. Herzog BA, Husmann L, Valenta I, et al. Long-term prognostic value of 13N-ammonia myocardial perfusion positron emission tomography added value of coronary flow reserve. J Am Coll Cardiol 2009; 54(2):150–6.
58. Beanlands R, Heller GV. Proceedings of the ASNC cardiac PET summit, 12 May 2014, Baltimore, MD: 1: the value of PET: integrating cardiovascular PET into the care continuum. J Nucl Cardiol 2015;22(3): 557–62.
59. Heller GV, Bateman TM, Cerqueira MD, et al. Proceedings of the ASNC cardiac PET summit, 12 May 2014, Baltimore, MD, quantitation of myocardial blood flow. J Nucl Cardiol 2015;22(3):555–6.
60. Kajander S, Joutsiniemi E, Saraste M, et al. Cardiac positron emission tomography/computed tomography imaging accurately detects anatomically and functionally significant coronary artery disease. Circulation 2010;122(6):603–13.

Long-Term Risk Assessment After the Performance of Stress Myocardial Perfusion Imaging

Alan Rozanski, MD[a,*], Daniel S. Berman, MD[b,c]

KEYWORDS

• Myocardial perfusion imaging • Myocardial ischemia • Coronary artery disease • SPECT

KEY POINTS

- Stress-rest myocardial perfusion imaging (MPI) is a potent method for assessing the presence and magnitude of inducible myocardial ischemia.
- Stress MPI currently faces increased scrutiny for its therapeutic effectiveness because of the emergence of other competing means for assessing clinical risk.
- Changing patterns of coronary artery disease (CAD) presentation are reshaping the optimal utility of MPI.
- New data have examined the usefulness of stress-rest-MPI as a predictor for long-term clinical outcomes, in contrast to its traditional role for assessing short-term cardiovascular risk.
- These data indicates that temporal risk is highly influenced by both the magnitude of ischemia and various baseline clinical factors.
- An optimized assessment of stress MPI, which includes long-term risk prediction, might improve the potential future clinical effectiveness of this imaging modality.

Stress-rest MPI is a strongly proved method for assessing the presence and magnitude of inducible myocardial ischemia. The technique is inherently quantitative and reproducible and has been shown to predict adverse outcomes in a wide variety of clinical settings. Nevertheless, stress MPI currently faces increased scrutiny for its therapeutic effectiveness because of the emergence of other competing means for assessing clinical risk. This article evaluates the historical evidence that first established the clinical utility of stress-rest MPI and then reviews changing patterns of CAD presentation that are reshaping the optimal utility of MPI. New data are then reviewed that have examined the usefulness of SPECT-MPI as a predictor for long-term clinical outcomes, in contrast to its traditional role for assessing short-term cardiovascular risk. Finally, how an optimized assessment of stress MPI to include long-term risk prediction might improve the potential future clinical effectiveness of this imaging modality is reviewed.

INITIAL VALIDATION STUDIES AND CLINICAL USES OF STRESS-REST MYOCARDIAL PERFUSION IMAGING

In the 1960s, a standardized protocol was widely adopted for the performance of graded treadmill exercise ECG, based on the work of Robert Bruce

[a] Division of Cardiology, Department of Medicine, Mt Sinai St. Lukes and Roosevelt Hospitals, 1111 Amsterdam Avenue, New York, NY 10025, USA; [b] Department of Imaging, Burns and Allen Research Institute, Cedars-Sinai Medical Center, Los Angeles, CA, USA; [c] Department of Medicine, Burns and Allen Research Institute, Cedars-Sinai Medical Center, 8700 Beverly Boulevard, Los Angeles, CA 90048, USA
* Corresponding author. Division of Cardiology, Mt Sinai St. Lukes and Roosevelt Hospitals, 1111 Amsterdam Avenue, New York, NY 10025.
E-mail address: arozanski@chpnet.org

Cardiol Clin 34 (2016) 87–99
http://dx.doi.org/10.1016/j.ccl.2015.07.016

and colleagues.[1] The same decade saw the advent of cardiac catheterization and coronary artery bypass surgery, and subsequent research demonstrated that the results of exercise ECG, such as exercise capacity and the ST segment response to exercise, could help identify which cardiac patients were at high risk and thus, presumably, most likely to benefit from bypass surgery. In the mid- to late 1970s, MPI, initially performed with planar imaging and subsequently using SPECT, was introduced into medicine. This test had a rapid and wide adoption across medical centers due to various innate characteristics of the test.

First, early research demonstrated that stress MPI had inherently greater sensitivity and specificity for the detection of angiographically significant CAD compared with exercise ECG. Subsequent work demonstrated that stress MPI provided incremental prognostic information when first assessing risk according to more readily available clinical information, such as CAD risk factors and the results of exercise ECG.[2–4] Moreover, whereas exercise ECG is an imprecise measure of the magnitude of inducible myocardial ischemia, stress MPI can precisely quantify the magnitude of ischemia according to its regional extent (eg, the number and location of reversible myocardial perfusion defects) and the severity of perfusion defects. In important early work, Ladenheim and colleagues[5] demonstrated the presence of an exponential relationship between the magnitude of ischemia as assessed by MPI and the likelihood of adverse cardiac events. The extent and severity of myocardial perfusion defects were found to provide independent and thus incremental information to each other for the prediction of cardiac events, as illustrated in **Fig. 1**. Thus, there was quick recognition that the results of stress

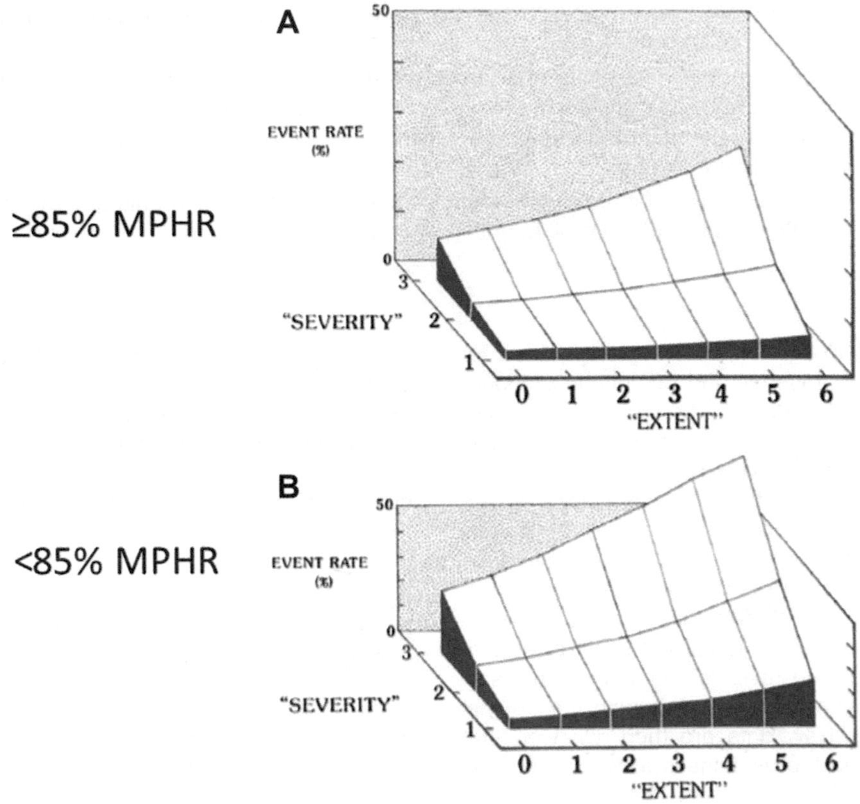

Fig. 1. Orthogonal axes show the number of perfusion defects, ranging from 1 to 6 regions; the severity of perfusion defects, ranging from none (score = 0) to severe (score = 3); and the frequency of cardiac events. (*A*) The graph is for patients achieving greater than or equal to 85% of maximal predicted heart rate and (*B*) the graph is for patients failing to achieve 85% of maximal predicted heart rate. In both cases, the event rate increased as a curvilinear function of the extent and severity of myocardial hypoperfusion. There was an at least 3-fold increase in cardiac events for the patients who could not achieve greater than or equal to 85% of maximal predicted heart rate. (*From* Ladenheim ML, Pollock BH, Rozanski A, et al. Extent and severity of myocardial hypoperfusion as predictors of prognosis in patients with suspected coronary artery disease. J Am Coll Cardiol 1986;7:469; with permission.)

MPI were best served by carefully characterizing the overall extent and severity of myocardial perfusion defects. Moreover, the work of Ladenheim and colleagues further demonstrated the important role of exercise capacity in modifying the risk associated with any given magnitude of myocardial perfusion defect (see **Fig. 1**).

One of the important bedrocks of applying exercise MPI was the recognition that a normal scan was associated with a low risk for adverse cardiac events, found to average only 0.45% per year in a meta-analysis conducted by Metz and colleagues.[6] Based on such studies, it became widely assumed that a normal exercise SPECT-MPI study provided a warranty period of low risk after testing, with varying length depending on a patient's clinical and historical factors.[7]

An important development that further increased the utility of stress MPI was the advent of pharmacologic stress testing, after research demonstrated that radiotracer uptake during the infusion of dipyridamole infusion was comparable to that induced with maximal exercise in the same patients. This approach thus allowed the extension of cardiac stress testing to many patients who could not be previously tested due to their inability to exercise.

Based on these characteristics of MPI, this test became widely used as a decision guide for clinical decision making in cardiology.

THE CHANGING PATTERN OF CLINICAL CORONARY ARTERY DISEASE AND ITS IMPLICATION FOR CARDIAC TESTING

In recent years, however, dynamic trends have begun to reshape some of the considerations regarding the optimal use of cardiac stress tests, including SPECT-MPI. These trends include a dynamic change in the clinical presentation of CAD. Since peaking as an epidemic in the 1960s, the mortality rate from CAD has declined dramatically.[8,9] This decline has been accompanied by a decline in the prevalence of myocardial infarction,[10] stroke,[11] and peripheral vascular disease.[12] It has been estimated that approximately half of this decline has been due to enhanced cardiovascular care and approximately half has been due to enhanced prevention, including lower rates of smoking, population level decrease in serum cholesterol levels and transfat ingestion, and enhanced treatment of hyperlipidemia, hypertension, and diabetes.[8,9,13,14]

Given these trends, the authors tested the hypothesis that the frequency of stress-induced myocardial ischemia has also declined over time, by assessing the temporal frequency of myocardial ischemia among 39,515 diagnostic patients who underwent stress-rest SPECT-MPI studies between 1991 and 2009.[15] The overall prevalence of abnormal studies fell from 40.9% to 8.7% during this time period, and the frequency of ischemia fell from 29.6% to 5.0% (**Fig. 2**). There was also a decline in the frequency of severe myocardial perfusion defects. This decline has been broad based, occurring in every age group, among men and women, in all symptom class and risk factor groups, and among those undergoing exercise or pharmacologic SPECT-MPI. This cause for this decline is likely multifactorial in origin, probably due in large part to the same preventive factors that have contributed to the temporal decline in cardiac mortality rates. In addition, earlier referral of patients with chest pain syndromes for testing, a lowered threshold for referral of sicker patients

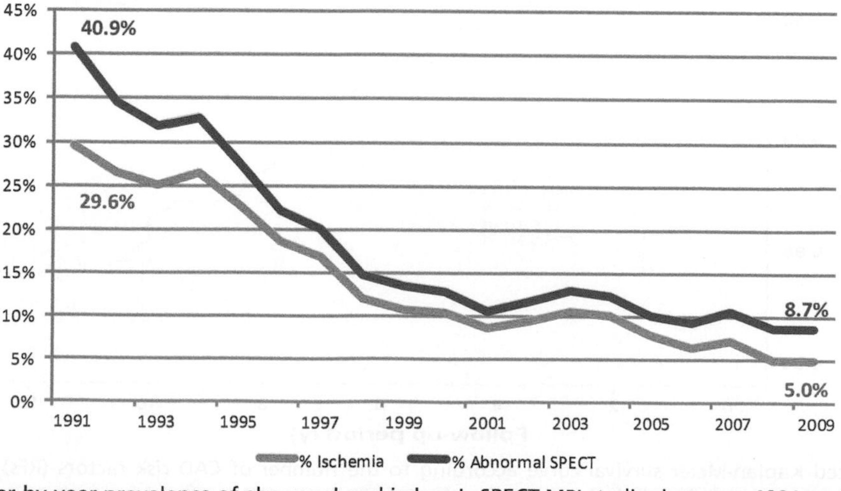

Fig. 2. The year-by-year prevalence of abnormal and ischemic SPECT-MPI studies between 1991 and 2009 among 39,515 diagnostic patients.

to cardiac catheterization, and other factors may also have been potential but as yet unsubstantiated contributors to this decline.

A reported temporal decline in myocardial ischemia has also been reported at other medical centers during this same time period, including a decline noted among 108,654 patients at 2 northeastern medical centers[16]; among 29,255 patients from the Mayo Clinic[17]; and among patients studied in Kansas City and in Cairo, Egypt.[18]

LONG-TERM OUTCOMES AFTER SINGLE-PHOTON EMISSION COMPUTED TOMOGRAPHY–MYOCARDIAL PERFUSION IMAGING

Until the past decade, outcome studies involving SPECT-MPI have focused on its ability to predict short-term outcomes, and follow-up periods in these studies were generally for 2 to 3 years. This made sense in an era where this test was primarily used for diagnostic purposes and short-term management decisions, such as deciding between the need for immediate revascularization versus medical therapy, evaluating recurrent symptoms after coronary bypass surgery or coronary angioplasty, assessing the hemodynamic significance of coronary angiographic findings, and assessing patients preoperatively for ischemic risk. With the declining rate of cardiac events and the decreasing frequency of inducible myocardial ischemia, there has been increased focus on also assessing long-term risk after cardiac testing.

To this end, increasing study has evaluated the long-term risk among patients undergoing SPECT-MPI, particularly among patients with normal MPI studies. Whereas, as discussed previously, the warranty period associated with an exercise SPECT-MPI study is low in the short term, increasing data have demonstrated that long-term risk is heterogeneous and influenced by a variety of clinical factors. One of the early studies in this regard, as reported by Supariwala and colleagues,[19] involved the follow-up of 2597 diagnostic patients with a normal exercise SPECT-MPI study for a mean of 6.8 years. Of the common CAD risk factors, 3 were significant predictors of long-term outcome: hypertension, smoking, and diabetes. Annualized mortality ranged from only 0.2% per year for those without any of these 3 risk factors to 1.8% per year when all 3 were present (**Fig. 3**).

A second study provided confirmatory findings.[20] In this study, 12,232 patients with a normal exercise SPECT-MPI study were followed for mean of 11.2 years. Among 6 commonly assessed CAD risk factors, 4 were significant predictors of long-term mortality: hypertension, smoking, diabetes, and exercise capacity (**Fig. 4**). When combining these 4 predictors, annualized mortality rates ranged from only 0.2% per year among those patients who exercised for greater than or equal to 9 minutes and had none of these 3 CAD risk factors to 1.6% per year for those who exercised less than 6 minutes and had greater than or equal to 2 of these risk factors (**Fig. 5**). Other clinical factors that modify long-term risk among the patients

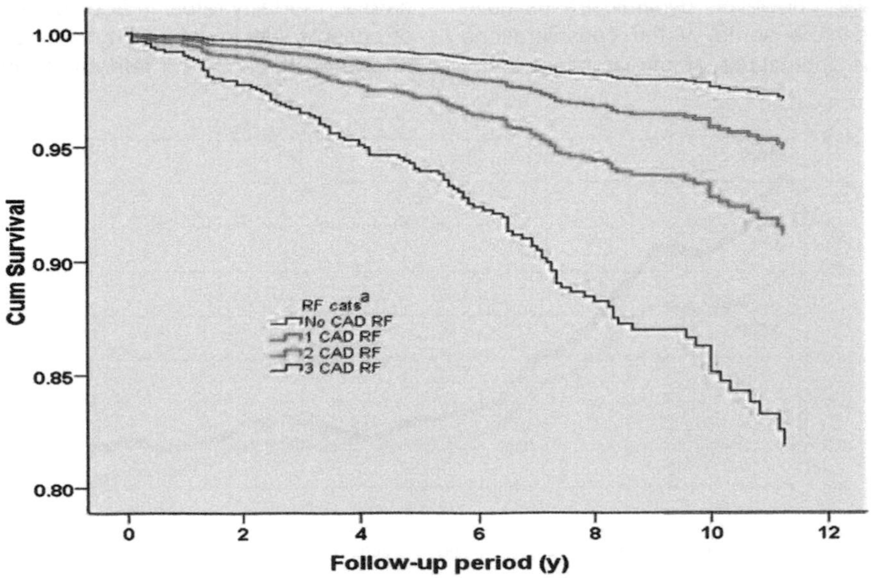

Fig. 3. Adjusted Kaplan-Meier survival curve according to the number of CAD risk factors (RFs) (from among hypertension, smoking, and diabetes) after adjustment for all covariates of outcome among 2567 patients with normal SPECT-MPI studies. [a] HT, diabetes, and smoking.

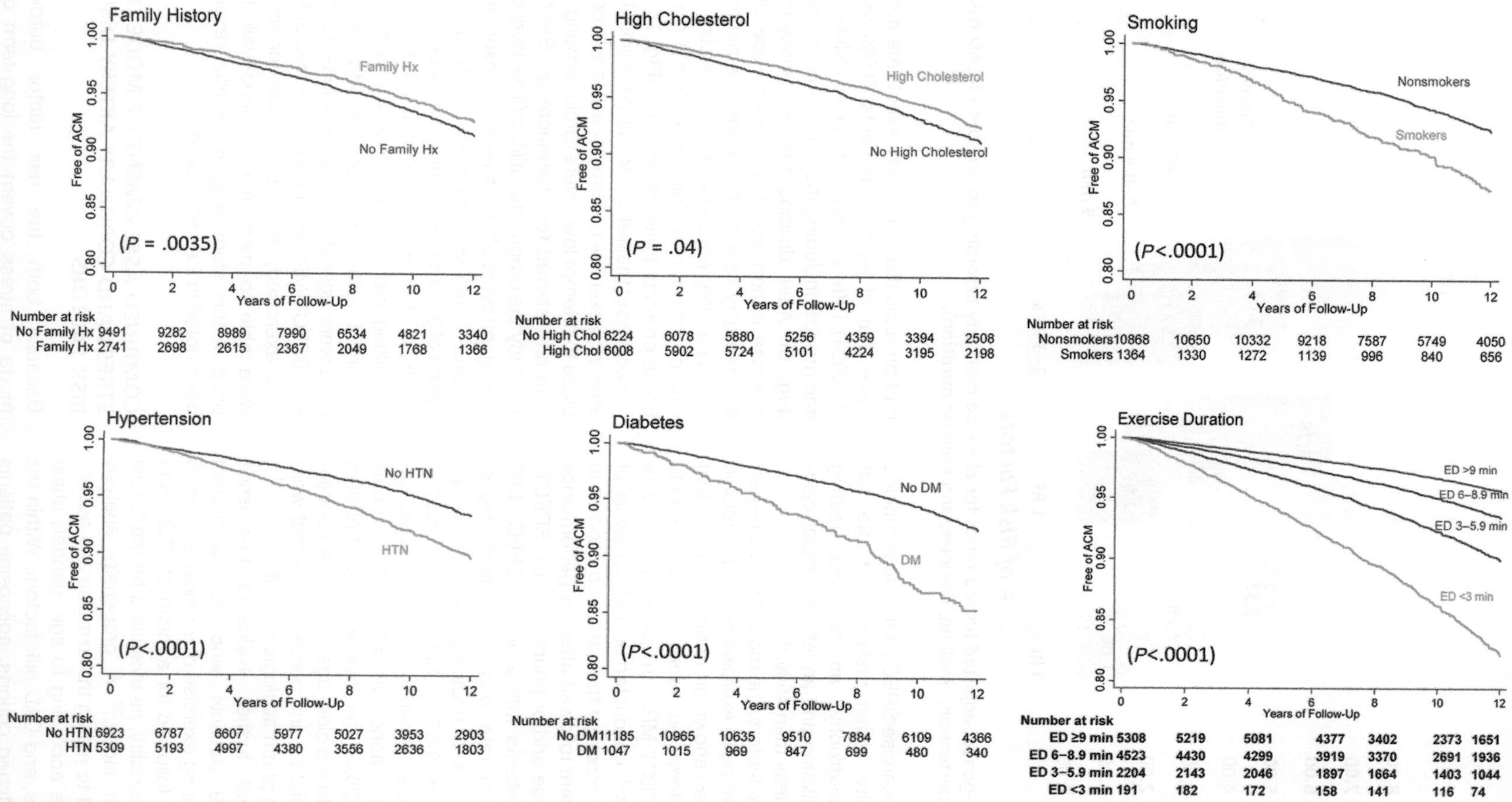

Fig. 4. Kaplan-Meier survival curves among 12,232 patients with normal SPECT-MPI studies followed for 11.2 ± 4.5 years, according to 6 CAD risk factors: family history, high cholesterol, smoking, hypertension, diabetes, and Cox-modeled survival curves of risk factor-adjusted exercise capacity (minutes of performed exercise). ACM, all-cause mortality; Chol, cholesterol; DM, diabetes mellitue; ED, emergency department; HX, history; HTN, hypertension.

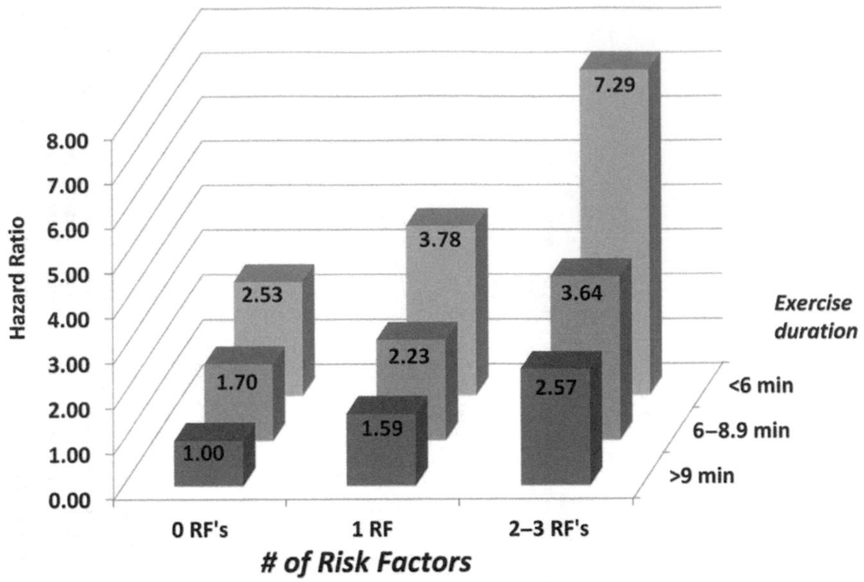

Fig. 5. Age- and gender-adjusted hazard ratios for all-cause mortality according to number of CAD risk factors (from among hypertension, smoking, diabetes, and exercise duration).

with a normal exercise SPECT-MPI study include dyspnea, obesity, higher resting heart rate, left ventricular hypertrophy, an abnormal resting ECG, atrial fibrillation and an left ventricular ejection fraction of less than 45%.[20]

Besides these factors, the mode of stress—performance according to exercise or pharmacologic stress—has been shown an important factor that modifies long-term outcomes among patients undergoing SPECT-MPI. In particular, Navare and colleagues[21] conducted a meta-analysis of 24 studies that reported the cardiac outcomes in patients who were followed after the performance of either exercise and/or pharmacologic SPECT-MPI. Among patients with a normal SPECT-MPI study, the event rate was substantially higher among patients who underwent pharmacologic stress (1.78% vs 0.65%). Similarly, the cardiac event rates were higher for pharmacologic patients with an abnormal SPECT-MPI study (9.98% vs 4.43%). The investigators attributed this difference to the older age and higher concentration of risk factors and comorbidities that were present among pharmacologic patients.

A study that further evaluated this issue analyzed 6069 patients who had a normal SPECT-MPI during exercise or adenosine infusion and were then followed for a mean of 10.2 years for all-cause mortality, as evaluated by the Social Security Death Index.[22] A propensity analysis was performed to match the exercise and adenosine subgroups according to age, gender, chest pain symptoms, and CAD risk factors. Within the propensity-matched cohorts, adenosine patients had an annualized mortality event rate more than twice that of exercise patients (3.9% vs 1.6%, $P<.0001$). Differences in mortality persisted among age groups, including those less than 55 years old (**Fig. 6**). After dividing the propensity-matched exercise cohort according to exercise duration, the mortality rate of the adenosine patients was approximately parallel to those exercise patients who could not complete more than 3 minutes of Bruce protocol treadmill exercise (**Fig. 7**).

Because of the well demonstrated clinical utility of analyzing exercise performance, it is now commonplace to attempt low-level exercise among patients who are referred for pharmacologic SPECT-MPI. To study the prognostic utility of low-level exercise during pharmacologic stress, Johnson and colleagues[23] assessed all-cause mortality among a cohort of 3479 patients who were divided according the type of stress test: exercise, adenosine with a walking protocol, or adenosine and unable to perform a walking protocol. Risk-adjusted mortality rates were highest for those who underwent adenosine SPECT-MPI without exercise, lowest for those who exercised, and intermediate for those who were able to perform the adeno-walk protocol used in this study (**Fig. 8**). Similar results have been noted in 2 recent studies.[24,25]

COMBINED ASSESSMENT OF MODE OF STRESS AND CORONARY ARTERY DISEASE RISK FACTORS

Because both the risk factor burden and mode of stress govern the long-term outcome

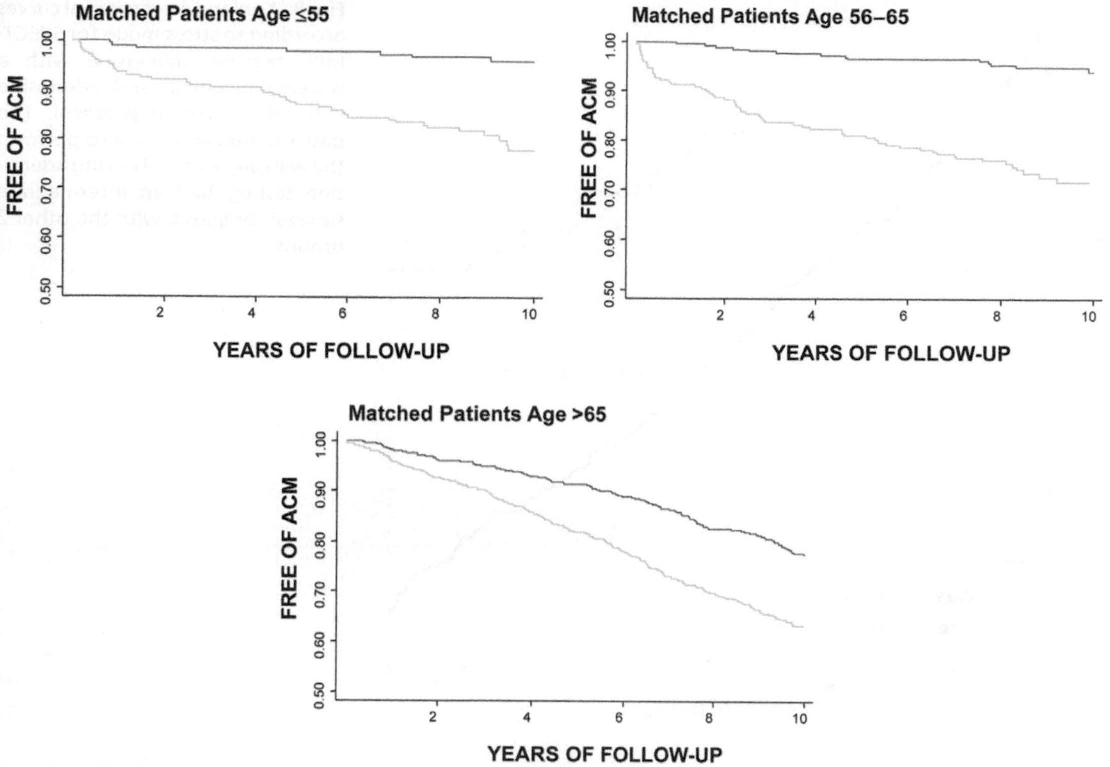

Fig. 6. Kaplan-Meier curves showing comparing survival from death among patients undergoing exercise vs adenosine SPECT, grouped into 3 age groups, after propensity matching to create similar groups on the basis of age, gender, cardiac risk factors, and chest pain symptoms.

among patients undergoing SPECT-MPI, the combined consideration of both factors should provide synergistic information as to long-term outcomes after cardiac stress testing. To assess this interaction, Supariwala and colleagues[26] evaluated long-term all-cause mortality among 5762 patients who had a normal stress-rest SPECT-MPI study at baseline. The patients

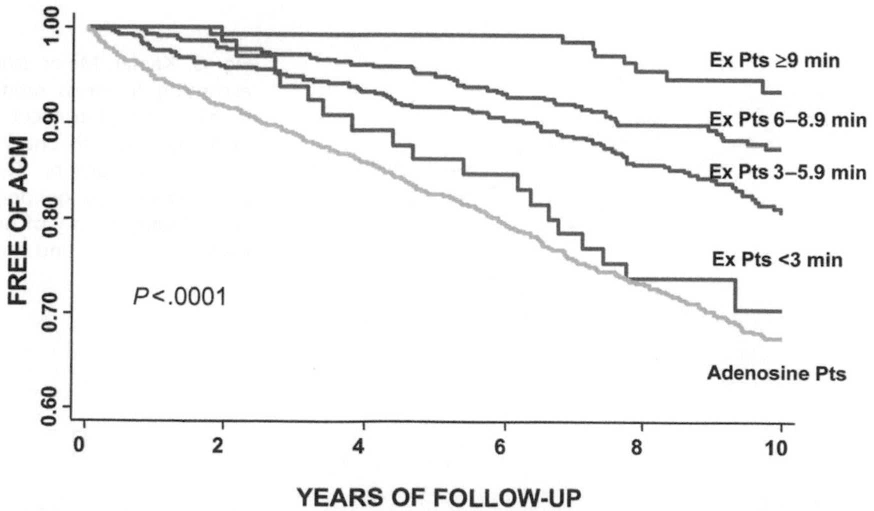

Fig. 7. Kaplan-Meier curves in the propensity-matched exercise (Ex) and adenosine patients (Pts). The exercise patients were divided according to exercise duration. All-cause mortality rate increased as exercise duration diminished. Mortality rates were similar among patients unable to exercise 3 min and patients who underwent adenosine SPECT.

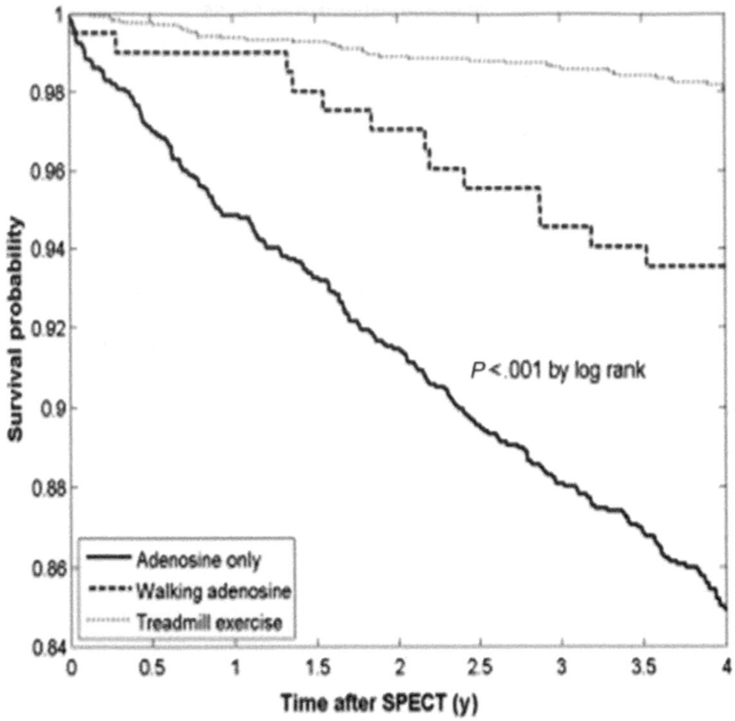

Fig. 8. Kaplan-Meier survival curves according to stress mode for SPECT-MPI: exercise, adenosine with a walking protocol, and adenosine without a walking protocol. The patients who were able to perform the walking protocol during adenosine testing had an intermediate survival compared with the other 2 groups.

were divided according to mode of stress testing (exercise or pharmacologic) and number of CAD risk factors. As shown in **Fig. 9**, Kaplan-Meier survival analysis revealed a marked heterogeneity in all-cause mortality rates, ranging from 0.8% per year in exercise patients and no CAD risk factors to 4.2% per year among pharmacologic patients with greater than or equal to 2 CAD risk factors.

Thus, among studies conducted primarily among patients with normal SPECT-MPI, consideration of clinical factors can differentiate between patients who are at very low risk (ie, high exercise tolerance and little CAD risk factor burden) and

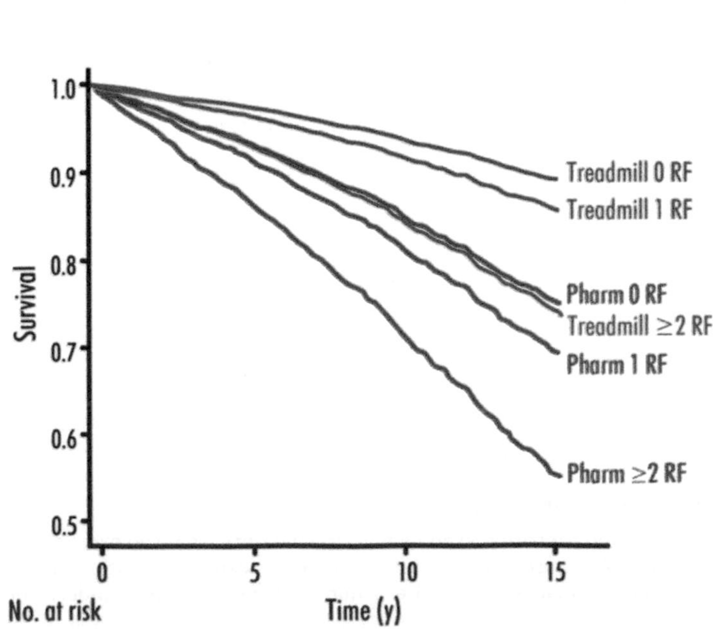

Fig. 9. Kaplan-Meier survival curves according to stress mode (treadmill in *blue* and pharmacologic [pharm] in *orange*) and coronary disease risk factor (RF) burden. The data are adjusted for age, gender, hyperlipidemia, family history of heart disease, body mass index, and chest pain.

groups at progressively greater long-term risk (ie, diminished exercise tolerance or inability to exercise and increasing CAD risk factor burden). Combining such data with assessment of the magnitude of stress induced myocardial ischemia should provide even greater fidelity in long-term risk prediction.

ASSESSMENT OF ANATOMIC BURDEN

Stress tests require the presence of hemodynamically significant disease for the detection of myocardial ischemia. Thus, a principal limitation of stress tests is their inability to characterize the presence and extent of subclinical atherosclerosis. This is borne out by many studies that have identified that atherosclerosis, as measured by coronary artery calcium (CAC) scanning is commonplace among patients with a normal SPECT-MPI study.[27,28] As shown in **Fig. 10**, the frequency of CAC abnormality can vary markedly among patients with a normal SPECT-MPI study, and the presence of even extensive CAC scores is common.

Chang and colleagues[29] evaluated whether the combined consideration of CAC score and MPI abnormality might provide incremental prognostic information. They evaluated 1216 generally asymptomatic diagnostic patients who underwent combined SPECT-MPI and CAC scanning. The patients were followed for a median of 6.9 years. As shown in **Fig. 11**, cardiac events increased with both increasing CAC abnormality and with MPI abnormality but the combined presence of both predicted those patients who were at highest risk. Of importance, in patients with a normal SPECT-MPI study, a high CAC score (>400) predicted elevated long-term cardiac risk.

POTENTIAL CLINICAL RELEVANCE

In recent years, consideration as to the optimal utilization of SPECT-MPI has been affected by 2 important trends. First, there has been an increase in the number of noninvasive methods that can be used to assess the presence and magnitude of coronary artery disease, including methods that can now be used to noninvasively assess atherosclerotic disease burden (**Box 1**). Second, there has been growing concern for the cost of cardiovascular health care. As a consequence, various approaches were introduced over the past decade to curb inappropriate testing and to make noninvasive cardiovascular testing more cost effective, such as the adoption of appropriateness criteria, practice guidelines, and precertification for SPECT-MPI tests.

In addition, there has been increasing call to compare the utility of cardiac tests according to a new bar (**Fig. 12**). Previously, the approved utilization of cardiac tests merely depended on demonstrating that a test could predict outcomes. Increasingly, however, there is a demand for research that examines how tests actually influence outcomes. This new standard has become the objective of comparative effectiveness research that assesses the ability of 2 tests or types of tests to influence outcomes in prospective randomized clinical trials.

An example of a comparative effectiveness research trial involving SPECT-MPI was the What is the Optimal Method for Ischemia Evaluation in

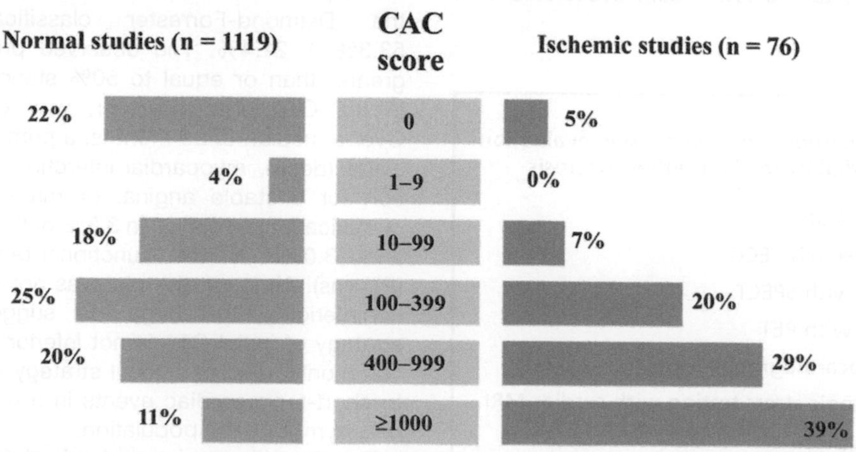

Fig. 10. The frequency of CAC scores, divided into 6 groups (from scores of 0 to >1000) among 1119 patients with as normal SPECT-MPI study (*on the left*) and among 76 patients with an abnormal study (*on the right*). Few patients with an abnormal SPECT-MPI had a low CAC score. Among the normal SPECT-MPI studies, CAC scores were heterogeneous, with only 22% having a normal CAC score and more than one-third having CAC scores greater than 400.

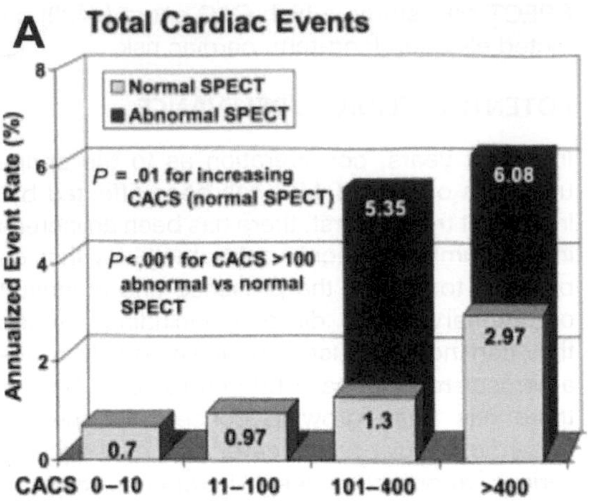

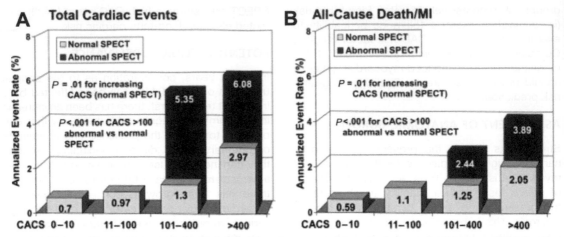

Fig. 11. Adjusted annualized event rates for total cardiac events (*A*) and all-cause death/myocardial infarction (MI) (*B*) according to CAC score (CACS) and the presence of a normal or abnormal stress SPECT-MPI study. Event rates increased with increasing CACs but event rates were further increased when SPECT-MPI was abnormal.

Women (WOMEN) trial.[30] In this trial, 824 women with chest pain, 61% who presented with typical angina, were randomized to either exercise ECG or exercise SPECT-MPI. All participants had an interpretable ECG. At the end of a 2-year follow-up, the frequency of cardiac events was comparable in both groups. The overall frequency of cardiac events was low (approximately 2%), indicative of the benign prognosis that is currently present among patients who have stable symptoms and can exercise adequately. Thus, whereas SPECT-MPI has greater intrinsic sensitivity and specificity for detection of ischemia than exercise ECG, in exercising women with stable chest pain symptoms and an interpretable ECG, exercise ECG testing alone seems a more optimal initial strategy due to the lower cost associated with this test.

Box 1
Common methods for noninvasive evaluation of myocardial ischemia or atherosclerosis

Functional tests

Treadmill exercise ECG

Stress MPI with SPECT

Stress MPI with PET

Stress echocardiography

Pharmacologic stress testing with cardiac MRI

Anatomic tests

CAC scanning

Carotid ultrasound

Coronary CTA

Recent comparative effectiveness research has focused particularly on the clinical utility of coronary CT angiography (CTA), which can characterize the presence and magnitude of calcified and noncalcified plaque and evaluate the magnitude of coronary stenoses. Two large multicenter randomized clinical trials have evaluated a strategy of using coronary CTA in stable symptomatic patients with suspected CAD. The PROMISE (PROspective Multicenter Imaging Study for Evaluation of Chest Pain) trial[31] evaluated 10,003 symptomatic patients with no prior CAD who were referred for noninvasive testing, randomizing them to CTA (4686) or functional testing (4692) with stress nuclear (67.3%), stress echo (22.5%), or stress ECG alone (10.2%). The mean pretest likelihood of obstructive CAD by the Diamond-Forrester classification was 53.3% $\pm$ 21.4%. The observed prevalence of greater than or equal to 50% stenosis on CTA in the CTA arm, however, was only 10.7%. Over a median of 25 months, a primary endpoint event (death, myocardial infarction, hospitalization for unstable angina, or major procedural complication) occurred in 3.3% of the CTA group and 3.0% in the functional-testing group (P = ns). Although the trial was not powered for noninferiority, this large trial suggests that a strategy of initial CTA is not inferior to the more commonly used functional strategy with respect to short-term cardiac events in a relatively low-risk, symptomatic population.

The Scot-Heart trial randomized 4146 patients presenting to 12 rapid access chest pain centers in Scotland to CTA versus a standard of care approach.[32] Of note, 85% of the patients had already had stress ECG testing at the time of

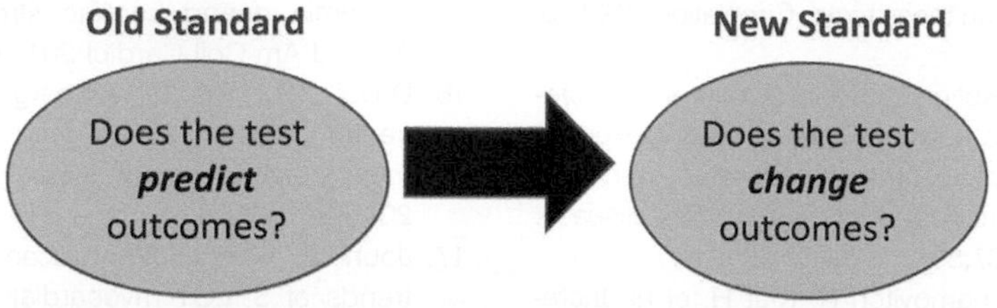

Fig. 12. Schematic representation for the changing bar for evaluating cardiac tests. Until recently, cardiac tests were assessed for their intrinsic ability to predict adverse clinical outcomes. More recently, tests are also evaluated for the direct and indirect impact they have on altering subsequent clinical outcomes, such as their potential impact on cardiac risk factor profiles, downstream utilization of medical resources, and reduction in adverse clinical events.

randomization. The primary endpoint was certainty of the diagnosis of angina secondary to coronary heart disease at 6 weeks. CTA reclassified the presence of CHD in 558 (27%) patients and a diagnosis of angina due to CHD in 481 (23%) patients ($P<.0001$). CTA was associated with increased physician certainty regarding the presence of CHD and diagnosis of angina ($P<.0001$) and changed medical treatment in 23% ($P<.0001$). After a median of 1.7 years, CTA was associated with a 38% reduction in fatal and nonfatal myocardial infarction, close to, but missing, statistical significance ($P = .0527$).

The potential comparative effectiveness of SPECT MPI when conducting such trials might be improved by considering not only short-term clinical risk but also the long-term clinical risk that is shaped not only by the presence or absence of ischemia but also by the mode of stress that was used for testing the presence and magnitude of CAD risk factors as well as other clinical determinants of long-term risk. Furthermore, in this regard, combining SPECT-MPI (or positron emission tomography [PET]-MPI) with CAC scanning—such as might be routine with SPECT/CT or PET/CT scanners—might add to the effectiveness of a strategy using these modalities.

CHANGE IN REPORTING SCHEMA FOR SINGLE-PHOTON EMISSION COMPUTED TOMOGRAPHY–MYOCARDIAL PERFUSION IMAGING

How might such long-term risk assessment be conveyed? Currently, it is common practice to issue a report of low risk among patients with absence of inducible ischemia on SPECT-MPI studies, regardless of the mode of stress and burden of CAD risk factors. From a long-term perspective, however, a nonischemic or mildly ischemic patient could be at low short-term risk and yet be at high long-term risk if the patient, for example, had 2 to 3 major CAD risk factors and required pharmacologic testing. Refinement in risk characterization in such cases could be achieved by adding an additional paragraph to the clinical report. For instance, if a highly sedentary patient with atypical angina and a normal SPECT-MPI study required pharmacologic stress, has hypertension, and is a present smoker, the clinical report might read as follows:

> *The stress-rest SPECT study shows normal radiotracer concentration throughout the myocardium on stress and rest imaging. Thus, short-term ischemic risk is low. Long-term clinical risk may still be elevated, however, in this patient due to the patient's inability to exercise (due to physical deconditioning) and the presence of multiple CAD risk factors, including hypertension and current smoking.*

As interest in comparative effectiveness research grows, increasing emphasis will be placed on maximizing the ability of tests to actually alter risk. Combining the assessment of myocardial ischemia, which is the inherent strength of SPECT-MPI, with assessment of the clinical predictors of long-term risk and with calcium scores (when available) represents a potential means for optimizing the ability of SPECT-MPI to favorably affect long-term outcomes, by better identifying who are the high-risk patients who require the most aggressive medical management. Prospective studies are indicated to test this possibility.

REFERENCES

1. Bruce RA, Blackmon JR, Jones JW, et al. Exercising testing in adult normal subjects and cardiac patients. Pediatrics 1963;32:742–56.
2. Pollock SG, Abbott RD, Boucher CA, et al. Independent and incremental prognostic value of tests performed in hierarchial order to evaluate patients with suspected coronary artery disease. Validation

of models based on these tests. Circulation 1992;85: 237–48.
3. Ladenheim ML, Kotler TS, Pollock BH, et al. Incremental prognostic power of clinical history, exercise electrocardiography and myocardial perfusion scintigraphy in suspected coronary artery disease. Am J Cardiol 1987;59:270–7.
4. Berman DS, Hachamovitch R, Kiat H, et al. Incremental value of prognostic testing in patients with known or suspected ischemic heart disease: a basis for optimal utilization of exercise technetium-99m sestamibi myocardial perfusion single-photon emission computed tomography. J Am Coll Cardiol 1995; 26:639–47.
5. Ladenheim ML, Pollock BH, Rozanski A, et al. Extent and severity of myocardial hypoperfusion as predictors of prognosis in patients with suspected coronary artery disease. J Am Coll Cardiol 1986;7: 464–71.
6. Metz LD, Beattie M, Hom R, et al. The prognostic value of normal exercise myocardial perfusion imaging and exercise echocardiography: a meta-analysis. J Am Coll Cardiol 2007;49:227–37.
7. Hachamovitch R, Hayes S, Friedman JD, et al. Determinants of risk and its temporal variation in patients with normal stress myocardial perfusion scans. What is the warranty period of a normal scan? J Am Coll Cardiol 2003;41:1329–40.
8. Fox CS, Evans JC, Larson MG, et al. Temporal trends in coronary heart disease mortality and sudden cardiac death from 1950 to 1999: the Framingham Heart Study. Circulation 2004;110:522–7.
9. Ford ES, Ajani UA, Croft JB, et al. Explaining the decrease in U.S. deaths from coronary disease, 1980-2000. N Engl J Med 2007;356:2388–98.
10. Yeh RW, Sidney S, Chandra M, et al. Population trends in the incidence and outcomes of acute myocardial infarction. N Engl J Med 2010;362: 2155–65.
11. Carandang R, Seshadri S, Beiser A, et al. Trends in incidence, lifetime risk, severity, and 30-day mortality of stroke over the past 50 years. JAMA 2006;296: 2939–46.
12. Murabito JM, Evans JC, D'Agostino RB Sr, et al. Temporal trends in the incidence of intermittent claudication from 1950 to 1999. Am J Epidemiol 2005; 162:430–7.
13. Carroll MD, Lacher DA, Sorlie PD, et al. Trends in serum lipids and lipoproteins of adults, 1960-2002. JAMA 2005;294:1773–81.
14. Cutler JA, Sorlie PD, Wolz M, et al. Trends in hypertension prevalence, awareness, treatment, and control rates in United States adults between 1988-1994 and 1999-2004. Hypertension 2008;52: 818–27.
15. Rozanski A, Gransar H, Hayes SW, et al. Temporal trends in the frequency of inducible myocardial ischemia during cardiac stress testing: 1991 to 2009. J Am Coll Cardiol 2013;61:1054–65.
16. Duvall WL, Rai M, Ahlberg AW, et al. A multicenter assessment of the temporal trends in myocardial perfusion imaging. J Nucl Cardiol 2015;22:539–51.
17. Jouni H, Askew JW, Crusan DJ, et al. Temporal trends of SPECT myocardial perfusion imaging in patients without coronary artery disease; a 17 year experience from a tertiary academic medical center. Circ Cardiovasc Oucomes 2013;6:A40.
18. Thompson RC, Allam AH. More risk factors, less ischemia, and the relevance of MPI testing. J Nucl Cardiol 2015;22:552–4.
19. Supariwala A, Uretsky S, Singh P, et al. Synergistic effect of coronary artery disease risk factors on long-term survival in patients with normal exercise SPECT studies. J Nucl Cardiol 2011;18:207–14.
20. Rozanski A, Gransar H, Min JK, et al. Long-term mortality following normal exercise myocardial perfusion SPECT according to coronary disease risk factors. J Nucl Cardiol 2014;21:341–50.
21. Navare S, Mather J, Shaw LJ, et al. Comparison of risk stratification with pharmacologic and exercise stress myocardial perfusion imaging: a meta-analysis. J Nucl Cardiol 2004;11:551–61.
22. Rozanski A, Gransar H, Hayes SW, et al. Comparison of long-term mortality risk following normal exercise vs adenosine myocardial perfusion SPECT. J Nucl Cardiol 2010;17:999–1008.
23. Johnson NP, Schimmel DR, Dyer SP, et al. Survival by stress modality in patients with a normal myocardial perfusion study. Am J Cardiol 2011;107:986–9.
24. Poulin MF, Alexander S, Doukky R. Prognostic implications of stress modality on mortality risk and cause of death in patients undergoing office-based SPECT myocardial perfusion imaging. J Nucl Cardiol 2015. [Epub ahead of print].
25. Nair SU, Ahlberg AW, Katten DM, et al. Does risk for major adverse cardiac events in patients undergoing vasodilator stress with adjunctive exercise differe from patients undergoing either standard exercise or vasodilator stress with myocardial perfusion imaging? J Nucl Cardiol 2015;22:22–35.
26. Supariwala A, Uretsky S, Depuey EG, et al. Influence of mode of stress and coronary risk factor burden upon long-term mortality following normal stress myocardial perfusion single-photon emission computed tomographic imaging. Am J Cardiol 2013;111:846–50.
27. He ZX, Hedrick TD, Pratt CM, et al. Severity of coronary artery calcification by electron beam computed tomography predicts silent myocardial ischemia. Circulation 2000;101:244–51.
28. Berman DS, Wong ND, Gransar H, et al. Relationship between stress-induced myocardial ischemia

and atherosclerosis measured by coronary calcium tomography. J Am Coll Cardiol 2004;44:923–30.
29. Chang SM, Nabi F, Xu J, et al. The coronary artery calcium score and stress myocardial perfusion imaging provide independent and complementary prediction of cardiac risk. J Am Coll Cardiol 2009; 54:1872–82.
30. Shaw LJ, Mieres JH, Hendel RH, et al. Comparative effectiveness of exercise electrocardiography with or without myocardial perfusion single photon emission computed tomography in women with suspected coronary artery disease. Results from the what is the optimal method for ischemia evaluation in Women (WOMEN) trial. Circulation 2011;124: 1239–49.
31. Douglas PS, Hoffmann U, Patel MR, et al. Outcomes of anatomical versus functional testing for coronary artery disease. N Engl J Med 2015;372: 1291–300.
32. SCOT-HEART Investigators. CT coronary angiography in patients with suspected angina due to coronary heart disease (SCOT-HEART): an open-label, parallel-group, multicentre trial. Lancet 2015;385: 2383–91.

Radionuclide Assessment of Left Ventricular Dyssynchrony

Hussein Abu Daya, MD[a], Saurabh Malhotra, MD, MPH[b], Prem Soman, MD, PhD, FRCP (UK)[a,*]

KEYWORDS

• Left ventricular dyssynchrony • Cardiac resynchronization therapy • Heart failure • Radionuclide • Site of latest activation • Myocardial scar • SPECT • Echo • LBBB • QRS

KEY POINTS

- Phase analysis of GMPS is a widely available and reproducible measure of LV dyssynchrony, which also provides comprehensive assessment of LV function, global and regional scar burden, and patterns of LV mechanical activation.
- Preliminary studies indicate potential use in predicting CRT response and elucidation of mechanisms.
- In contemporary CRT, patients selected for the presence of a wide QRS and LBBB are likely to have a septal to lateral wall activation delay, which is amenable to resynchronization by biventricular pacing. In these patients, imaging may be helpful in identifying scar and extensive LV remodeling, which may suggest lack of potential for functional improvement with CRT.
- Because advances in technology may expand capabilities for precise LV lead placement in the future, identification of specific patterns of dyssynchrony may have a critical role in guiding CRT.

DEFINITION AND PREVALENCE

Dyssynchrony refers to a temporal dispersion in the activation and contraction of the normally coordinate ventricle. Minor differences in the amplitude and timing of left ventricular (LV) contraction exist in normally functioning hearts,[1] thus pathophysiologic dyssynchrony needs to be defined using threshold rarely encountered in the normal population.[2] LV dyssynchrony is not an all-or-nothing phenomenon, but represents a continuum of different grades of severity.[1]

LV dyssynchrony can manifest in several different ways: electrical versus mechanical, systolic versus diastolic, intraventricular versus interventricular, and normal versus pathologic dyssynchrony. Currently the QRS duration on a 12-lead electrocardiogram is used as a surrogate for electromechanical dyssynchrony and a wide QRS duration taken to denote a prolonged ventricular conduction time and nonsimultaneous ventricular wall contraction.[3,4] However, there is increasing evidence about the limitations of using the QRS duration as the sole marker of mechanical dyssynchrony.[5,6] Mechanical dyssynchrony can occur between the atria and the ventricles (atrioventricular dyssynchrony), the left and the right ventricles (interventricular dyssynchrony), or among different myocardial segments of the left ventricle (intraventricular dyssynchrony).[7,8] Intraventricular dyssynchrony has been shown to strongly correlate with cardiac hemodynamic parameters and adverse cardiac events, as opposed to interventricular dyssynchrony,[9] and the term is

[a] Division of Cardiology, Department of Medicine, University of Pittsburgh Medical Center, 200 Lothrop Street, Pittsburgh, PA 15213, USA; [b] Division of Cardiology, University at Buffalo, 875 Ellicott Street, Suite 7030, Buffalo, NY 14203, USA
* Corresponding author. A-429 Scaife Hall, 200 Lothrop Street, Pittsburgh, PA 15213.
E-mail address: somanp@upmc.edu

Cardiol Clin 34 (2016) 101–118
http://dx.doi.org/10.1016/j.ccl.2015.08.006
0733-8651/16/$ – see front matter

used interchangeably with mechanical dyssynchrony. Much of the current knowledge on LV dyssynchrony comes from echocardiographic studies, which have traditionally quantified LV dyssynchrony as either greater than 60 to 65 millisecond (ms) delay in time to peak systolic contraction between the septum and posterolateral walls of the left ventricle, or by the Yu index, defined as the standard deviation (SD) of the time to peak systolic velocity in a 12-segment LV model (>33 ms represents dyssynchrony).[2] Diastolic dyssynchrony is less clearly defined compared with its systolic counterpart.

The mechanisms underlying LV dyssynchrony are poorly understood, but known to depend on a complex interplay of numerous factors including LV systolic dysfunction, electrical abnormality (QRS widening), and LV scar burden. In general, the prevalence of dyssynchrony increases with worsening systolic dysfunction and increasing QRS duration. Among patients with severely reduced LV systolic function, dyssynchrony has been reported in up to 75% of the patients.[10] Similarly, among patients with systolic heart failure, the prevalence of dyssynchrony reportedly varies from 27% in patients with narrow QRS (<120 ms) to 89% in those with QRS duration greater than 150 ms.[1,11] In diastolic heart failure, however, the prevalence of systolic dyssynchrony is reported to be 33% to 60%, whereas diastolic dyssynchrony is 40% to 58%.[12,13]

PATHOPHYSIOLOGY

Ventricular contraction occurs by a geographically coordinated process where myocardial fibers shorten synchronously and by the same amount throughout the ventricle. This highly coordinated process is maintained by an endocardial electrical conduction system that carries the cardiac action potential from the endocardium to the epicardium and from the apex to the base, facilitating synchronized ventricular myocardial contraction.[14–16] Any disruption of this conduction or contraction pattern leads to dyssynchronous ventricular contraction. A classic example of such pathophysiology is seen in left bundle branch block (LBBB), where the early systolic contraction of the LV septum followed by late systolic activation of the lateral free wall results in dyssynchronous contraction, producing regional heterogeneity in myocardial work load and blood flow.[17–19] These are thought to result in LV remodeling (increased LV end-systolic volume) and increasing wall stress, a rightward shift of the end-systolic pressure-volume relationship,[20] a reduction in net LV ejection pressure,[20,21] an increase in the rate of LV pressure (dP/dt_{max}),[22] and a reduced stroke work and volume.[21] This mechanical inefficiency is further exacerbated by functional mitral regurgitation, which is caused by dyssynchronous papillary muscle contraction, annular dilation, and atrioventricular conduction delay.[17,23] The end result is reduced net cardiac output and symptomatic heart failure that is often refractory to conventional medical therapy.[24,25]

CLINICAL IMPLICATIONS IN HEART FAILURE

An association between LV dyssynchrony and mortality has been demonstrated in patients with heart failure.[26] Sustained LV dyssynchrony has been shown to lead to LV systolic dysfunction,[27] whereas dyssynchrony promotes progression of established heart failure, and is an independent predictor of adverse cardiac events.[26,28,29] Cardiac resynchronization therapy (CRT) improves the net systolic function and cardiac mechanical efficiency by resynchronizing biventricular contraction, without increasing myocardial oxygen consumption.[30–32] Simultaneous biventricular preexcitation by CRT and the associated reduction in dyssynchronous contraction improves functional mitral regurgitation, eventually resulting in smaller LV volumes (reverse remodeling).[33,34] Several large, randomized controlled trials have shown that CRT reduces mortality and morbidity in patients with drug-refractory heart failure, particularly in the presence of LV dyssynchrony.[35–38] However, applying CRT to patients with heart failure with no underlying dyssynchrony may lead to poor clinical outcomes.[39]

Initial guidelines for CRT were based on studies that were performed in patients with New York Heart Association (NYHA) class III or IV heart failure, LBBB, QRS greater than 120 ms, and LV ejection fraction (LVEF) less than or equal to 35%.[40] Subsequent studies have shown benefit in patients with milder heart failure.[41–43] A recent meta-analysis of five randomized clinical trials involving 4317 patients with NYHA class I to II heart failure, LVEF less than 40%, and QRS greater than 120 ms showed that CRT with implantable cardioverter defibrillator (ICD) therapy decreased all-cause mortality, heart failure hospitalizations, and improved LVEF compared with ICD alone.[44] More specifically, in NYHA functional class I patients, heart failure hospitalization risk remained lower with CRT, whereas there was no difference in mortality. Following these new data, the guidelines were updated and CRT is now indicated for patients with NYHA class II heart failure with LVEF less than or equal to 35%, LBBB, and a QRS duration greater than or equal to 150 ms (class I recommendation) or QRS equal or greater than 120 but less than 150 ms (class IIa recommendation), and may be considered for patients with NYHA class I heart failure with LVEF less than or equal to 30%, LBBB, with ischemic cause and a QRS duration greater than or equal to 150 ms (class IIb recommendation), and may be considered for patients with NYHA class I heart failure with LVEF less than or equal to 30%, LBBB, with ischemic cause and a QRS duration greater than or equal to 150 ms (class IIb recommendation).[45] CRT implantation is an invasive procedure and not without complications.[46] In addition, CRT implantation based on the current criteria is not optimally cost effective,[47] because two-thirds of recipients do not derive symptomatic or functional benefit from the procedure.[48] Although randomized controlled trials have highlighted that the greatest benefit from CRT is in patients with an LBBB and a wide QRS duration,[49] other studies and meta-analyses have reported either modest or no correlation between QRS duration and response to CRT.[50,51] Thus, there is interest in identifying parameters that might improve prediction of CRT response including the use of multimodality imaging. This article discusses the different modalities used to assess mechanical dyssynchrony, with a focus on gated myocardial perfusion single-photon emission computed tomography (SPECT) and its use in predicting response and prognosis after CRT.

Current Methods of Assessing Ventricular Dyssynchrony

Echocardiography

Echocardiographic techniques have traditionally formed the backbone of dyssynchrony assessment and have been widely used because of wide availability, noninvasiveness, and low cost. Dyssynchrony on echocardiography can be assessed from M-mode, two-dimensional (2D), and three-dimensional (3D) image acquisitions. However, the most contemporaneous approach is to use Doppler-based techniques, such as tissue Doppler or speckle tracking. The use of Doppler-based techniques allows for data acquisition in radial and longitudinal directions, and during rest and exercise.[1,8] The currently used parameters of systolic or diastolic dyssynchrony were mostly derived from cutoff values used in clinical trials. Cutoff values for systolic dyssynchrony range from greater than or equal to 33 ms for the Yu index (SD of the six basal and six mid LV segments in ejection phase) using the tissue Doppler imaging parameter of time to systolic peak velocity,[52] to greater than or equal to 130 ms for septal-to-posterior wall mechanical delay using the M-mode[53] or for the septal-to-posterior delay using time to peak systolic strain on 2D speckle tracking.[54] Using the 3D echo parameter of time to minimal regional volume, the cutoff value used is 10.4% for the SD of the 16 LV segments.[55] Assessment of diastolic dyssynchrony is less frequently performed and not well studied; however, a value of greater than 34 ms for the time to peak early diastolic velocity from six basal and six mid-LV segments has been used as a measure of diastolic dyssynchrony.[13]

Several attempts to use echocardiographic techniques to enhance patient selection for CRT have been discouraging. Early studies may have been affected by the low repeatability of echo-based parameters, as was demonstrated in the Predictors of the Response to CRT (PROSPECT) trial.[56] However, even contemporary approaches, such as speckle tracking imaging and real-time 3D echocardiography, have not proved effective in improving prediction of CRT response. The recently published Echocardiography Guided Cardiac Resynchronization Therapy (EchoCRT) study included 809 patients with narrow QRS (<130 ms) and echocardiographic evidence of LV dyssynchrony (using speckle tracking and other contemporary techniques). In this randomized trial CRT based on the presence of LV dyssynchrony did not reduce the composite outcome of death or hospitalization for heart failure; in fact, the trial was terminated early for increased mortality in the CRT arm.[57] Notably, in all of these studies, the prediction of CRT response was based primarily on dyssynchrony parameters, and other factors known to influence CRT response, such as the location and size of myocardial scar[58] and LV lead placement in relation to the latest activated myocardial segment[59,60] were not included in the prediction algorithms.

Cardiac MRI

Dyssynchrony is assessed by cardiac MRI (CMR) using multiple techniques including myocardial tagging, 3D-tagged CMR, strain-coded CMR, and CMR tissue resynchronization imaging.[38,61–64] Studies using CMR to assess mechanical dyssynchrony and to predict response to CRT have been promising. Bilchick and colleagues[62] showed that CMR tagging circumferential uniformity ratio estimate derived from magnetic resonance myocardial tagging predicted improvement in functional class in patients undergoing CRT with 90% accuracy (positive and negative predictive values, 87% and 100%, respectively). In this same study, adding delayed enhancement CMR (% total scar <15%) further improved this predictive value and accuracy increased to 95% (positive and negative predictive values, 93% and 100%, respectively). In another study, Chalil and colleagues[38] showed that patients with baseline CMR tissue resynchronization imaging value greater than or equal to 110 ms before CRT were 5.2 times more likely to experience death or hospitalization for a major cardiovascular event within a short-term follow-up period. Recently, it has been shown that CMR mechanical dyssynchrony measures together with scar quantification and measures of strain at the LV lead position can accurately predict response to CRT.[65] Because of its high resolution and excellent tissue characterization (presence of scar) CMR is emerging as a valuable tool for the assessment of cardiac dyssynchrony. However, its cost, limited availability, longer examination times, and inability to image patients with implanted devices precludes the routine application of CMR for assessment of dyssynchrony.[66]

Myocardial Single-Photon Emission Computed Tomography

Mechanical dyssynchrony is determined from radionuclide cardiac Imaging techniques and is based on the assessment of regional LV thickening by phase analysis. This has been classically done through phase analysis of equilibrium radionuclide-gated blood-pool angiography (ERNA) and relies on the assessment of regional changes in blood-pool tracer activity during a cardiac cycle.[67] Intraventricular and interventricular dyssynchrony indices are calculated from blood-pool time activity curves, after subjecting the curves to a first-harmonic Fourier transformation. Using ERNA, CRT has been shown to improve interventricular and intraventricular dyssynchrony within 6 months following implantation.[68] Seminal work on dyssynchrony assessment among patients with nonischemic cardiomyopathy (NICM) using ERNA has highlighted the importance of intra-LV dyssynchrony over interventricular dyssynchrony in predicting changes in cardiac hemodynamics.[9] The advantage of ERNA over SPECT is its relatively higher temporal resolution. The limitation of poor anatomic localization of planar (2D) ERNA is addressed by 3D acquisition using gated blood-pool SPECT. In a recent study on 28 patients with dilated cardiomyopathy and heart failure, CRT improved interventricular and intraventricular dyssynchrony in those who responded to this therapy.[69]

Contrary to ERNA, dyssynchrony assessment by phase analysis of gated myocardial perfusion SPECT (GMPS) is based on determining the timing of wall thickening during a cardiac cycle. The poor spatial resolution of SPECT makes it subject to the partial volume effect, based on which there is a relatively linear relationship between myocardial thickening and myocardial count density in any segment of the myocardium.[70] This is evident in standard gated SPECT myocardial perfusion images where the myocardium is brighter in systole. The time activity curve of a myocardial segment is therefore essentially its thickening curve, albeit with poor temporal fidelity because of the 8- or 16-bin gating that is generally used for myocardial SPECT. Application of Fourier transformation to the time-activity curve of the myocardium improves the temporal resolution of the gated SPECT images, and generates a continuous thickening curve that delineates the timing of segmental myocardial contraction (**Fig. 1**).[67,71] During a standard myocardial perfusion SPECT acquisition, information from many (>600) myocardial segments is collected, and the phase of initial or peak contraction is determined and compared among segments. The commonly used software packages for myocardial perfusion image interpretation including quantitative gated SPECT (QGS; Cedars-Sinai Medical Center, Los Angeles, CA) (**Fig. 2**), Emory Cardiac Toolbox (ECTb; Emory University, Atlanta, GA), and 4DM SPECT (INVIA Medical Imaging Solutions, Ann Arbor, MI) all now offer phase analysis capabilities in their standard offerings.[72,73]

Despite its inherent low temporal resolution compared with ERNA, its widespread availability and the ability to derive comprehensive information on perfusion, function, and dyssynchrony from a standard perfusion study, makes GMPS an attractive tool for dyssynchrony assessment.

The most commonly used and validated indices of LV dyssynchrony from GMPS are the phase histogram band width (HBW), the range of degree of the cardiac cycle that encompasses 95% of the phase distribution, and the phase SD (PSD), which is the SD of the phase distribution. Additional software-specific indices are (1) entropy, a measure of variability that is normalized to its maximum value and reported as a percentage[72,74]; (2) phase histogram skewness, which indicates the symmetry of the histogram; and (3) the phase histogram kurtosis, which represents the degree to which the histogram is peaked.[73] PSD and HBW values from GMPS have been validated against echo-derived measures using tissue Doppler imaging[72,75] or more contemporary techniques, such as speckle tracking[76] and 3D echo.[77,78] The most rigorously determined cutoffs for LV dyssynchrony have been described by Chen and colleagues[73] using ECTb, where a PSD value of greater than 24.4° in men and greater

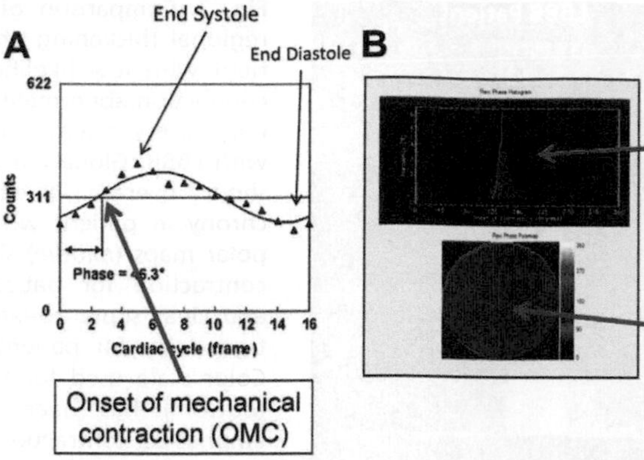

Fig. 1. Phase analysis by gated myocardial perfusion SPECT. (*A*) Example of a time-activity curve for a single myocardial sample volume generated by 16-bin gating. The data points (▲) are then fitted to a continuous curve, using a Fourier transform. Based on the partial volume effect, this time-activity curve represents the thickening curve of this particular myocardial sample during a cardiac cycle. The point at which the continuous thickening curve intersects with the average count density of this voxel (*horizontal line*) is considered the onset of mechanical contraction (OMC) for this region. The software computes the OMC for all LV myocardial samples collected (>600) and then displays the composite result as a phase histogram and phase polar map (*B*). The phase histogram shows the percentage of myocardium contracting (y-axis) at each point in the cardiac cycle (x-axis). The phase polar map is a bull's-eye representation of the LV, showing the sequence of mechanical activation, using a color-coded scheme. This is an example of synchronous LV contraction with a narrow and highly peaked histogram and a uniform color on the phase polar map. (*Adapted from* Friehling M, Chen J, Saba S, et al. A prospective pilot study to evaluate the relationship between acute change in left ventricular synchrony after cardiac resynchronization therapy and patient outcome using a single-injection gated SPECT protocol. Circ Cardiovasc Imaging 2011;4(5):533; with permission.)

than 22.2° in women or an HBW value of greater than 62.2° in men and greater than 49.8° in women identifies presence of dyssynchrony.[73] These cut-offs represent mean + 2 SD of PSD and HBW determined from GMPS of healthy men and women. Sampling differences between commercially available software packages result in differences in PSD and HBW values.[72,79] In a recent study, Rastgou and colleagues[80] compared the ECTb and QGS software in a population of patients with heart failure. PSD and HBW values derived from ECTb and QGS were compared with each other and with the Yu index and septal-lateral wall delay on echocardiography. Although there was good correlation between QGS and ECTb derived PSD and HBW, the mean values obtained from ECTb were significantly higher. The authors also found no correlation between dyssynchrony measures by ECTb and QGS and the Yu index; however, PSD and HBW significantly correlated with the septal-lateral wall delay, suggesting a systematic difference is dyssynchrony assessment by GMPS and echocardiographic methods. Given the computational differences among GMPS analysis software, it is generally recommended to use software-specific cut-offs when evaluating dyssynchrony in a fashion similar to that routinely applied to other GMPS variables, such as LV volumes, mass, and LVEF. GMPS has several advantages over echocardiography, such as high repeatability and reproducibility,[81,82] universal availability of SPECT without the need for specialized image acquisition, and ability to provide information on perfusion (scar and site of latest activation), and provides a 3D representation of LV contraction, unlike echocardiography in which dyssynchrony assessment is directional, either longitudinal or radial or opposing wall delay depending on the approach used. This has led some authors to consider GMPS a "one-stop shop" for LV dyssynchrony assessment.[71]

Dyssynchrony Assessment by Gated Myocardial Perfusion Single-Photon Emission Computed Tomography As a Diagnostic and Risk Stratification Tool

Predicting response to cardiac resynchronization therapy

GMPS has now become an established tool for assessing LV dyssynchrony and multiple observational studies have explored its use in predicting response to CRT (**Table 1**).[72,79,83–87] Henneman and colleagues[79] were the first to evaluate the ability of LV dyssynchrony measures derived from

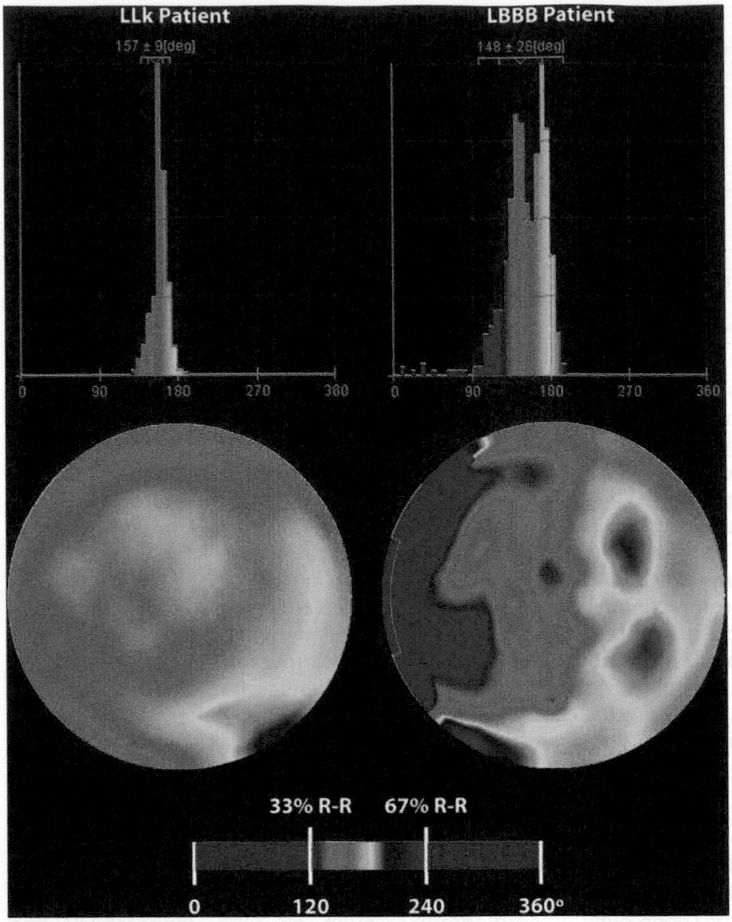

Fig. 2. Comparison of global and regional thickening phase in a patient with low likelihood (LLk) of conduction abnormalities and coronary artery disease and a patient with LBBB. Global histograms (*top*) show overall increased dyssynchrony in patient with LBBB, and polar maps (*middle*) show uniform contraction for patient with LLk and clear septal-to-lateral contraction delay for patient with LBBB. Color scale used for both patients (*bottom*) has been adjusted to emphasize contraction timing differences in middle third of R-R cycle. deg, degrees. (*Adapted from* Van Kriekinge SD, Nishina H, Ohba M, et al. Automatic global and regional phase analysis from gated myocardial perfusion SPECT imaging: application to the characterization of ventricular contraction in patients with left bundle branch block. J Nucl Med 2008;49(11):1792; with permission.)

phase analysis of GMPS to predict CRT response in a population with ischemic cardiomyopathy (ICM) and NICM. They found that a value of 135° for phase HBW (70% sensitivity and specificity, receiver operating characteristic [ROC] area under the curve 0.78) and 43° for PSD (74% sensitivity and specificity, ROC area under the curve 0.81) predicted response to CRT defined as an improvement by greater than or equal to one NYHA class.[79] Similar results were obtained by Mukherjee and colleagues[84] in a small study of 32 NICM patients with NYHA class III to IV, 63% with LBBB, LVEF 23 ± 5%, and QRS 150 ± 18 ms in whom GMPS was performed before and 3 months after CRT. On follow-up, 69% of the patients responded to CRT, defined as an improvement in NYHA class by greater than or equal to one grade and in LVEF by greater than 5%. Responders had significantly worse dyssynchrony indices PSD (64 ± 17 vs 39 ± 13°; $P<.01$) and HBW (215 ± 64 vs 110 ± 44°; $P<.01$) when compared with nonresponders. ROC curve analysis demonstrated that the maximum accuracy for prediction of CRT response was obtained with values of 128° for HBW and 43° for PSD (86% sensitivity and 80% specificity with ROC 0.89 for both).[84] Similar findings have been reported by other studies,[72,85] all of which suggest that a threshold level of dyssynchrony may be necessary at baseline for CRT benefit to accrue. In addition to the value of PSD and HBW for predicting response to CRT, Azizian and colleagues[85] showed that an entropy cut-off of 52% predicted CRT response with 90% sensitivity and 80% specificity. More recently, Kiso and colleagues[83] used GMPS to develop a new variable for assessing dyssynchrony, called the dyssynchrony index, calculated as the maximum difference in time to end-systole among four myocardial segments (anterior, lateral, inferior, and septal) corrected for R-R interval. In a small cohort of 44 NICM patients, dyssynchrony index at baseline correlated significantly with time to peak velocity measured by tissue Doppler imaging, and it was significantly larger in responders than in nonresponders (response defined as LVEF increase by >10% or LVESV decrease

Table 1
Studies of radionuclide imaging–based approaches to predict CRT response

Author (Ref)	Patient (N)	Patient Criteria	Follow-Up, mo	Imaging	Phase Analysis Software	CRT Response Definition	Major Findings
Mukherjee et al,[84] 2015	32 (all with NICM)	NYHA class III–IV, 63% with LBBB, LVEF 23 ± 5%, QRS 150 ± 18 ms	3–4	^{99m}Tc GMPS	Emory Cardiac Toolbox	Improvement of NYHA class by ≥1 and LVEF by >5%	Phase HBW 128° and PSD 43° (Sen 86% and Spec 80%, ROC AUC 0.89 for both) predicted CRT response
Azizian et al,[85] 2014	30 (86% with ICM)	NYHA class III–IV, LVEF 19 ± 4%, QRS 156 ± 22 ms	6	^{99m}Tc GMPS	Cedars Sinai SPECT-QGS	LVESV decreased by >15%	Phase HBW 112° (Sen 72% and Spec 70%), PSD 21° (Sen 90% and Spec 74%), and entropy 52% (Sen 90% and Spec 80%) predicted CRT response Patients with concordant LV lead position were more likely to respond to CRT compared with those with discordant LV lead position
Kiso et al,[83] 2011	33 (6% with ICM)	NYHA class II–IV, LVEF 25 ± 12%, QRS 160 ± 30 ms	6	^{99m}Tc GMPS	Cedars Sinai SPECT-QGS; novel algorithm using DI as a measure of LV dyssynchrony	LVEF increase by >10% or LVESV decrease by >10%	DI at baseline measured by SPECT correlated significantly with time to peak velocity measured by TDI DI before CRT was significantly larger in responders vs nonresponders DI showed a significant decrease after CRT in the responder group

(*continued on next page*)

Table 1
(continued)

Author (Ref)	Patient (N)	Patient Criteria	Follow-Up, mo	Imaging	Phase Analysis Software	CRT Response Definition	Major Findings
Friehling et al,[86] 2011	44 (43% with ICM)	NYHA class II–IV, 96% with LBBB, LVEF 25 ± 9%, QRS 178 ± 34 ms	9.6 ± 6.8	^{99m}Tc GMPS	Emory Cardiac Toolbox	Algorithm incorporating the presence of baseline dyssynchrony, myocardial scar burden, and lead concordance predicted acute change in LV synchrony	The algorithm predicted acute improvement or no change in LV synchrony with Sen 72%, Spec 93%, PPV 96%, and NPV 64% and had NPV 96% for acute deterioration in synchrony Patients who had an acute deterioration in synchrony after CRT had a higher composite event rate of death, HHF, appropriate defibrillator discharges, and CRT device deactivation for worsening heart failure symptoms
Nakamura et al,[87] 2011	24 (all with NICM)	NYHA class III–IV, LVEF <35%, 33% with QRS <120 ms	6	^{99m}Tc GMPS	cardioGRAPH, Tokyo, Japan	Plasma brain natriuretic peptide level decrease by >50%	The standard deviation of time to end systole (TES-SD) >49 ms predicted responders (Sen 100% and Spec 78.8%, ROC AUC 0.881)
Boogers et al,[60] 2011	40 (70% with ICM)	NYHA class III–IV, LVEF 25 ± 8%, QRS 156 ± 34 ms	6	^{99m}Tc GMPS	Cedars Sinai SPECT-QGS	Improvement by ≥1 NYHA class	Phase HBW 72.5° (Sen 83% and Spec 81%, ROC 0.83) and PSD 19.6° (Sen 83% and Spec 81%, ROC 0.85) predicted CRT response
Henneman et al,[79] 2007	42 (67% with ICM)	NYHA class III–IV, LVEF 24 ± 7%, QRS 153 ± 32 ms	6	^{99m}Tc GMPS	Emory Cardiac Toolbox	Improvement by ≥1 NYHA class	Phase HBW 135° (Sen and Spec of 70%, ROC AUC 0.78) and PSD 43° (Sen and Spec of 74%, ROC AUC 0.81) predicted CRT response

Lalonde et al,[103] 2014	49 (55% with ICM)	NYHA class II–III, 80% with LBBB, LVEF <35% QRS >120 ms	3	^{99m}Tc-gated SPECT RNA and PET perfusion and viability scans	NA; time- activity curves were subject to cluster analysis to produce global and segmental cluster size and scores as measures of dyssynchrony	Improvement in LVEF by >5% or LVESV decreased by >10%	In patients with ICM, the septal wall predicted CRT outcome (ROC AUC 0.73 vs equal chance ROC AUC 0.5, *P*<.05) with an optimal operating point of 71% sensitivity and 60% specificity Cluster analysis results were equivalent to SPECT RNA phase analysis and PET scar size analysis
Lishmanov et al,[69] 2013	28 (all with NICM)	NYHA class III–IV, LBBB, LVEF 24 ± 6%, QRS 183 ± 32 ms	12 ± 3	^{99m}Tc-MIBI and ^{123}I-BMIPP gated SPECT, and blood-pool SPECT	QPS and QBS Cedars-Sinai	Hyperresponders: LVEF increase by ≥10% Responders: LVEF increase by >5% but <10%	Hyperresponders and responders had an increase in LVEF, decrease in inter/intraventricular dyssynchrony, and decrease in average size of perfusion defects following CRT Nonresponders had more pronounced disturbance of myocardial metabolism compared with hyperresponders on SPECT with (123)I-BMIPP before CRT
Toussaint et al,[68] 2003	34 (53% with ICM)	NYHA class III–IV, LVEF 20 ± 8%, QRS 179 ± 18 ms	20 ± 3	^{99m}Tc-gated blood-pool RNA	NA	Improvement in LVEF >5%	The baseline combination of LVEF >15% and interventricular dyssynchrony >60 ms have Sen 78%, Spec 79%, NPV 73%, and PPV 82% to predict response to CRT

Abbreviations: AUC, area under the curve; DI, dyssynchrony index; HHF, hospitalization for heart failure; ICM, ischemic cardiomyopathy; LVESV, left ventricular end systolic volume; NA, not applicable; NPV, negative predictive value; PPV, positive predictive value; ROC, receiver operating characteristic curve; Sen, sensitivity; Spec, specificity; TDI, tissue Doppler imaging.

by >10%). Dyssynchrony index decreased significantly after CRT among responders (25.9 ± 22.2 before CRT vs 13.6 ± 10.9 after CRT; $P<.05$) and this tended to correlate with the improvement in LV function.

Because of its widespread use for myocardial perfusion imaging, most of the recent evidence on the use of cardiac radionuclide imaging for prediction of CRT response comes from GMPS-based studies. However, other non-GMPS radionuclide imaging approaches have shown promising results. In one of the earlier studies using ERNA, Toussaint and colleagues[68] showed that the combination of baseline LVEF greater than 15% and interventricular dyssynchrony greater than 60 ms had 78% sensitivity, 79% specificity, and 82% positive predictive value to predict response to CRT. Lalonde and colleagues[88] recently proposed a new algorithm that subjects the time-activity curves obtained by SPECT RNA images to cluster analysis to produce global and segmental cluster size and scores as measures of dyssynchrony. They reported a similar value for predicting CRT response from the cluster analysis technique and the Fourier transform method used by phase analysis. Lishmanov and colleagues[69] expanded the application of cardiac radionuclide imaging by studying the role of myocardial metabolism as a predictor of CRT response. They studied 28 patients with NICM and heart failure who were undergoing CRT, with GMPS, gated blood-pool SPECT, and (^{123}I-beta-methyl-p-iodophenylpentadecanoic acid [123I-BMIPP]) imaging. They found that responders and hyperresponders to CRT had significantly less severe myocardial metabolic abnormality on 123I-BMIPP scans compared with nonresponders (14% vs 20%; $P<.05$) and that metabolic imaging could also identify myocardium that is more likely to positively respond to CRT.

Assessment of the Site of Latest Activated Segment and Myocardial Scar Burden

Although the presence of LV intraventricular dyssynchrony seems to be essential for clinical improvement following CRT, CRT response is a complex phenomenon that can be influenced by several other parameters. Important considerations in this regard include global and regional myocardial scar, the pattern of LV dyssynchrony as regards the segments of activation delay in the LV, and the location of the LV lead in relation to segments with delayed activation.

Earlier studies using GMPS to evaluate myocardial scar burden and its effect on response to CRT in patients with ICM showed that nonresponders were more likely to have higher overall scar burden, a larger number of severely scarred segments, and greater scar density near the LV lead tip[89] or with viable tissue in the region of the LV lead but with extensive scar tissue.[90] This was systematically studied by Adelstein and colleagues[58] in a population of 620 patients with NYHA class III to IV, LVEF less than 35%, and QRS greater than 120 ms who were referred for CRT. In this study, scar burden was assessed by rest-redistribution Tl-201 myocardial perfusion SPECT, and it showed a lack of functional improvement and poorer survival among those with a summed rest score greater than 27 (40% LV myocardium involved).[58] Another smaller study of 213 patients undergoing CRT also showed a greater burden of myocardial scar among nonresponders compared with CRT responders (18% vs 6%; $P<.001$).[91] These results suggest that a high myocardial scar burden precludes a favorable response to CRT and this important aspect should be accounted for when evaluating the predictive value of dyssynchrony measures.

LV lead placement at the site of latest mechanical activation using echocardiographic techniques has been shown to predict response to CRT with improved outcomes in patients with NICM or ICM.[59,92] More recently, efforts have shifted toward identifying the LV site of latest activation and optimizing LV lead placement using phase analysis of GMPS.[60,93,94] Boogers and colleagues[60] showed that patients with a concordant LV lead placement at the site of latest activation as assessed by GMPS were significantly more likely to have CRT response (improvement in LV volumes and systolic function) compared with patients with discordant LV lead placement. Similar findings were also reported by Azizian and colleagues[85] in their study of 44 patients with NICM. Contemporary CRT with biventricular pacing in the right ventricle and coronary sinus allows limited operator discretion in the position of the LV lead, which is predominantly determined by the anatomy of the coronary sinus.[45] Nevertheless, most patients with LBBB have a septal to lateral delay in activation that can be assumed to be amenable to biventricular pacing. Using phase analysis of GMPS to assess the site of latest mechanical activation in patients with LBBB and either ICM or NICM, Lin and colleagues[94] showed that this assumption is more likely true in dilated cardiomyopathy patients with prolonged QRS greater than 150 ms rather than those with QRS 120 to 150 ms. This association was not observed in patients with ICM where the site of latest activation could be scar, irrespective of QRS duration.[94]

These findings support the localization of scar and the site of latest activation in a viable segment of the myocardium to guide optimal LV lead placement for CRT response.

The combined predictive value of these important determinants of CRT response was evaluated by our group in a population of CRT recipients.[86] Predictors of response to CRT were prospectively studied in a population of 44 patients with NYHA class II to IV heart failure (96% with LBBB), severely reduced LVEF, and a mean QRS duration of 178 ms. Using a novel single-injection protocol, GMPS images were acquired and dyssynchrony assessed before and immediately following biventricular pacing.[86] An algorithm incorporating the presence of dyssynchrony at baseline, scar burden of less than 40%, and concordance of the LV lead with the site of latest activation was used to predict response to CRT (**Fig. 3**). This algorithm predicted acute improvement in LV synchrony with 72% sensitivity, 93% specificity, 96% positive predictive value, and 96% negative predictive value for acute deterioration in synchrony (**Fig. 4**). Patients who had acute improvement or no change in LV synchrony following CRT had lower composite outcome of death, heart failure hospitalization, and ventricular arrhythmia compared with those who had acute deterioration (**Fig. 5**).[86]

These recent findings may explain the lack of symptomatic or functional improvement in a proportion of patients selected for CRT using clinical criteria alone. The contemporary knowledgebase suggests futility in attempts to predict CRT response using dyssynchrony parameters alone. Available literature strongly supports an in-depth assessment of several parameters (presence and pattern of dyssynchrony, location and extent of scar, site of latest activation) to identify myocardial substrate that is amenable to improvement after CRT.

Other Applications

Although the main application of LV dyssynchrony assessment by phase analysis of GMPS has been in heart failure patients receiving CRT, it has been also studied in other patient populations (**Table 2**). Phase analysis of GMPS has been applied to patients with NICM with narrow QRS and mildly decreased LVEF,[95] ICD,[96] end-stage renal disease (ESRD),[97,98] suspected or known coronary artery disease (CAD),[99,100] hypertension,[101] and Wolff-Parkinson-White syndrome.[102]

Goldberg and colleagues[95] evaluated the prognostic value of LV dyssynchrony assessment by phase analysis GMPS in 324 patients with NICM with mildly depressed LVEF (44 $\pm$ 5%) and narrow QRS 100 $\pm$ 17 ms who were followed for a mean of 4.6 years. They found that dyssynchrony measures (PSD and HBW) were independent predictors of all-cause mortality after adjusting for age, comorbidities, QRS, and LVEF and that PSD itself added incremental prognostic value.[95] Exploring the effect of dyssynchrony on outcomes in patients with ICD, Aljaroudi and colleagues[96] found higher PSD and HBW in patients who experienced death or appropriate ICD shock, and a cutoff value of greater than 50° for PSD predicted these outcomes. In a similar study by the same group, a phase HBW greater than or equal to 62° was associated with higher mortality in patients with ESRD, and LV dyssynchrony was an independent predictor of death.[97] These findings were supported by a larger study that included 828 patients with ESRD where patients with median PSD greater than or

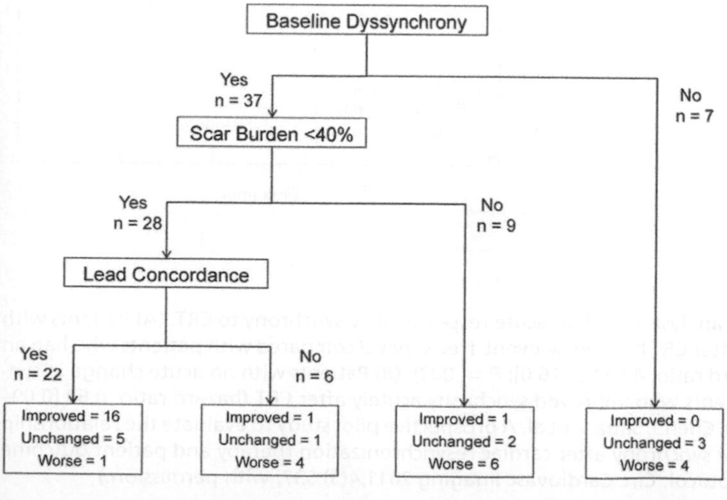

Fig. 3. The algorithm used by Friehling and colleagues for prediction of acute change in synchrony. (*Adapted from* Friehling M, Chen J, Saba S, et al. A prospective pilot study to evaluate the relationship between acute change in left ventricular synchrony after cardiac resynchronization therapy and patient outcome using a single-injection gated SPECT protocol. Circ Cardiovasc Imaging 2011;4(5):536; with permission.)

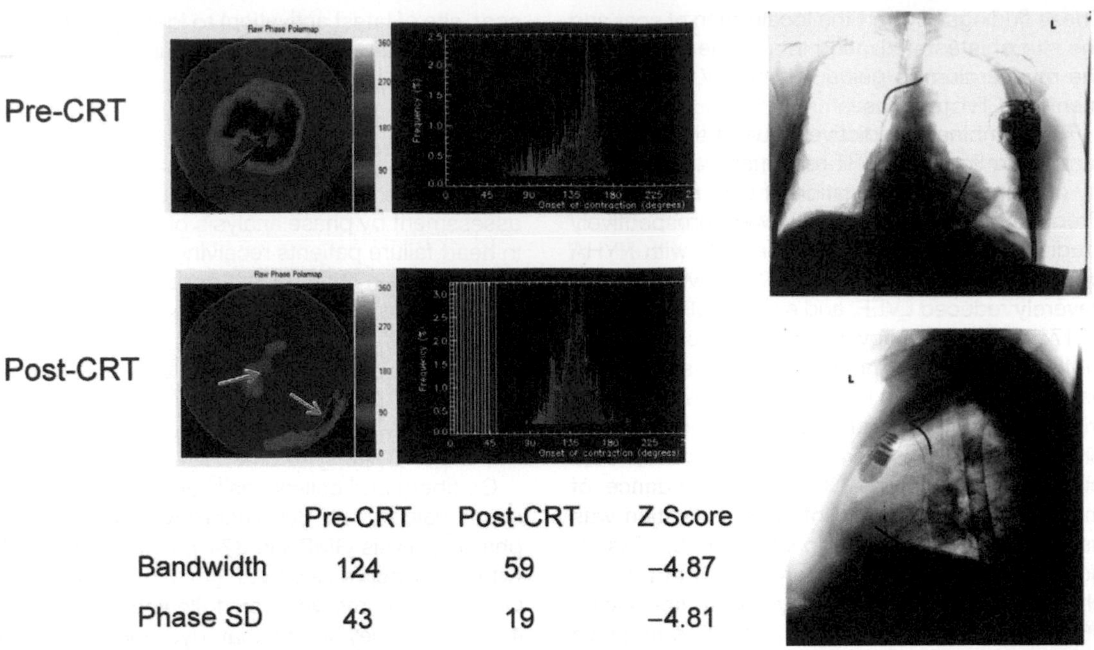

Fig. 4. Example of a patient with chronic right ventricular (RV) pacing and scar burden of less than 40% who was expected to have an improvement in synchrony after CRT based on the algorithm by Friehling and colleagues. The pre-CRT phase polarmap shows an early area of activation at the LV apex (*black arrow*); there is significant dyssynchrony, as evidenced by the wide histogram bandwidth and the large phase SD. Chest radiograph shows the LV lead positioned in the mid posterior wall, which is concordant with an area of delayed activation. This patient was expected to have an improvement in synchrony after CRT, based on our algorithm described in the text (also see **Fig. 3**). The post-CRT phase polarmap now shows two areas of early activation (*yellow arrows*) corresponding to LV (*lateral yellow arrow*) and RV (*apical yellow arrow*) activation wave fronts, and the histogram shows significant improvement in the bandwidth and PSD. (*Adapted from* Friehling M, Chen J, Saba S, et al. A prospective pilot study to evaluate the relationship between acute change in left ventricular synchrony after cardiac resynchronization therapy and patient outcome using a single-injection gated SPECT protocol. Circ Cardiovasc Imaging 2011;4(5):535; with permission.)

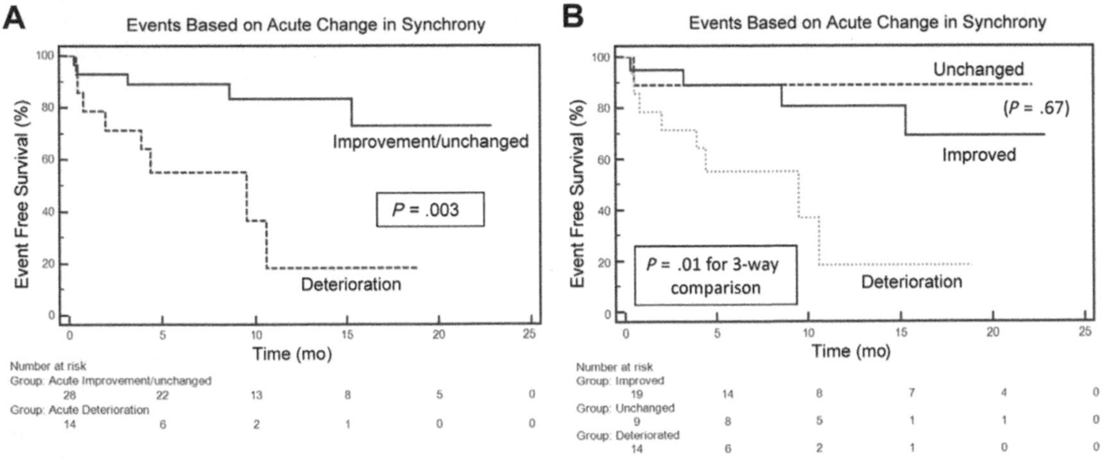

Fig. 5. Kaplan-Meier event-free survival analysis based on acute response of LV synchrony to CRT. (*A*) Patients with an acute deterioration in LV synchrony after CRT had worse event-free survival compared with patients who had an acute improvement or no change (hazard ratio, 4.6 [1.3–16.0]; $P = .003$). (*B*) Patients with no acute change in synchrony were similar in prognosis to patients who improved synchrony acutely after CRT (hazard ratio, 0.62 [0.09–4.4]; $P = .67$). (*Adapted from* Friehling M, Chen J, Saba S, et al. A prospective pilot study to evaluate the relationship between acute change in left ventricular synchrony after cardiac resynchronization therapy and patient outcome using a single-injection gated SPECT protocol. Circ Cardiovasc Imaging 2011;4(5):537; with permission.)

Table 2
Risk stratification application of LV dyssynchrony assessment by SPECT

Author (Ref)	Study Settings	Major Findings
Aggarwal et al,[98] 2014	828 patients with ESRD, LVEF 55 ± 0.4%, followed for 61 ± 0.9 mo	Patients with median PSD ≥21° or phase HBW >56° had worse 5-y survival LV dyssynchrony by phase analysis of gated SPECT MPI (mainly phase HBW >56°) provides prognostic value in ESRD beyond myocardial perfusion and LVEF
AlJaroudi et al,[97] 2010	144 patients with ESRD, LVEF 48 ± 12%, followed for 41 ± 28 mo	2-y mortality was higher in those with phase HBW ≥62° in the entire cohort, and in the subsets of patients with normal LVEF, coronary artery disease by angiography, QRS <110 ms, and perfusion defect size <20% of the LV LV dyssynchrony by phase analysis is a predictor of mortality in patients with ESRD
Aljaroudi et al,[96] 2010	70 patients with ICD, LVEF 26 ± 8%, QRS 135 ± 38 ms, LBBB 26%, followed for 1 y	PSD and HBW were higher in patients who experienced death or appropriate ICD shock PSD >50° predicted death or ICD shock
Goldberg et al,[95] 2014	324 patients with NICM, LVEF 44 ± 5%, QRS 100 ± 17 ms, followed for 1689 ± 843 d	PSD and HBW were independent predictors of all-cause mortality PSD added incremental prognostic value to a clinical model of age, DM, and other comorbidities
Hida et al,[99] 2012	278 patients with suspected or known CAD who underwent exercise stress-gated SPECT MPI and coronary angiography; Emory Cardiac Toolbox used	An increase in PSD of ≥4.4° and phase HBW of ≥14° after exercise detected patients with multivessel CAD with Sen of 74% and 68%, and Spec of 84% and 91%, respectively The addition of poststress increases in PSD and HBW to the conventional perfusion analysis parameters better identified multivessel CAD (Sen 77%, Spec 88%) compared with the conventional method alone (Sen 70%, Spec 76%)
Huang et al,[100] 2014	144 patients with suspected CAD who underwent dipyridamole stress/rest T1-201 gated SPECT MPI and coronary angiography; QGS Cedars-Sinai used	Patients with multivessel CAD had significantly more global dyssynchrony than the patients without ≥70% stenosis at stress, and more global and territorial dyssynchrony on stress images than on rest More patients with three-vessel CAD were correctly classified as multivessel disease when combining visual interpretation and dyssynchrony assessment
Ozdemir et al,[101] 2015	196 patients who underwent SPECT MPI for CAD with (63%) and without HTN; Emory Cardiac Toolbox used	PSD and phase HBW were significantly different between the patients with and without HTN Echocardiographic findings were significantly correlated with the result of the phase analysis
Chen et al,[102] 2012	45 patients with WPW who underwent SPECT MPI pre- and post-RFA; Emory Cardiac Toolbox used	LV dyssynchrony was most prominent in the patients with septal accessory pathways and RFA improved LV synchrony in these patients
Zafrir et al,[104] 2014	787 patients who underwent SPECT MPI, followed for 18.3 ± 6.2 mo; composite end point included cardiac death, new-onset or worsening heart failure, and life-threatening arrhythmias	PSD (for each 10° increment) was an independent predictor for cardiac mortality (hazard ratio, 1.2; 95% confidence interval, 1.01–1.45; $P = .04$)

Abbreviations: CAD, coronary artery disease; DM, diabetes mellitus; ESRD, end-stage renal disease; HTN, hypertension; MPI, myocardial perfusion imaging; RFA, radiofrequency catheter ablation; Sen, sensitivity; Spec, specificity; WPW, Wolff-Parkinson-White.

equal to 21° or phase HBW greater than 56° had worse 5-year survival and a phase HBW greater than 56° was found to have a prognostic value beyond myocardial perfusion and LVEF.[98]

Interesting attempts to evaluate the ability of phase analysis of GMPS to identify disease processes have been promising. Hida and colleagues[99] evaluated LV dyssynchrony using ECTb software in 278 patients with suspected or known CAD and found that an increase in PSD of greater than or equal to 4.4° and HBW of greater than or equal to 14° after exercise detected patients with multivessel CAD with approximately 70% sensitivity and approximately 90% specificity for both. The addition of poststress increases in dyssynchrony measures to the conventional perfusion analysis parameters improved the detection of multivessel CAD compared with the conventional method alone (77 vs 70% sensitivity and 88 vs 76% specificity, respectively).[99] Similar findings have been reported using the QGS software.[100]

SUMMARY AND FUTURE DIRECTIONS

Phase analysis of GMPS is a widely available and reproducible measure of LV dyssynchrony that also provides comprehensive assessment of LV function, global and regional scar burden, and patterns of LV mechanical activation. Preliminary studies indicate potential use in predicting CRT response and elucidation of mechanisms. In contemporary CRT, patients selected for the presence of a wide QRS LBBB are likely to have a septal to lateral wall activation delay, which is amenable to resynchronization by biventricular pacing. In these patients, imaging may be helpful in identifying scar and extensive LV remodeling, which may suggest lack of potential for functional improvement with CRT. Because advances in technology may expand capabilities for precise LV lead placement in the future, identification of specific patterns of dyssynchrony may have a critical role in guiding CRT.

REFERENCES

1. Nagueh SF. Mechanical dyssynchrony in congestive heart failure: diagnostic and therapeutic implications. J Am Coll Cardiol 2008;51(1):18–22.
2. Bax JJ, Abraham T, Barold SS, et al. Cardiac resynchronization therapy: Part 1–issues before device implantation. J Am Coll Cardiol 2005;46(12):2153–67.
3. Cazeau S, Ritter P, Bakdach S, et al. Four chamber pacing in dilated cardiomyopathy. Pacing Clin Electrophysiol 1994;17(11 Pt 2):1974–9.
4. Freemantle N, Tharmanathan P, Calvert MJ, et al. Cardiac resynchronisation for patients with heart failure due to left ventricular systolic dysfunction: a systematic review and meta-analysis. Eur J Heart Fail 2006;8(4):433–40.
5. Nelson GS, Curry CW, Wyman BT, et al. Predictors of systolic augmentation from left ventricular preexcitation in patients with dilated cardiomyopathy and intraventricular conduction delay. Circulation 2000;101(23):2703–9.
6. Leclercq C, Faris O, Tunin R, et al. Systolic improvement and mechanical resynchronization does not require electrical synchrony in the dilated failing heart with left bundle-branch block. Circulation 2002;106(14):1760–3.
7. Cazeau S, Leclercq C, Lavergne T, et al. Effects of multisite biventricular pacing in patients with heart failure and intraventricular conduction delay. N Engl J Med 2001;344(12):873–80.
8. Zhang Q, Yu CM. Clinical implication of mechanical dyssynchrony in heart failure. J Cardiovasc Ultrasound 2012;20(3):117–23.
9. Fauchier L, Marie O, Casset-Senon D, et al. Interventricular and intraventricular dyssynchrony in idiopathic dilated cardiomyopathy: a prognostic study with Fourier phase analysis of radionuclide angioscintigraphy. J Am Coll Cardiol 2002;40(11):2022–30.
10. Malhotra S, Pasupula D, Sharma R, et al. Left ventricular dyssynchrony predicts ventricular tachyarrhythmias in patients with severely reduced left ventricular systolic function. J Am Coll Cardiol 2013;61(10):E1003.
11. Hawkins NM, Petrie MC, MacDonald MR, et al. Selecting patients for cardiac resynchronization therapy: electrical or mechanical dyssynchrony? Eur Heart J 2006;27(11):1270–81.
12. Kwon BJ, Lee SH, Park CS, et al. Left ventricular diastolic dyssynchrony in patients with treatment-naive hypertension and the effects of antihypertensive therapy. J Hypertens 2015;33(2):354–65.
13. Yu CM, Zhang Q, Yip GW, et al. Diastolic and systolic asynchrony in patients with diastolic heart failure: a common but ignored condition. J Am Coll Cardiol 2007;49(1):97–105.
14. Uhley HN, Rivkin L. Peripheral distribution of the canine A-V conduction system; observations on gross morphology. Am J Cardiol 1960;5:688–91.
15. Spach MS, Barr RC. Ventricular intramural and epicardial potential distributions during ventricular activation and repolarization in the intact dog. Circ Res 1975;37(2):243–57.
16. Durrer D, van Dam RT, Freud GE, et al. Total excitation of the isolated human heart. Circulation 1970;41(6):899–912.
17. Helm RH, Spragg DD, Chakir K, et al. Pathobiology of left ventricular dyssynchrony and

resynchronization. In: Ellenbogen KA, Auricchio A, editors. Pacing to support the failing heart. Oxford: Wiley-Blackwell; 2009. p. 31–56.

18. Rosen BD, Fernandes VR, Nasir K, et al. Age, increased left ventricular mass, and lower regional myocardial perfusion are related to greater extent of myocardial dyssynchrony in asymptomatic individuals: the multi-ethnic study of atherosclerosis. Circulation 2009;120(10):859–66.
19. Vernooy K, Verbeek XA, Peschar M, et al. Left bundle branch block induces ventricular remodelling and functional septal hypoperfusion. Eur Heart J 2005;26(1):91–8.
20. Burkhoff D, Oikawa RY, Sagawa K. Influence of pacing site on canine left ventricular contraction. Am J Physiol 1986;251(2 Pt 2):H428–35.
21. Park RC, Little WC, O'Rourke RA. Effect of alteration of left ventricular activation sequence on the left ventricular end-systolic pressure-volume relation in closed-chest dogs. Circ Res 1985;57(5): 706–17.
22. Liu L, Tockman B, Girouard S, et al. Left ventricular resynchronization therapy in a canine model of left bundle branch block. Am J Physiol Heart Circ Physiol 2002;282(6):H2238–44.
23. Brecker SJ, Xiao HB, Sparrow J, et al. Effects of dual-chamber pacing with short atrioventricular delay in dilated cardiomyopathy. Lancet 1992; 340(8831):1308–12.
24. Aiba T, Hesketh GG, Barth AS, et al. Electrophysiological consequences of dyssynchronous heart failure and its restoration by resynchronization therapy. Circulation 2009;119(9):1220–30.
25. Chakir K, Daya SK, Tunin RS, et al. Reversal of global apoptosis and regional stress kinase activation by cardiac resynchronization. Circulation 2008; 117(11):1369–77.
26. Bader H, Garrigue S, Lafitte S, et al. Intra-left ventricular electromechanical asynchrony. A new independent predictor of severe cardiac events in heart failure patients. J Am Coll Cardiol 2004;43(2):248–56.
27. Lieberman R, Padeletti L, Schreuder J, et al. Ventricular pacing lead location alters systemic hemodynamics and left ventricular function in patients with and without reduced ejection fraction. J Am Coll Cardiol 2006;48(8):1634–41.
28. Cho GY, Song JK, Park WJ, et al. Mechanical dyssynchrony assessed by tissue Doppler imaging is a powerful predictor of mortality in congestive heart failure with normal QRS duration. J Am Coll Cardiol 2005;46(12):2237–43.
29. Fauchier L, Marie O, Casset-Senon D, et al. Ventricular dyssynchrony and risk markers of ventricular arrhythmias in nonischemic dilated cardiomyopathy: a study with phase analysis of angioscintigraphy. Pacing Clin Electrophysiol 2003; 26(1 Pt 2):352–6.
30. Nelson GS, Berger RD, Fetics BJ, et al. Left ventricular or biventricular pacing improves cardiac function at diminished energy cost in patients with dilated cardiomyopathy and left bundle-branch block. Circulation 2000;102(25):3053–9.
31. Ukkonen H, Beanlands RS, Burwash IG, et al. Effect of cardiac resynchronization on myocardial efficiency and regional oxidative metabolism. Circulation 2003;107(1):28–31.
32. Kyriacou A, Whinnett ZI, Sen S, et al. Improvement in coronary blood flow velocity with acute biventricular pacing is predominantly due to an increase in a diastolic backward-travelling decompression (suction) wave. Circulation 2012;126(11):1334–44.
33. van Bommel RJ, Marsan NA, Delgado V, et al. Cardiac resynchronization therapy as a therapeutic option in patients with moderate-severe functional mitral regurgitation and high operative risk. Circulation 2011;124(8):912–9.
34. Sutton MG, Plappert T, Hilpisch KE, et al. Sustained reverse left ventricular structural remodeling with cardiac resynchronization at one year is a function of etiology: quantitative Doppler echocardiographic evidence from the Multicenter InSync Randomized Clinical Evaluation (MIRACLE). Circulation 2006;113(2):266–72.
35. Bristow MR, Saxon LA, Boehmer J, et al. Cardiac-resynchronization therapy with or without an implantable defibrillator in advanced chronic heart failure. N Engl J Med 2004;350(21):2140–50.
36. Cleland JGF, Daubert JC, Erdmann E, et al, For the Cardiac Resynchronization-Heart Failure (Care-HF) Study Investigators. The effect of cardiac resynchronization on morbidity and mortality in heart failure. N Engl J Med 2005;352(15):1539–49.
37. Gorcsan J III, Oyenuga O, Habib PJ, et al. Relationship of echocardiographic dyssynchrony to long-term survival after cardiac resynchronization therapy. Circulation 2010;122(19):1910–8.
38. Chalil S, Stegemann B, Muhyaldeen S, et al. Intraventricular dyssynchrony predicts mortality and morbidity after cardiac resynchronization therapy: a study using cardiovascular magnetic resonance tissue synchronization imaging. J Am Coll Cardiol 2007;50(3):243–52.
39. Auger D, Bleeker GB, Bertini M, et al. Effect of cardiac resynchronization therapy in patients without left intraventricular dyssynchrony. Eur Heart J 2012;33(7):913–20.
40. Epstein AE, DiMarco JP, Ellenbogen KA, et al. ACC/AHA/HRS 2008 guidelines for device-based therapy of cardiac rhythm abnormalities: a report of the American College of Cardiology/American Heart Association Task Force on Practice Guidelines (Writing Committee to Revise the ACC/AHA/NASPE 2002 guideline update for implantation of cardiac pacemakers and antiarrhythmia devices)

developed in collaboration with the American Association for Thoracic Surgery and Society of Thoracic Surgeons. J Am Coll Cardiol 2008; 51(21):e1–62.
41. Tang AS, Wells GA, Talajic M, et al. Cardiac-resynchronization therapy for mild-to-moderate heart failure. N Engl J Med 2010;363(25):2385–95.
42. Moss AJ, Hall WJ, Cannom DS, et al. Cardiac-resynchronization therapy for the prevention of heart-failure events. N Engl J Med 2009;361(14): 1329–38.
43. Linde C, Abraham WT, Gold MR, et al. Randomized trial of cardiac resynchronization in mildly symptomatic heart failure patients and in asymptomatic patients with left ventricular dysfunction and previous heart failure symptoms. J Am Coll Cardiol 2008;52(23):1834–43.
44. Adabag S, Roukoz H, Anand IS, et al. Cardiac resynchronization therapy in patients with minimal heart failure: a systematic review and meta-analysis. J Am Coll Cardiol 2011;58(9):935–41.
45. Tracy CM, Epstein AE, Darbar D, et al. 2012 ACCF/AHA/HRS focused update of the 2008 guidelines for device-based therapy of cardiac rhythm abnormalities: a report of the American College of Cardiology Foundation/American Heart Association Task Force on Practice Guidelines. J Am Coll Cardiol 2012;60(14):1297–313.
46. Palmisano P, Accogli M, Zaccaria M, et al. Rate, causes, and impact on patient outcome of implantable device complications requiring surgical revision: large population survey from two centres in Italy. Europace 2013;15(4):531–40.
47. Nichol G, Kaul P, Huszti E, et al. Cost-effectiveness of cardiac resynchronization therapy in patients with symptomatic heart failure. Ann Intern Med 2004;141(5):343–51.
48. Yu CM, Hayes DL. Cardiac resynchronization therapy: state of the art 2013. Eur Heart J 2013;34(19): 1396–403.
49. Zareba W, Klein H, Cygankiewicz I, et al. Effectiveness of cardiac resynchronization therapy by QRS morphology in the multicenter automatic defibrillator implantation trial-cardiac resynchronization therapy (MADIT-CRT). Circulation 2011;123(10): 1061–72.
50. Yu CM, Bleeker GB, Fung JW, et al. Left ventricular reverse remodeling but not clinical improvement predicts long-term survival after cardiac resynchronization therapy. Circulation 2005;112(11):1580–6.
51. Mollema SA, Bleeker GB, van der Wall EE, et al. Usefulness of QRS duration to predict response to cardiac resynchronization therapy in patients with end-stage heart failure. Am J Cardiol 2007; 100(11):1665–70.
52. Yu CM, Gorcsan J III, Bleeker GB, et al. Usefulness of tissue Doppler velocity and strain dyssynchrony for predicting left ventricular reverse remodeling response after cardiac resynchronization therapy. Am J Cardiol 2007;100(8):1263–70.
53. Pitzalis MV, Iacoviello M, Romito R, et al. Cardiac resynchronization therapy tailored by echocardiographic evaluation of ventricular asynchrony. J Am Coll Cardiol 2002;40(9):1615–22.
54. Suffoletto MS, Dohi K, Cannesson M, et al. Novel speckle-tracking radial strain from routine black-and-white echocardiographic images to quantify dyssynchrony and predict response to cardiac resynchronization therapy. Circulation 2006;113(7):960–8.
55. Kapetanakis S, Bhan A, Murgatroyd F, et al. Real-time 3D echo in patient selection for cardiac resynchronization therapy. JACC Cardiovasc Imaging 2011;4(1):16–26.
56. Chung ES, Leon AR, Tavazzi L, et al. Results of the predictors of response to CRT (PROSPECT) trial. Circulation 2008;117(20):2608–16.
57. Ruschitzka F, Abraham WT, Singh JP, et al. Cardiac-resynchronization therapy in heart failure with a narrow QRS complex. N Engl J Med 2013; 369(15):1395–405.
58. Adelstein EC, Tanaka H, Soman P, et al. Impact of scar burden by single-photon emission computed tomography myocardial perfusion imaging on patient outcomes following cardiac resynchronization therapy. Eur Heart J 2011;32(1):93–103.
59. Daya HA, Alam MB, Adelstein E, et al. Echocardiography-guided left ventricular lead placement for cardiac resynchronization therapy in ischemic vs nonischemic cardiomyopathy patients. Heart Rhythm 2014;11(4):614–9.
60. Boogers MJ, Chen J, van Bommel RJ, et al. Optimal left ventricular lead position assessed with phase analysis on gated myocardial perfusion SPECT. Eur J Nucl Med Mol Imaging 2011;38(2): 230–8.
61. White JA, Yee R, Yuan X, et al. Delayed enhancement magnetic resonance imaging predicts response to cardiac resynchronization therapy in patients with intraventricular dyssynchrony. J Am Coll Cardiol 2006;48(10):1953–60.
62. Bilchick KC, Dimaano V, Wu KC, et al. Cardiac magnetic resonance assessment of dyssynchrony and myocardial scar predicts function class improvement following cardiac resynchronization therapy. JACC Cardiovasc Imaging 2008;1(5): 561–8.
63. Marsan NA, Westenberg JJ, Ypenburg C, et al. Magnetic resonance imaging and response to cardiac resynchronization therapy: relative merits of left ventricular dyssynchrony and scar tissue. Eur Heart J 2009;30(19):2360–7.
64. Taylor AJ, Elsik M, Broughton A, et al. Combined dyssynchrony and scar imaging with cardiac

magnetic resonance imaging predicts clinical response and long-term prognosis following cardiac resynchronization therapy. Europace 2010; 12(5):708–13.

65. Bilchick KC, Kuruvilla S, Hamirani YS, et al. Impact of mechanical activation, scar, and electrical timing on cardiac resynchronization therapy response and clinical outcomes. J Am Coll Cardiol 2014; 63(16):1657–66.
66. Lardo AC, Abraham TP, Kass DA. Magnetic resonance imaging assessment of ventricular dyssynchrony: current and emerging concepts. J Am Coll Cardiol 2005;46(12):2223–8.
67. Chen J, Boogers MJ, Bax JJ, et al. The use of nuclear imaging for cardiac resynchronization therapy. Curr Cardiol Rep 2010;12(2):185–91.
68. Toussaint JF, Lavergne T, Kerrou K, et al. Basal asynchrony and resynchronization with biventricular pacing predict long-term improvement of LV function in heart failure patients. Pacing Clin Electrophysiol 2003;26(9):1815–23.
69. Lishmanov Y, Minin S, Efimova I, et al. The possible role of nuclear imaging in assessment of the cardiac resynchronization therapy effectiveness in patients with moderate heart failure. Ann Nucl Med 2013;27(4):378–85.
70. Galt JR, Garcia EV, Robbins WL. Effects of myocardial wall thickness on SPECT quantification. IEEE Trans Med Imaging 1990;9(2):144–50.
71. Soman P, Chen J. Left ventricular dyssynchrony assessment using myocardial single-photon emission CT. Semin Nucl Med 2014;44(4):314–9.
72. Boogers MM, Van Kriekinge SD, Henneman MM, et al. Quantitative gated SPECT-derived phase analysis on gated myocardial perfusion SPECT detects left ventricular dyssynchrony and predicts response to cardiac resynchronization therapy. J Nucl Med 2009;50(5):718–25.
73. Chen J, Garcia EV, Folks RD, et al. Onset of left ventricular mechanical contraction as determined by phase analysis of ECG-gated myocardial perfusion SPECT imaging: development of a diagnostic tool for assessment of cardiac mechanical dyssynchrony. J Nucl Cardiol 2005; 12(6):687–95.
74. Van Kriekinge SD, Nishina H, Ohba M, et al. Automatic global and regional phase analysis from gated myocardial perfusion SPECT imaging: application to the characterization of ventricular contraction in patients with left bundle branch block. J Nucl Med 2008;49(11):1790–7.
75. Henneman MM, Chen J, Ypenburg C, et al. Phase analysis of gated myocardial perfusion single-photon emission computed tomography compared with tissue Doppler imaging for the assessment of left ventricular dyssynchrony. J Am Coll Cardiol 2007;49(16):1708–14.
76. Hsu TH, Huang WS, Chen CC, et al. Left ventricular systolic and diastolic dyssynchrony assessed by phase analysis of gated SPECT myocardial perfusion imaging: a comparison with speckle tracking echocardiography. Ann Nucl Med 2013;27(8): 764–71.
77. Marsan NA, Henneman MM, Chen J, et al. Real-time three-dimensional echocardiography as a novel approach to quantify left ventricular dyssynchrony: a comparison study with phase analysis of gated myocardial perfusion single photon emission computed tomography. J Am Soc Echocardiogr 2008;21(7):801–7.
78. Marsan NA, Henneman MM, Chen J, et al. Left ventricular dyssynchrony assessed by two three-dimensional imaging modalities: phase analysis of gated myocardial perfusion SPECT and tri-plane tissue Doppler imaging. Eur J Nucl Med Mol Imaging 2008;35(1):166–73.
79. Henneman MM, Chen J, bbets-Schneider P, et al. Can LV dyssynchrony as assessed with phase analysis on gated myocardial perfusion SPECT predict response to CRT? J Nucl Med 2007;48(7):1104–11.
80. Rastgou F, Shojaeifard M, Amin A, et al. Assessment of left ventricular mechanical dyssynchrony by phase analysis of gated-SPECT myocardial perfusion imaging and tissue Doppler imaging: comparison between QGS and ECTb software packages. J Nucl Cardiol 2014;21(6):1062–71.
81. Lin X, Xu H, Zhao X, et al. Repeatability of left ventricular dyssynchrony and function parameters in serial gated myocardial perfusion SPECT studies. J Nucl Cardiol 2010;17(5):811–6.
82. Trimble MA, Velazquez EJ, Adams GL, et al. Repeatability and reproducibility of phase analysis of gated single-photon emission computed tomography myocardial perfusion imaging used to quantify cardiac dyssynchrony. Nucl Med Commun 2008;29(4):374–81.
83. Kiso K, Imoto A, Nishimura Y, et al. Novel algorithm for quantitative assessment of left ventricular dyssynchrony with ECG-gated myocardial perfusion SPECT: useful technique for management of cardiac resynchronization therapy. Ann Nucl Med 2011;25(10):768–76.
84. Mukherjee A, Patel CD, Naik N, et al. Quantitative assessment of cardiac mechanical dyssynchrony and prediction of response to cardiac resynchronization therapy in patients with nonischaemic dilated cardiomyopathy using gated myocardial perfusion SPECT. Nucl Med Commun 2015;36(5): 494–501.
85. Azizian N, Rastgou F, Ghaedian T, et al. LV dyssynchrony assessed with phase analysis on gated myocardial perfusion SPECT can predict response to CRT in patients with end-stage heart failure. Res Cardiovasc Med 2014;3(4):e20720.

86. Friehling M, Chen J, Saba S, et al. A prospective pilot study to evaluate the relationship between acute change in left ventricular synchrony after cardiac resynchronization therapy and patient outcome using a single-injection gated SPECT protocol. Circ Cardiovasc Imaging 2011;4(5):532–9.
87. Nakamura K, Takami M, Shimabukuro M, et al. Effective prediction of response to cardiac resynchronization therapy using a novel program of gated myocardial perfusion single photon emission computed tomography. Europace 2011;13(12):1731–7.
88. Lalonde M, Wells RG, Birnie D, et al. Development and optimization of SPECT gated blood pool cluster analysis for the prediction of CRT outcome. Med Phys 2014;41(7):072506.
89. Adelstein EC, Saba S. Scar burden by myocardial perfusion imaging predicts echocardiographic response to cardiac resynchronization therapy in ischemic cardiomyopathy. Am Heart J 2007;153(1):105–12.
90. Ypenburg C, Schalij MJ, Bleeker GB, et al. Impact of viability and scar tissue on response to cardiac resynchronization therapy in ischaemic heart failure patients. Eur Heart J 2007;28(1):33–41.
91. Xu YZ, Cha YM, Feng D, et al. Impact of myocardial scarring on outcomes of cardiac resynchronization therapy: extent or location? J Nucl Med 2012;53(1):47–54.
92. Saba S, Marek J, Schwartzman D, et al. Echocardiography-guided left ventricular lead placement for cardiac resynchronization therapy: results of the speckle tracking assisted resynchronization therapy for electrode region trial. Circ Heart Fail 2013;6(3):427–34.
93. Hung GU, Huang JL, Lin WY, et al. Impact of right-ventricular apical pacing on the optimal left-ventricular lead positions measured by phase analysis of SPECT myocardial perfusion imaging. Eur J Nucl Med Mol Imaging 2014;41(6):1224–31.
94. Lin X, Xu H, Zhao X, et al. Sites of latest mechanical activation as assessed by SPECT myocardial perfusion imaging in ischemic and dilated cardiomyopathy patients with LBBB. Eur J Nucl Med Mol Imaging 2014;41(6):1232–9.
95. Goldberg AS, Alraies MC, Cerqueira MD, et al. Prognostic value of left ventricular mechanical dyssynchrony by phase analysis in patients with non-ischemic cardiomyopathy with ejection fraction 35-50% and QRS <150 ms. J Nucl Cardiol 2014;21(1):57–66.
96. Aljaroudi WA, Hage FG, Hermann D, et al. Relation of left-ventricular dyssynchrony by phase analysis of gated SPECT images and cardiovascular events in patients with implantable cardiac defibrillators. J Nucl Cardiol 2010;17(3):398–404.
97. AlJaroudi W, Aggarwal H, Venkataraman R, et al. Impact of left ventricular dyssynchrony by phase analysis on cardiovascular outcomes in patients with end-stage renal disease. J Nucl Cardiol 2010;17(6):1058–64.
98. Aggarwal H, AlJaroudi WA, Mehta S, et al. The prognostic value of left ventricular mechanical dyssynchrony using gated myocardial perfusion imaging in patients with end-stage renal disease. J Nucl Cardiol 2014;21(4):739–46.
99. Hida S, Chikamori T, Tanaka H, et al. Diagnostic value of left ventricular dyssynchrony after exercise and at rest in the detection of multivessel coronary artery disease on single-photon emission computed tomography. Circ J 2012;76(8):1942–52.
100. Huang WS, Huang CH, Lee CL, et al. Relation of early post-stress left ventricular dyssynchrony and the extent of angiographic coronary artery disease. J Nucl Cardiol 2014;21(6):1048–56.
101. Ozdemir S, Kirilmaz B, Barutcu A, et al. The evaluation of left ventricular dyssynchronization in patients with hypertension by phase analysis of myocardial perfusion-gated SPECT. Ann Nucl Med 2015;29(3):240–7.
102. Chen C, Li D, Miao C, et al. LV dyssynchrony as assessed by phase analysis of gated SPECT myocardial perfusion imaging in patients with Wolff-Parkinson-White syndrome. Eur J Nucl Med Mol Imaging 2012;39(7):1191–8.
103. Lalonde M, Birnie D, Ruddy TD, et al. SPECT gated blood pool phase analysis of lateral wall motion for prediction of CRT response. Int J Cardiovasc Imaging 2014;30(3):559–69.
104. Zafrir N, Nevzorov R, Bental T, et al. Prognostic value of left ventricular dyssynchrony by myocardial perfusion-gated SPECT in patients with normal and abnormal left ventricular functions. J Nucl Cardiol 2014;21(3):532–40.

Radionuclide Imaging in Congestive Heart Failure

Assessment of Viability, Sarcoidosis, and Amyloidosis

John P. Bois, MD, Panithaya Chareonthaitawee, MD*

KEYWORDS

- Amyloidosis • Cardiac imaging • Radionuclide • Sarcoidosis • Viability

KEY POINTS

- ^{18}F-fluorodeoxyglucose (^{18}F-FDG) PET has the highest sensitivity for detection of myocardial viability.
- Viability assessment helps to guide clinical decision making in patients with moderate-to-severe ischemic cardiomyopathy but its exact role and impact on revascularization outcomes remain uncertain.
- Cardiac PET with ^{18}F-FDG and myocardial "perfusion" imaging has tremendous diagnostic and prognostic potential for cardiac sarcoidosis.
- 99m-Technetium pyrophosphate and 3,3-diphosphono-1,2-propanodicarboxylic acid demonstrate preferential transthyretin-related amyloidosis (ATTR) uptake and may be helpful in distinguishing between ATTR and amyloid light-chain amyloidosis.

INTRODUCTION

The diverse etiologies of myocardial diseases pose diagnostic and therapeutic challenges in patients with congestive heart failure. In specific cardiomyopathies, such as sarcoidosis and amyloidosis, precise identification of the underlying etiology is paramount to treatment choice and outcome. In other situations, such as moderate-to-severe ischemic cardiomyopathy, myocardial viability assessment has important implications for revascularization (**Box 1**). The need for precise identification of these entities has led to intense efforts to develop and refine radionuclide imaging techniques for their assessment. The current review outlines the pathophysiology of each entity, highlights the associated clinical challenges, describes established and emerging radionuclide imaging techniques, and compares them with nonradionuclide imaging modalities.

ASSESSMENT OF MYOCARDIAL VIABILITY IN ISCHEMIC CARDIOMYOPATHY

Despite therapeutic advances, the high morbidity and mortality of ischemic cardiomyopathy persist.[1] At the same time, potential revascularization benefits on survival, functional status, and myocardial contraction must be weighed against the greater periprocedural risks and possible lack of benefit in these patients. Past studies have demonstrated better outcomes with revascularization in patients with versus without viability by noninvasive imaging,[1] but recent trials have not confirmed these prior observations. Although controversy lingers

Disclosures: The authors have nothing to disclose.
Division of Cardiovascular Diseases, Mayo Clinic, 200 First Street Southwest, Rochester, MN 55905, USA
* Corresponding author.
E-mail address: Chareonthaitawee.Panithaya@mayo.edu

Cardiol Clin 34 (2016) 119–132
http://dx.doi.org/10.1016/j.ccl.2015.07.014

Box 1
Myocardial viability assessment

- Fluorine-18 deoxyglucose PET has the highest sensitivity for detection of myocardial viability.
- Each imaging modality has inherent strengths and weaknesses.
- Viability assessment helps to guide clinical decision making in patients with moderate-to-severe ischemic cardiomyopathy, but its exact role and impact on revascularization outcomes remain uncertain.

on the role of noninvasive viability testing, the pathophysiology of dysfunctional but viable myocardium and the available techniques for its assessment are discussed herein.

Pathophysiology of Dysfunctional but Viable Myocardium

Both hibernating and stunned myocardium exhibit reversible contractile dysfunction and have distinct pathophysiologic definitions. In hibernation, chronically reduced myocardial blood flow leads to adaptive or protective left ventricular (LV) systolic dysfunction, which may improve with revascularization. In myocardial stunning, the pathophysiologic mechanism is the temporary impediment of coronary blood flow that leads to transient contractile dysfunction, which may persist for hours to months even after restoration of flow.[1] Although these 2 entities have distinct pathophysiologic and histologic definitions, in the clinical setting, they may represent the same pathophysiologic process, and may be indistinguishable. Their potential improvement in function with revascularization underscores the role of noninvasive imaging to differentiate between viable myocardium and scar.

Single Photon Emission Computed Tomography

The most common single photon emission computed tomography (SPECT) tracers for viability assessment are thallium-201 (^{201}Tl)[2] and technetium-99m (^{99m}Tc)-based agents.[3] Viability assessment with ^{201}Tl relies on an electromechanical gradient across the intact (viable) cell membrane,[4,5] and on redistribution, whereby ^{201}Tl uptake is initially high in normal myocytes but decreases rapidly within hours as ^{201}Tl returns to the blood pool and becomes available for hibernating/ischemic segments. Two main ^{201}Tl protocols are used for viability: rest–redistribution and stress–redistribution. The definition of viability by ^{201}Tl requires at least 1 of the following: (1) 50% or greater radioactivity in the hypocontractile segments relative to the maximal radioactivity (usually in a normally contracting area), and/or (2) an increase in the relative radioactivity between the initial and redistribution images of at least 1 grade on a standard 5-point semiquantitative visual scale. The ^{201}Tl rest–redistribution protocol has greater sensitivity than the stress–redistribution protocol for predicting contractile recovery after revascularization, but specificity is low (**Fig. 1**, **Table 1**). Over the past decade, use of ^{201}Tl for viability assessment has decreased, likely related to the lower specificity, higher patient radiation exposure (approximately 20–30 mSV), longer duration of the complete study, and lower image quality, especially in patients with a larger body habitus.

Similar to ^{201}Tl, myocardial cellular uptake and retention of ^{99m}Tc requires maintenance of an electrochemical gradient across the cell membrane.[13] Two main ^{99m}Tc viability protocols have been developed: the rest with nitrate enhancement and the rest–stress protocols. Sensitivity of ^{99m}Tc to identify contractile recovery after revascularization is less than that of other noninvasive techniques (see **Fig. 1**, **Table 1**), but specificity is higher than that of ^{201}Tl. Similar to ^{201}Tl, ^{99m}Tc use for viability assessment has also been declining, likely related to similar reasons as for ^{201}Tl, although the radiation exposure associated with ^{99m}Tc is less. Major advantages and disadvantages of SPECT are listed in **Table 1**.

PET

Positron Emission Tomography (PET) with the glucose analog, ^{18}F-fluorodeoxyglucose (^{18}F-FDG), has traditionally been considered the gold standard for the identification of viable myocardium. Viability assessment with ^{18}F-FDG depends on the shift in substrate metabolism from free fatty acids, when flow is normal, to the use of glucose, when oxygen supply is compromised by reduced flow. Ischemic and hibernating cells, therefore, demonstrate relatively increased ^{18}F-FDG uptake compared with scar tissue, and to normal myocytes. ^{18}F-FDG PET viability imaging requires concomitant myocardial perfusion imaging, usually with either ^{13}N-ammonia, or rubidium-82 (^{82}Rb). Proper patient preparation is crucial to diagnostic ^{18}F-FDG image quality, and usually requires a combination of insulin and glucose administration to decrease free fatty acid levels and maximize myocardial ^{18}F-FDG uptake.[14]

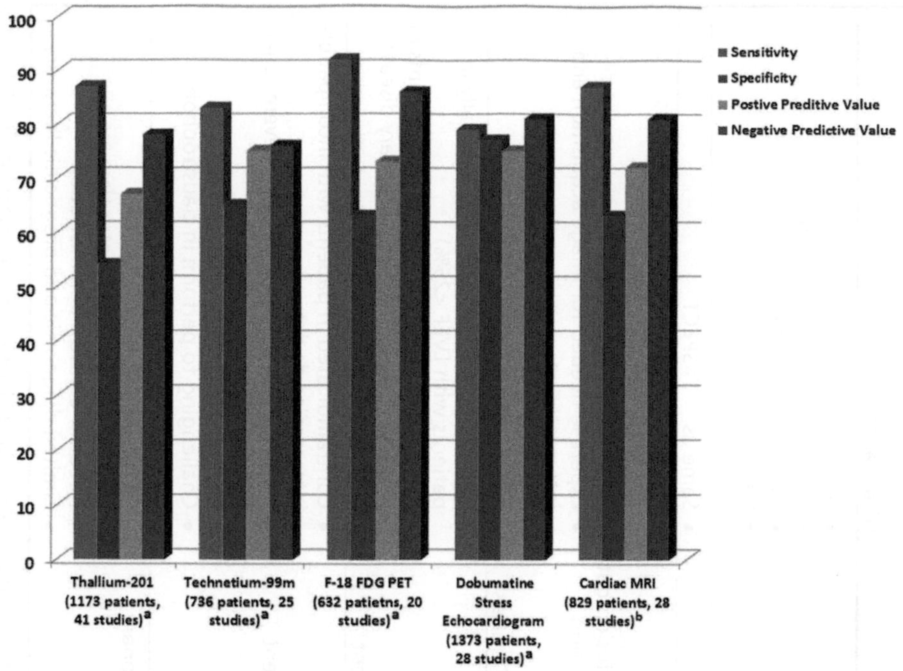

Fig. 1. Sensitivity, specificity, negative predictive value, and positive predictive value for detecting myocardial viability. Pooled, unweighted analysis of 5 imaging modalities that assess for cardiac viability as defined as improvement of regional contractility after revascularization. Note that ^{18}F-FDG PET has highest sensitivity and negative predictive value. Additional studies (see Refs.[6–9]) were included If they were prospective, patients were revascularized, and data were provided that allowed calculation of sensitivity, specificity, positive predictive value, and negative predictive value. ^{18}F-FDG, fluorine-18 deoxyglucose. [a] Studies identified by prior metaanalysis by Ref.[10] [b] Studies identified by a prior 2012 metaanalysis by Ref.[11]

Patterns of resting perfusion, metabolism, and contractile function and their interpretation are shown in **Table 2**. Among the patterns, the classical PET mismatch of decreased perfusion with preserved or enhanced ^{18}F-FDG uptake consistent with hibernating myocardium has the highest likelihood of contractile recovery after revascularization (**Fig. 2**). Other approaches to image analysis include (1) 50% or greater radioactivity in the hypocontractile segments relative to the radioactivity in a normally contracting segment, and (2) absolute glucose utilization, which requires dynamic imaging and kinetic modeling. These additional approaches have relatively high sensitivity but low specificity for contractile recovery after revascularization.

The limitations of PET viability assessment are listed in **Table 1**. Lack of protocol standardization and variability in PET viability definition[15] may, in part, explain the variable sensitivity (71%–100%) and specificity (33%–91%) of PET for contractile recovery after revascularization. Limitations withstanding, a pooled analysis of 20 studies including 632 patients undergoing PET viability assessment, demonstrated a sensitivity of 92%, specificity of 63%, positive predicative value of 73%, and negative predictive value of 86% for determination of regional contractile recovery after revascularization (see **Fig. 1**).

Comparison with Nonradionuclide Imaging Modalities for Viability Assessment

Low-dose dobutamine echocardiography (LDDE) identifies dysfunctional but viable myocardium by the biphasic response, the initial contractile improvement with subsequent deterioration during increasing doses of dobutamine infusion from 5 to 10 μg/kg/min (see **Fig. 1**, **Table 1**). A nonweighted assessment of 1373 patients in 28 studies report a lower sensitivity (79%) and higher specificity (77%), compared with PET (see **Table 1**), for predicting regional contractile recovery after revascularization. The advantages and disadvantages of LDDE for viability assessment are listed in **Table 1**.

Cardiac MRI (cMRI) may be used to assess viability with either dobutamine stress, similar to LDDE, delayed contrast enhancement, or measurement of LV end-diastolic wall thickness (<5.5 mm). In 28 studies of 829 patients who had at least 1 of these approaches, sensitivity (87%) of cMRI was slightly lower than that of PET

Table 1
Comparison of imaging modalities to assess myocardial viability

Imaging Modality	Sensitivity (%), Specificity (%), PPV (%), NPV (%)	Radiation Dose (mSv)[a]	Advantages	Disadvantages
^{201}Tl SPECT	87, 54, 67, 78	22.0–31.4[12,b]	• Widely accessible • Ease of patient preparation • Perfusion data • Standardized protocols • High sensitivity	• Low specificity • Limited anatomic information • Attenuation artifacts • Radiation exposure
^{99m}Tc SPECT	83, 65, 75, 76	11.3[12]	• Same as ^{201}Tl SPECT	• Same as ^{201}Tl SPECT
^{18}F-FDG PET/CT	92, 63, 73, 86	7.0[12]	• Highest sensitivity • High NPV • Concomitant metabolic and perfusion data • High spatial and temporal resolution • Robust attenuation correction • Lower radiation exposure • Increasing access to PET and PET tracers	• Complex patient preparation • Higher cost • Less standardized protocols • Expertise needed for image acquisition and interpretation
DSE echocardiography	79, 77, 75, 81	NA	• Widely accessible • Versatile • High temporal resolution • No radiation exposure • Comprehensive cardiac assessment	• High interobserver variability (especially in patients with LVEF <25%) • Limited acoustic windows in obese patients or patients with obstructive pulmonary disease
Cardiac MRI	87, 63, 72, 81	NA	• High spatial resolution • No radiation exposure • Simultaneous anatomic assessment	• Contraindicated in patients with incompatible intracardiac device • Contraindicated in patients with severe renal failure • Not widely accessible • Challenging to perform in claustrophobic patients
Cardiac CT	Studies needed	13–21.4[12,c]	• Simultaneous assessment of coronary anatomy	• Increased radiation exposure • Limited standardized protocols • Need for contrast administration • Limited diagnostic and prognostic literature

Abbreviations: ^{18}F-FDG, fluorine-18 deoxyglucose; ^{99m}Tc, technetium-99m; ^{201}Tl, thallium-201; CT, computed tomography; DSE, dobutamine stress echocardiography; LVEF, left ventricular ejection fraction; mSv, milliSieverts; NA, not applicable; NPV, negative predictive value; PPV, positive predictive value; SPECT, single-photon emission tomography.

[a] Effective dose.

[b] ^{201}Tl stress-redistribution 22.0 mSv, ^{201}Tl stress-reinjection 31.4 mSv.

[c] Reflects 64 slice CT coronary angiogram, coronary artery calcium score only reported as 1.3 to 1.7 mSv.

Table 2
Positron emission tomography (PET) perfusion patterns in viability assessment

Myocardial State	Resting Perfusion	Resting Metabolism	Contractile Function
Normal myocardium	Normal	Normal	Normal
Stunned myocardium	Normal	Normal or mildly reduced	Reduced
Hibernating myocardium	Reduced	Normal or increased	Reduced
Partially viable myocardium	Reduced	Mildly to moderately reduced	Reduced
Scar/nonviable myocardium	Severely reduced to absent	Severely reduced to absent	Reduced

but higher than other techniques, and specificity (63%) was similar between the 2 techniques (see **Fig. 1**). Furthermore, lack of hyperenhancement (representing scar) on cMRI correlated with LV ejection fraction improvement after revascularization.[16] In a prospective analysis of 144 ischemic cardiomyopathy patients undergoing cMRI, the presence of dysfunctional viable myocardium by cMRI delayed enhancement was an independent predictor of mortality in those without revascularization.[17] The advantages and disadvantages of cMRI for viability assessment are listed in **Table 1**.

Delayed hyperenhancement multidetector computed tomography (DE-MDCT) may reflect viability when demonstrating areas of absent or limited hyperenhancement. Initial comparison of DE-MDCT with SPECT and LDDE report an agreement of 87.8% and 92.2%, respectively.[18] Further evaluation by Koyama and colleagues[19] demonstrated that DE-MDCT holds promise in predicting contractile recovery after revascularization. Potential advantages of DE-MDCT include the ability to evaluate both coronary anatomy and viability in a single session, although the former may be less useful in this patient population with probable severe obstructive coronary artery disease, coronary calcification, and prior revascularization. Disadvantages of DE-MDCT are listed in **Table 1**.

Hybrid Imaging

The majority of current PET systems are hybrid PET/computed tomography scanners, whose main advantage compared with PET-only systems is faster throughput owing to the more rapid computed tomography transmission acquisition (30 seconds vs up to 15 minutes for PET-only

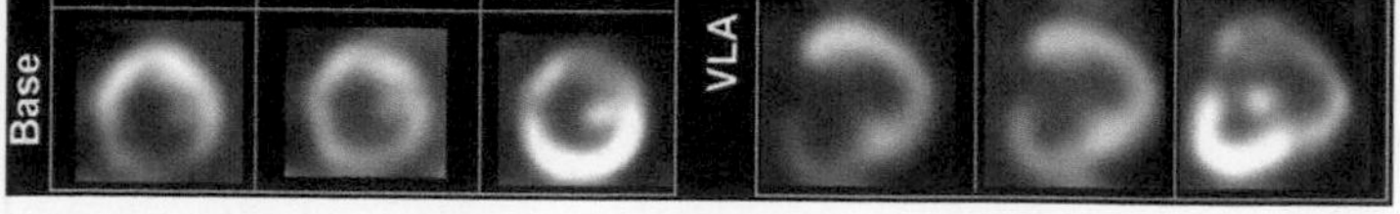

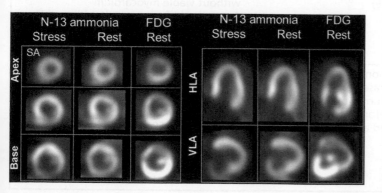

Fig. 2. ^{13}N-ammonia ^{18}F-fluorodeoxyglucose (^{18}F-FDG) PET viability study. Standard reconstructed views of rest–stress ^{13}N ammonia and resting ^{18}F-FDG PET images in a 58-year-old woman with recent cardiac arrest and multivessel coronary artery disease with 100% occlusion of the right coronary artery with collaterals. Initial echocardiogram demonstrated severe left ventricular (LV) enlargement with an ejection fraction of 20% but subsequent LV ejection fraction by echocardiogram was 29% and later by gated PET images 41%. The rest–stress ^{13}N-ammonia PET images (*first 2 columns of each panel*) demonstrate a large defect that is completely reversible in parts of the apex and partially reversible defect in the rest of the apical, inferior, inferoseptal, and inferolateral segments, consistent with ischemia, infarction, and partial viability. ^{18}F-FDG PET images obtained during the hyperinsulinemic euglycemic clamp protocol demonstrate substantially increased uptake in the areas with a residual resting perfusion defect, particularly the mid to basal inferior, inferoseptal, and inferolateral areas. This PET perfusion–metabolism mismatch pattern with contractile dysfunction is consistent with hibernating myocardium and has a high likelihood of contractile recovery after revascularization. HLA, horizontal long axis; SA, short axis; VLA, vertical long axis.

systems). Investigations of hybrid PET/MRI systems should consider assessment of viability as a possible indication for this emerging technology. The advantages and disadvantages of hybrid imaging for viability assessment are listed in **Table 1**.

Landmark Trials

The benefits of revascularization on global LV systolic function and patient outcomes in moderate-to-severe ischemic cardiomyopathy are the most important clinical considerations, but remain uncertain (**Table 3**). Results of observational studies and the few prospective clinical trials are incongruent. Observational studies suggest that there are revascularization benefits in the presence of viable myocardium identified by noninvasive imaging. On the other hand, the Positron Emission Tomography and Revascularization (PARR-2) and the STICH viability substudy[20,21] did not demonstrate a reduction in the primary endpoints in the presence of viability by noninvasive imaging. These studies are summarized in **Table 3**. PARR-2 reported "no significant reduction in cardiac events in patients with LV dysfunction and suspected coronary disease for ^{18}F-FDG

Table 3
Landmark myocardial viability trials

Study	PARR-2 (2007)[20]	STICH Viability (2011)[21]
Aim	• Determine if ^{18}F-FDG PET results improved clinical outcomes in patients being considered for revascularization	• Determine if myocardial viability impacts survival in patients with coronary artery disease and LV dysfunction
Methods	• Multicenter, randomized (to PET or no PET) prospective trial of 430 patients considered for revascularization • All patients with cardiomyopathy (LVEF ≤35%) suspected to be ischemic • Baseline PET or standard care then followed for 1 y	• Substudy of STICH (trial of patients with ischemic cardiomyopathy, LVEF <35% randomized to medical therapy or CABG) • 601 eligible patients underwent DSE or SPECT viability testing before revascularization • Median follow-up of 5.1 y • DSE viable if >5 segments demonstrate contractile reserve. SPECT viable if >11 viable segments based on relative tracer activity
Results	• Composite endpoint (cardiac death, MI, hospitalization for cardiac cause) not different between groups (RR, 0.82; 95% CI, 0.59–1.14; *P*=0.16)	• After adjustment for baseline variables no significant association with mortality (*P* = .21) between patients with and without viable myocardium • Assessment of myocardial viability did not identify patients with a differential survival benefit from CABG, compared with medical therapy alone
Critiques	• High rate (25%) of nonadherence to study recommendations based on PET • High rate of other form of functional testing within or before randomization may have introduced a bias against PET	• Viability substudy not randomized • Binary definition of viability • Only one-half of overall study population underwent viability testing • Only DSE and SPECT were included in the STICH viability substudy and not the more sensitive PET or MRI techniques • 20% of study population actually had a LVEF of >35% at baseline[22,a]

Abbreviations: cMRI, cardiac MRI; DSE, dobutamine stress echocardiography; LV, left ventricle; LVEF, left ventricular ejection fraction; MI, myocardial infarction; PARR-1, Positron Emission Tomography and Recovery Following Revascularization (PARR-1): The Importance of Scar and the Development of a Prediction Rule for the Degree of Recovery of Left Ventricular Function; PARR-2, F-18-Fluorodeoxyglucose Positron Emission Tomography Imaging-Assisted Management of Patients with Severe Left Ventricular Dysfunction and Suspected Coronary Artery Disease; RNA, radionuclide angiogram/angiography; RR, relative risk; SPECT, single photon emission tomography; STICH, Surgical Treatment for Ischemic Heart Failure.

[a] This discrepancy was discovered when studies were reanalyzed. The resultant concern is that the population the study was designed for and that would most likely benefit from revascularization, a LVEF of ≤35%, was not represented sufficiently in the trial.

PET-assisted management versus standard care".[23] Low adherence to the PET-guided recommendations and the use of other forms of functional testing before randomization[23] have been cited as limitations of the study. The STICH viability substudy reported no difference with revascularization versus medical therapy in the primary endpoint of mortality in the presence or absence of viability in patients with severe ischemic cardiomyopathy. Limitations of the STICH viability substudy are listed in **Table 3**.[24]

SARCOIDOSIS

Sarcoidosis is a noncaseating granulomas disease of unknown etiology most commonly affecting the pulmonary system but which can manifest in nearly every any organ, including the heart. The prevalence of cardiac sarcoid (CS) involvement in sarcoidosis ranges from 20% to 76%,[25,26] and accounts for up to 25% and 85% of sarcoid-related deaths in the United States[25] and in Japan,[27] respectively. CS diagnosis remains challenging for 2 reasons. First, despite pathologic evidence of disease, nearly one-half of patients remain clinically asymptomatic.[25] Second, CS is often focal, with very low detection by endomyocardial biopsy of only 20% to 30%.[28] The diagnostic guidelines outlined by the Ministry of Health, Labor and Welfare of Japan[27] are the most commonly used and cited, but have not been "clearly validated" and have been criticized for not incorporating ^{18}F-FDG PET imaging as a diagnostic criterion.[27] In contrast, more recent guidelines purported by the Heart Rhythm Society in 2014 incorporate ^{18}F-FDG PET into their diagnostic algorithm (**Table 4**).[30]

Pathophysiologic Basis for Radionuclide Imaging

Radionuclide imaging for CS assessment relies on detection of either or both inflammatory changes and granulomatous formation in CS. Inflamed tissue and activated macrophages, both characteristic of the active phase of sarcoidosis, can be detected by ^{18}F-FDG and gallium-67 (^{67}Ga).[31–33] Microvascular constriction in coronary arterioles around the granulomas and in later

Table 4
Comparison of current diagnostic guidelines for cardiac sarcoidosis

Guideline Variables	Japanese Ministry of Health and Welfare (2010)[29]	Heart Rhythm Society (2014)[30]
Histologic diagnosis	• EMB demonstrating noncaseatinggranulomas *and* • Histologic or clinical diagnosis of extracardiac sarcoidosis	• EMB demonstrating noncaseating granuloma
Clinical diagnosis	• ≥2 major criteria • 1 major and ≥2 minor criteria	• Histologic diagnosis of extracardiac sarcoidosis *and* • ≥1 clinical criteria

Clinical criteria	• Major
	  ○ Advanced AV block
	  ○ Basal thinning of IVS septum
	  ○ Positive ^{67}Ga cardiac uptake
	  ○ LVEF <50%
	• Minor
	  ○ Abnormal ECG: ventricular arrhythmias (VT, multifocal PVCs), RBBB, axis deviation or abnormal Q-wave
	  ○ Abnormal echocardiogram: RWMA, ventricular aneurysm
	  ○ ^{201}Tl or ^{9m}Tc perfusion defect
	  ○ Gadolinium-enhanced CMR imaging: DME
	  ○ EMB: interstitial fibrosis or monocyte infiltration > moderate grade.
		• CHB responsive to steroid or immunosuppressive therapy.
		• Mobitz type II second-degree or third-degree heart block
		• LVEF <40%
		• Spontaneous or induced VT
		• Positive ^{67}Ga cardiac uptake
		• Gadolinium-enhanced CMR imaging: DME
		• PET demonstrating patchy myocardial uptake

Abbreviations: ^{18}F-FDG, fluorine-18 deoxyglucose; ^{67}Ga, gallium-67; ^{99m}Tc, technetium 99m; ^{201}Tl, thallium-201; AV, atrioventricular block; CHB, complete heart block; CMR, cardiac MRI; DME, delayed myocardial enhancement; ECG, electrocardiogram; EMB, endomyocardial biopsy; IVS, interventricular septum; LVEF, left ventricular ejection fraction; PVC, premature ventricular contraction; RBBB, right bundle branch block; RWMA, regional wall motion abnormalities; VT, ventricular tachycardia.

stages, scar tissue, can be also be detected by myocardial "perfusion" imaging with SPECT or PET.

Single Photon Emission Computed Tomography

In the early stages of inflammation, ^{201}Tl and ^{99m}Tc SPECT images are typically grossly normal, but as the disease progresses, ^{201}Tl and ^{99m}Tc defects, which correlate histopathologically with the presence of myocardial granulomas and fibrosis, become more prevalent. Moreover, unlike ischemic abnormalities owing to obstructive coronary artery disease, ^{201}Tl and ^{99m}Tc defects owing to CS remain stable or improve during vasodilator stress. The latter, termed "reverse redistribution," is likely owing to focal reversible microvascular constriction in coronary arterioles around the granulomas[34] and predict response to steroid therapy in a small cohort of patients.[35] Although ^{99m}Tc is more sensitive in than ^{201}Tl in detecting CS,[16,17] both tracers tend to be effective only in symptomatic stages of the disease and are limited in their diagnostic sensitivity.

^{67}Ga uptake presumably by activated macrophages in inflammatory tissue[36] correlates with both clinical and histologic evidence of sarcoidosis[36–38] and is a marker of steroid-responsive CS.[39] Although relatively specific, the sensitivity of ^{67}Ga for CS is less than 40%,[40] which may be partly attributed to nearby extracardiac sarcoid, obscuring ^{67}Ga myocardial uptake.[41] Use of ^{99m}Tc in concert with ^{67}Ga outline the cardiac silhouette and reduce false-negative results has been proposed,[42] with a pilot study showing modest sensitivity (68%).[41] Ultimately, given the low sensitivity, even with combined perfusion imaging, and the greater patient radiation exposure, future use of ^{67}Ga in the diagnostic algorithm of CS is likely to decline further.

Cardiac PET

PET is a promising technique for CS detection and requires a combination of "perfusion" and ^{18}F-FDG imaging. In active CS with ongoing inflammation, ^{18}F-FDG accumulation is up to 8-fold greater in inflamed tissues, activated macrophages, and reactive lymphocytes, than in normal myocytes (**Fig. 3**). However, as CS progresses, scarring may occur, progressing to reduced or absent ^{18}F-FDG accumulation, along with "perfusion" abnormalities in the same segments. A prior metaanalysis of 7 studies using ^{18}F-FDG PET encompassing 164 patients demonstrated a sensitivity of 89% and a specificity of 78% for CS.[43] Incorporation of quantitative PET, which allows calculation of standard uptake value ([decay-corrected radiotracer concentration, mCi/mL]/[mCi of tracer injected dose into the patient][body weight]), markedly increases the specificity of PET from 46% to 97% without compromising sensitivity.[29] Standardization of standard uptake value analysis for CS, however, is necessary for meaningful interpretation and serial assessment, especially after treatment, and should be validated across different PET systems, protocols, and institutions.

Patient metabolic preparation is necessary to suppress physiologic myocardial ^{18}F-FDG uptake and one or more of the following protocols is currently in use for CS: (1) prolonged (>12 hours) fasting, shifting myocardial metabolism from glucose to free fatty acids, (2) high-fat, low-carbohydrate meal(s), and/or (3) intravenous heparin administration.[44] However, despite appropriate patient preparation, a few studies suggest that

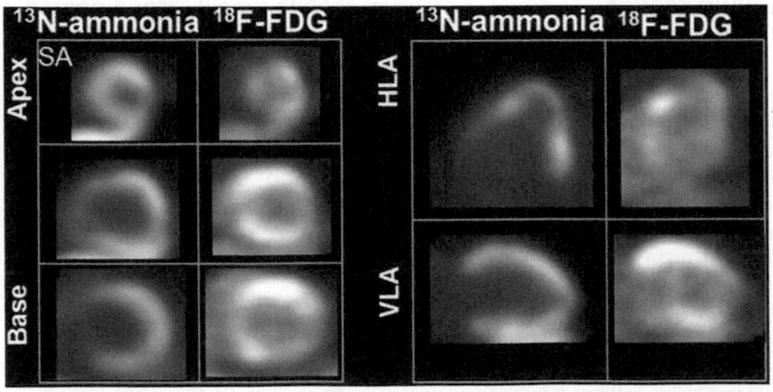

Fig. 3. ^{13}N-ammonia ^{18}F-fluorodeoxyglucose (^{18}F-FDG) PET sarcoid study. A 59-year-old woman presented with ventricular tachycardia and a dilated cardiomyopathy (left ventricular ejection fraction, 35%). Coronary angiogram was negative for atherosclerotic disease. A cardiac biopsy was negative for sarcoidosis. However, a ^{13}N-ammonia ^{18}F-FDG PET sarcoid study noted decreased perfusion along the ventricular septum with scattered FDG uptake particularly along the apex, anterior, anteroseptum, inferior, and inferospetum, suggestive of cardiac sarcoidoses. Regional wall motion abnormalities were noted along the septum. She demonstrated clinical improvement after treatment with high-dose prednisone. HLA, horizontal long axis; SA, short axis; VLA, vertical long axis.

only a minority of subjects have complete suppression of physiologic myocardial ^{18}F-FDG uptake.[45]

^{18}F-FDG PET may also provide assessment of both prognosis and therapeutic response in CS. Specifically, ventricular tachycardia has been documented in patients who develop recurrent ^{18}F-FDG uptake after stopping therapy.[46] Yamagishi and colleagues[47] also noted reduced ^{18}F-FDG uptake after initiation of corticosteroids. Further standardization of quantitative ^{18}F-FDG PET would enhance its role in diagnosis, risk stratification, and disease-monitoring in CS.

Comparison with Nonradionuclide Imaging Modalities for Cardiac Sarcoidosis

Echocardiographic features of CS include thinning of the basal interventricular septum, aneurysm formation (most commonly in the inferior–posterior wall), and regional wall motion abnormalities,[26,27] but are generally nonspecific and often not detected until the advanced stages of CS. This shortcoming has been demonstrated in 1 study that reported a 25% sensitivity for echocardiographic diagnosis of CS.[28]

cMRI assesses sarcoid-induced inflammation via T2-weighted imaging and scarring with T1-weighted analysis (**Fig. 4**). Both the sensitivity and specificity of cMRI for CS is 75%.[48] Greulich and colleagues[49] reported a 20-fold increased risk of death or appropriate defibrillator discharge in sarcoid patients with evidence of late gadolinium enhancement, whereas Sekiguchi and colleagues[50,51] and Vignaux and associates[51] reported an association between a decrease in gadolinium enhancement and a positive response to steroid therapy. Limitations of cMRI for CS are similar to those for viability assessment (see **Table 1**).

Hybrid Imaging

The use of emerging hybrid technology via the coupling of PET and MRI in a single session may allow "coregistration of metabolic/molecular probe imaging with morphologic, functional and tissue imaging."[52] A sentinel CS case of hybrid PET-MRI imaging reported by White and colleagues[52] demonstrated the feasibility of using this emerging technology for CS, which is anticipated to be an active area of investigation that may alter the recommended diagnostic approach and subsequent management of CS (**Box 2**).

AMYLOIDOSIS

Amyloidosis results from the extracellular deposition of proteinaceous materials into various organ systems with resultant deleterious effects. Two specific subtypes of amyloidosis, amyloid light-chain (AL) and transthyretin-related amyloidosis (ATTR, which includes familial ATTR and systemic senile amyloidosis), predominate when evaluating cardiac amyloidosis. AL amyloidosis has an incidence of approximately 2500 cases annually in the United States,[53] with one-half demonstrating cardiac involvement.[54] Cardiac AL amyloidosis carries a very poor prognosis with a median survival of only 15 months if left untreated.[55] ATTR amyloidosis has a much lower rate of cardiac involvement[56] and much higher median survival rate (43–75 months) compared with AL amyloid.[57] Systemic senile amyloidosis amyloid is almost exclusively seen in elderly men with a median survival of nearly 90 months. Establishing the

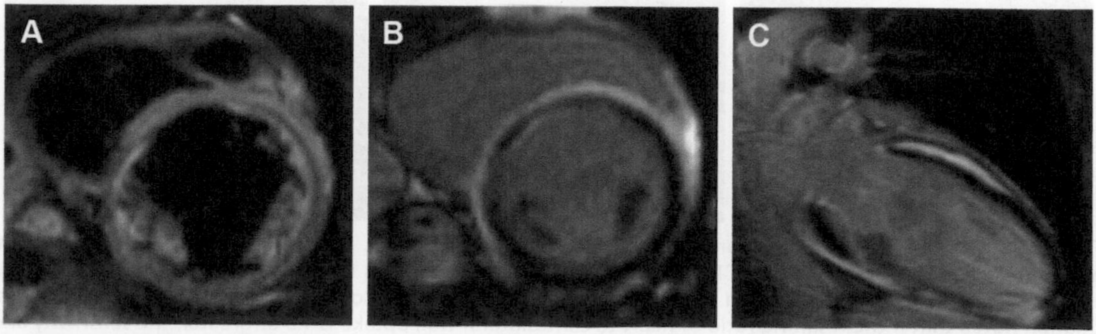

Fig. 4. Cardiac MRI in 37 year-old woman with cardiac sarcoidosis. Short-axis T2-weighted imaging (*A*) demonstrating subepicardial high signal suggestive of active inflammation, on the right ventricular side of the anterior basal septum extending into the right ventricular outflow tract. Delayed enhancement short axis imaging (*B*; appears slightly different to image *A* because it was obtained during a different phase of the cardiac cycle) and 2-chamber long-axis imaging (*C*) noting enhancement along the ventricular septum and anterior wall consistent with fibrosis and/or inflammation. (*Courtesy of* P.M. Young, MD, Rochester, MN.)

Box 2
Sarcoidosis

- Detection of CS is challenged by its focal nature (EMB yield 20%–30%) and varied and nonspecific presentation.
- Cardiac PET with ^{18}F-FDG and myocardial "perfusion" imaging has tremendous diagnostic and prognostic potential.
- Specific ^{18}F-FDG PET patient preparation protocols (prolonged fasting, high-fat, low-carbohydrate diet, and/or heparin) should be followed in to minimize physiologic myocardial ^{18}F-FDG uptake when imaging to detect CS.
- Perfusion imaging is necessary for interpretation of cardiac ^{18}F-FDG PET images for CS.
- Cardiac PET imaging has high sensitivity and modest specificity for the diagnosis of CS.

Abbreviations: ^{18}F-FDG, fluorine-18 deoxyglucose; CS, cardiac sarcoid; EMB, endomyocardial biopsy.

diagnosis of cardiac amyloidosis and differentiating which subtype is present are, therefore, critical for both prognostic and therapeutic implications.[58]

99m-Technetium Pyrophosphate

Recent interest in 99m-technetium pyrophosphate (^{99m}Tc-PYP) has resulted from reports[59] demonstrating the high discriminatory value in differentiating ATTR from AL amyloidosis with semi-quantitative ^{99m}Tc-PYP assessment. ^{99m}Tc-PYP uptake can also be visualized in subacute myocardial infarction and therefore accuracy can be enhanced with concurrent SPECT perfusion imaging (**Fig. 5**).

3,3-Diphosphono-1,2-Propanodicarboxylic Acid

Initial investigations using 3,3-diphosphono-1,2-propanodicarboxylic acid (^{99m}Tc-DPD) are also promising for diagnosing cardiac ATTR amyloidosis. In 2005, 15 patients with ATTR amyloidosis and 10 with AL amyloidosis underwent ^{99m}TC-DPD imaging with 100% of ATTR patients demonstrating uptake compared with 0% of AL amyloid patients.[60] A more recent investigation by Rapezzi and colleagues[42] demonstrated excellent agreement between echocardiography and ^{99m}Tc-DPD uptake for amyloid in ATTR patients. Furthermore, this study demonstrated that ^{99m}Tc-DPD uptake negatively correlated with LV ejection fraction ($r = 0.368$; $P = .004$) and was a predictor of major adverse cardiac outcomes.

Technetium-99m Aprotinin, Iodine-123 Serum Amyloid P, and Iodine-123 Meta-Iodobenzylguanidine Scintigraphy

Aprotinin is a serine protease inhibitor that was noted to be a component of amyloid matrix. It was therefore hoped that radiolabeled aprotinin (^{99m}Tc-aprotinin) might have prognostic benefits. However, sensitivity of ^{99m}Tc-aprotinin proved to be low (40%), thereby limiting its diagnostic utility.[42]

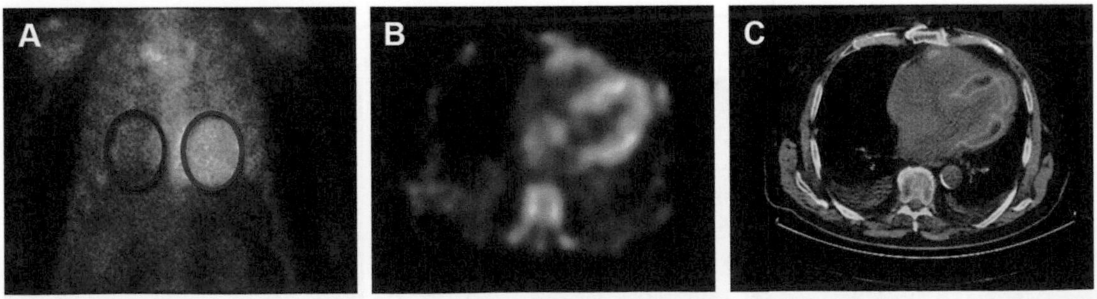

Fig. 5. ^{99m}Tc-PYP SPECT/computed tomography (CT) imaging for cardiac amyloidosis. Planar scintigraphy (*A*) allows quantitative assessment of ^{99m}Tc-PYP uptake by comparing counts in a selected region of interest over the heart (*red circle*) compared with a region of identical size (*blue circle*) on the contralateral chest. One investigation noted that if the resulting ratio of heart to contralateral wall uptake is 1.5 or greater, the sensitivity and specificity for differentiating ATTR from AL is near 100%.[59] Axial SPECT imaging (*B*) demonstrating ^{99m}Tc-PYP uptake in the myocardium. Fused SPECT/CT imaging (*C*) reveals diffuse ^{99m}Tc-PYP uptake in the left and right ventricle, highly suggestive of ATTR amyloidosis rather than myocardial infarction, which would be relegated to a specific vascular territory. ^{99m}Tc-PYP, 99m-technetium pyrophosphate; AL, amyloid light-chain; ATTR, transthyretin-related amyloidosis; CT, computed tomography; SPECT, single-photon emission CT. (*Courtesy of* G.B. Johnson, MD, PhD and J.W. Askew III, MD, Rochester, MN.)

Box 3
Amyloidosis

- AL cardiac amyloidosis has a poor prognosis (median survival of 15 months).
- F-18 florbetapir PET may be a useful emerging diagnostic modality in AL and ATTR amyloidosis.
- ^{99m}Tc-DPD and ^{99m}Tc-PYP demonstrate preferential ATTR uptake and may be helpful in distinguishing between ATTR and AL amyloidosis.
- A summary of noninvasive imaging in cardiac amyloidosis is provided in **Table 5**.

Abbreviations: ^{99m}Tc-DPD, 3,3-diphosphono-1,2-propanodicarboxylic acid; ^{99m}Tc-PYP, 99m-technetium pyrophosphate; AL, amyloid light-chain; ATTR, transthyretin-related amyloidosis.

Similarly, serum amyloid P is a component of amyloid deposits and thus was labeled with iodine-123 (^{123}I-SAP). Unfortunately further investigative work revealed an insufficient myocardial signal in ^{123}I-SAP scans.[61] Iodine-123 meta-iodobenzylguanidine scintigraphy has demonstrated both diagnostic and prognostic promise by identifying early myocardial denervation in patients with familial amyloid polyneuropathy.[62]

PET with F-18 Florbetapir

The potential diagnostic use of PET imaging in cardiac amyloidosis is an active area of investigation. A recent pilot study of 14 patients using F-18 florbetapir (^{18}F-florbetapir) PET demonstrated positive uptake in all 9 cardiac amyloid patients (including both AL and ATTR) and no uptake in the 5 control cases.[63] Further trials are anticipated to provide more evidence as to the diagnostic usefulness of PET in cardiac amyloidosis.

Comparison with Nonradionuclide Imaging Modalities for Cardiac Amyloidosis

Transthoracic echocardiography has been considered the "gold standard for noninvasive diagnosis of amyloidosis."[43] Classic echocardiographic features include wall thickness of greater than 12 mm, small LV cavity, restrictive LV filling pressures, and pericardial effusion.[64] A worse prognosis is associated with wall thickness of greater than 15 mm, marked left atrial enlargement, presence of pericardial effusion, and reduced longitudinal

Table 5
Comparison of imaging modalities to assess cardiac amyloidosis

Imaging Modality	Advantages	Disadvantages
^{99m}Tc-PYP SPECT	• High sensitivity for ATTR • Can combine with SPECT imaging to differentiate from subacute MI • FDA approval	• Also see uptake in subacute MI • Further investigation needed • Not diagnostic of AL
^{99m}Tc-DPD SPECT	• High sensitivity for ATTR • Correlates with LVEF • Predictor of MACE	• Further investigation needed • Not diagnostic of AL • Not FDA approved
^{99m}Tc-aprotinin SPECT	• Limited	• Low sensitivity (40%)
1231-SAP	• Limited	• Low sensitivity
123-MIBG	• Limited	• Low sensitivity
^{18}F-florbetapir PET	• Initial studies demonstrate high sensitivity and specificity for ATTR and AL	• May not be able to differentiate AL and ATTR • Further investigation needed
Echocardiography	• Considered diagnostic "gold standard"	• Decreased sensitivity early in disease process • Cannot differentiate amyloid subtypes
Cardiac MRI	• Detect early stages of disease • High sensitivity and specificity	• Contraindicated with implantable device • Further investigation needed

Abbreviations: ^{18}F-florbetapir, F-18 Florbetapir; ^{99m}TC, technetium-99m; ^{123}I-SAP, iodine-123 serum amyloid P; 123-MIBG, iodine-123 meta-iodobenzylguanidine scintigraphy; AL, amyloid light-chain; ATTR, transthyretin related amyloidosis; DPD, 3,3-diphosphono-1,2-propanodicarboxylic Acid; FDA, US Food and Drug Administration; LVEF, left ventricular ejection fraction; MACE, major adverse cardiac events; MI, myocardial infarction; PYP, pyrophosphate; SPECT, single-photon emission computed tomography.

strain.[64] Shortcomings of echocardiography include limited earlier stage diagnosis and difficulty distinguishing between a familiar and AL amyloid.

cMRI with gadolinium enhancement may be able to detect amyloid infiltration before wall thickening. Gadolinium distributes interstitially within the heart directly where amyloid fibrils are being deposited. Therefore, as the interstitial space increases with fibril deposition, gadolinium persists longer and delayed gadolinium enhancement is noted. Using this technique, cMRI has been noted to have a sensitivity and specificity of 86% for detecting amyloidosis.[65,66] Sensitivity was similar between cMRI and to ^{99m}Tc-DPD for detecting ATTR amyloid (**Box 3**, **Table 5**).[67]

SUMMARY

Myocardial viability, CS, and cardiac amyloidosis present unique diagnostic, prognostic and therapeutic dilemmas. As reflected in this review, the role of noninvasive imaging, particularly radionuclide imaging, continues to evolve. For myocardial viability, cardiac PET imaging has the greatest sensitivity and negative predictive value among the noninvasive techniques for predicting contractile recovery after revascularization. Despite this strength and those of other techniques, the exact role of viability testing and impact on revascularization outcomes have not been confirmed by recent clinical trials. For CS, cardiac PET imaging with myocardial "perfusion" and ^{18}F-FDG has tremendous diagnostic and prognostic potential, but further studies and standardization of techniques are needed. With respect to amyloidosis, radionuclide imaging has the potential to help establish the diagnosis and differentiate among the subtypes, which have diverse clinical presentations, natural histories, treatments, and prognoses. Development of standardized imaging protocols, proliferation of the necessary technology and expertise, managing financial considerations, and addressing radiation exposure are anticipated. Forthcoming investigations are critical to further define the role of radionuclide imaging in aiding the clinician in these challenging patient scenarios.

REFERENCES

1. Hunt S, Abraham WT, Chin MH, et al. 2009 Focused update incorporated into the ACC/AHA 2005 guidelines for the diagnosis and management of heart failure in adults. J Am Coll Cardiol 2009;53(15):e1–90.
2. Gibson RS, Watson DD, Taylor GJ, et al. Prospective assessment of regional myocardial perfusion before and after coronary revascularization surgery by quantitative thallium-201 scintigraphy. J Am Coll Cardiol 1983;1:804–15.
3. Udelson JE, Coleman PS, Metherall J, et al. Predicting recovery of severe regional ventricular dysfunction: comparison of resting scintigraphy with ^{201}Tl and ^{99m}Tc-sestamibi. Circulation 1994;89:2552–61.
4. Gutman J, Berman DS, Freeman M, et al. Time to completed redistribution of thallium-201 in exercise myocardial scintigraphy: relationship to the degree of coronary artery stenosis. Am Heart J 1983;106:989–95.
5. Dilsizian V, Rocco TP, Freedman NM, et al. Enhanced detection of ischemic but viable myocardium by the reinjection of thallium after stress-redistribution imaging. N Engl J Med 1990;323:141–6.
6. Regenfus M, Schlundt C, von Erffa J, et al. Head-to-head comparison of contrast-enhanced cardiovascular magnetic resonance and ^{201}thallium single photon emission computed tomography for prediction of reversible left ventricular dysfunction in chronic ischaemic heart disease. Int J Cardiovasc Imaging 2012;28(6):1427–34.
7. Iida H, Ruotsalainen U, Mäki M, et al. F-18 fluorodeoxyglucose uptake and water-perfusable tissue fraction in assessment of myocardial viability. Ann Nucl Med 2012;26:644–55.
8. Bansal M, Jeffriess L, Leano R, et al. Assessment of myocardial viability at dobutamine echocardiography by deformation analysis using tissue velocity and speckle-tracking. JACC Cardiovasc Imaging 2010;3(2):121–31.
9. Cianfrocca C, Pelliccia F, Pasceri V, et al. Strain rate analysis and levosimendan improve detection of myocardial viability by dobutamine echocardiography in patients with post-infarction left ventricular dysfunction: a pilot study. J Am Soc Echocardiogr 2008;21(9):1068–74.
10. Schinkel AF, Bax JJ, Poldermans D, et al. Hibernating myocardium: diagnosis and patient outcomes. Curr Probl Cardiol 2007;32:375–410.
11. Romero J, Xue X, Gonzalez W, et al. CMR imaging assessing viability in patients with chronic ventricular dysfunction due to coronary artery disease: a meta-analysis of prospective trials. JACC Cardiovasc Imaging 2012;5(5):494–508.
12. Einstein AJ, Moser KW, Thompson RC. Radiation dose to patients from cardiac diagnostic imaging. Circulation 2007;116:1290–305.
13. Freeman I, Grunwald AM, Hoory S, et al. Effect of coronary occlusion and myocardial activity of technetium-99m-sestamibi. J Nucl Med 1991;32:292–8.
14. Schoder H, Campisi R, Ohtake T, et al. Blood flow-metabolism imaging with positron emission tomography in patients with diabetes mellitus for the assessment of reversible left ventricular contractile dysfunction. J Am Coll Cardiol 1999;33:1328–37.

15. Knuuti J, Schelbert HR, Bax JJ. The need for standardization of cardiac FDG PET imaging in the evaluation of myocardial viability in patients with chronic ischemic left ventricular dysfunction. Eur J Nucl Med Mol Imaging 2002;29:1257–66.
16. Kim RJ, Wu E, Rafael A, et al. The use of contrast-enhanced magnetic resonance imaging to identify reversible myocardial dysfunction. N Engl J Med 2000;343(20):1445–53.
17. Gerber BL, Rousseau MF, Ahn SA, et al. Prognostic value of myocardial viability by delayed-enhancement magnetic resonance in patients with coronary artery disease with low ejection fraction: impact of revascularization therapy. J Am Coll Cardiol 2012;59(9):825–35.
18. Nikolaou K, Knez A, Sagmeister S, et al. Assessment of myocardial infarctions using multidetector-row computed tomography. Am J Cardiol 2006;98:303–8.
19. Koyama Y, Matsuoka H, Mochizuki T, et al. Assessment of reperfused acute myocardial infarction with two-phase contrast-enhanced helical CT: prediction of left ventricular function and wall thickness. Radiology 2005;235:804–11.
20. Beanlands RS, Nichol G, Huszti E, et al. F-18-fluorodeoxyglocose positron emission tomography imaging-assisted management of patients with severe left ventricular dysfunction and suspected coronary disease: a randomized, controlled trial (PARR-2). J Am Coll Cardiol 2007;50:2002–12.
21. Bonow RO, Maurer G, Lee KL, et al. Myocardial viability and survival in ischemic left ventricular dysfunction. N Engl J Med 2011;364:1617–25.
22. Oh JK, Pellikka PA, Panza JA, et al. Core lab analysis of baseline echocardiographic studies in the STICH trial and recommendation for use of echocardiography in future clinical trials. J Am Soc Echocardiogr 2012;25:327–36.
23. Leonici M, Marcucci G, Sciagra R, et al. Prediction of functional recovery in patients with chronic coronary artery disease and left ventricular dysfunction combining the evaluation of myocardial perfusion and of contractile reserve using nitrate-enhanced technetium-99m sestamibi gated single-photon emission computed tomography and dobutamine stress. Am J Cardiol 2001;87:1346–50.
24. Srichai MB, Jaber WA. Viability by MRI or PET would have changed the results of the STICH trial. Prog Cardiovasc Dis 2013;55(5):487–93.
25. Silverman KJ, Hutchins GM, Bulkley BH. Cardiac sarcoid: a clinicopathologic study of 84 unselected patients with systemic sarcoidosis. Circulation 1978;58(6):1204–11.
26. Perry A, Vuitch F. Causes of death in patients with sarcoidosis. A morphologic study of 38 autopsies with clinicopathologic correlations. Arch Pathol Lab Med 1995;119(2):167–72.
27. Doughan AR, Williams BR. Cardiac sarcoidosis. Heart 2006;92(2):282–8.
28. Cooper LT, Baughman KL, Feldman AM, et al. The role of endomyocardial biopsy in the management of cardiovascular disease. Circulation 2007;1216:2216–33.
29. Tahara N, Tahara A, Nitta Y, et al. Heterogenous myocardial FDG uptake and the disease activity in cardiac sarcoidosis. JACC Cardiovasc Imaging 2010;3(12):1219–28.
30. Birnie DH, Sauer WH, Bogun F, et al. HRS expert consensus statement on the diagnosis and management of arrhythmias associated with cardiac sarcoidosis. Heart Rhythm 2014;11:1304–23.
31. Amaral JF, Shearer JD, Mastrofrancesco B, et al. Can lactate be used as fuel by wounded tissue? Surgery 1986;100(2):252–61.
32. Daley JM, Shearer JD, Mastrofrancesco B, et al. Glucose metabolism in injured tissue: a longitudinal study. Surgery 1990;107(2):187–92.
33. Mauël J. Macrophage activation by OM-85 BV. Respiration 1992;59:14–8.
34. Tawarahara K, Kurata C, Okayama K, et al. Thallium-201 and gallium 67 single photon emission computed tomographic imaging in cardiac sarcoidosis. Am Heart J 1992;124(5):1383–4.
35. Matsui Y, Iwai K, Tachibana T, et al. Clinicopathological study of fatal myocardial sarcoidosis. Ann N Y Acad Sci 1976;278:455–69.
36. Mañá J, van Kroonebburgh M. Clinical usefulness of nuclear imaging techniques in cardiac sarcoidosis. Eur Respir Mon 2005;32:284–300.
37. Hirose Y, Ishida Y, Hayashida K, et al. Myocardial involvement in patients with sarcoidosis. An analysis of 75 patients. Clin Nucl Med 1994;19(6):522–6.
38. Okamoto H, Mizuno K, Ohtoshi E. Cutaneous sarcoidosis with cardiac involvement. Eur J Dermatol 1999;9(6):466–9.
39. Okayama K, Kurata C, Tawarahara K, et al. Diagnostic and prognostic value of myocardial scintigraphy with thallium-201 and gallium-67 in cardiac sarcoidosis. Chest 1995;107(2):330–4.
40. Mañá J, Gamez C. Molecular imaging in sarcoidosis. Curr Opin Pulm Med 2011;17:325–31.
41. Nakazawa A, Ikeda K, Ito Y, et al. Usefulness of dual 67Ga and 99mcTc-sestamibi single-photon-emission CT scanning in the diagnosis of cardiac sarcoidosis. Chest 2004;126:1372–6.
42. Rapezzi C, Quarta CC, Guidalotti PL, et al. Role of (99m)Tc-DPD scintigraphy in diagnosis and prognosis of hereditary transthyretin-related cardiac amyloidosis. JACC Cardiovasc Imaging 2011;4(6):659–70.
43. Youssef G, Leung E, Mylonas I, et al. The use of ^{18}F-FDG PET in the diagnosis of cardiac sarcoidosis: a systematic review and meta-analysis including the Ontario experience. J Nucl Med 2012;52(2):241–8, 55.

44. Williams G, Kolodny GM. Suppression of myocardial 18F-FDG uptake by preparing patients with high-fat, low-carbohydrate diet. AJR Am J Roentgenol 2008; 190(2):W151–6.
45. Maurer AH, Burshteyn M, Adler LP, et al. Variable cardiac ^{18}FDG patterns seen in oncologic positron emission tomography computed tomography importance for differentiating normal physiology from cardiac and paracardiac disease. J Thorac Imaging 2012;27:263–8.
46. Pandya C, Brunken RC, Tchou P, et al. Detecting cardiac involvement in sarcoidosis: a call for prospective studies of newer imaging techniques. Eur Respir J 2007;113(20):418–22.
47. Yamagishi H, Shirai N, Takagi M, et al. Identification of cardiac sarcoidosis with 12N-NH 3/18F-FDG PET. J Nucl Med 2003;44(7):1030–6.
48. Ohira H, Tsujino I, Ishimaru S, et al. Myocardial imaging with ^{18}F-fluoro-2-deoxyglucose positron emission tomography and magnetic resonance imaging in sarcoidosis. Eur J Nucl Med Mol Imaging 2008; 35(5):933–41.
49. Greulich S, Deluigi CC, Gloekler S, et al. CMR imaging predicts death and other adverse events in suspected cardiac sarcoidosis. JACC Cardiovasc Imaging 2013;6(4):501–11.
50. Sekiguchi M, Yazaki Y, Isobe M, et al. Cardiac sarcoidosis: diagnostic, prognostic, and therapeutic considerations. Cardiovasc Drugs Ther 1996;10(5): 495–510.
51. Vignaux O, Dhote R, Duboc D, et al. Clinical significance of myocardial magnetic resonance abnormalities in patients with sarcoidosis: a 1-year follow-up study. Chest 2002;122(6):1895–901.
52. White JA, Rajchl M, Butler J, et al. Active cardiac sarcoidosis: first clinical experience of simultaneous positron emission tomography-magnetic resonance imaging for the diagnosis of cardiac disease. Circulation 2013;127(22):639–41.
53. Gertz MA, Lacy MQ, Dispenzieri A. Amyloidosis. Hematol Oncol Clin North Am 1999;13(6):1211–33.
54. Dubrey SW, Cha K, Anderson J, et al. The clinical features of immunoglobulin light-chain (AL) amyloidosis with heart involvement. QJM 1998;91(2):141–57.
55. Ng B, Connors LH, Davidoff R, et al. Senile systemic amyloidosis presenting with heart failure: a comparison with light chain-associated amyloidosis. Arch Intern Med 2005;165(12):1425–9.
56. Nakamura M, Satoh M, Kowada S, et al. Reversible restrictive cardiomyopathy due to light-chain deposition disease. Mayo Clin Proc 2002;77(2):193–6.
57. Ruberg FL, Maurer MS, Judge DP, et al. Prospective evaluation of morbidity and mortality of wild-type and V122I mutant transthyretin amyloid cardiomyopathy: the transthyretin amyloidosis cardiac study (TRACS). Am Heart J 2012;164(2): 222–8.
58. Guidelines Working Group of UK Myeloma Forum, British Committee for Standards on Haematology, British Society for Haematology. Guidelines on the diagnosis and management of AL amyloidosis. Br J Haematol 2004;125(6):681–700.
59. Bokhari S, Castaño A, Pozniakoff T, et al. ^{99m}Tc-Pyrophosphate scintigraphy for differentiating light-chain cardiac amyloidosis from the transthyretin-related familial and senile cardiac amyloidoses. Circ Cardiovasc Imaging 2013;6(2):195–201.
60. Perugini E, Guidalotti PL, Salvi F, et al. Noninvasive etiologic diagnosis of cardiac amyloidosis using 99mTc-3,3-diphosphono-1,2-propanodicarboxylic acid scintigraphy. J Am Coll Cardiol 2005;46(6): 1076–84.
61. Hazenberg BP, van Rijswijk MH, Lub-de Hooge MN, et al. Diagnostic performance and prognostic value of extravascular retention of ^{123}I-labeled serum amyloid P component in systemic amyloidosis. J Nucl Med 2007;48:865–72.
62. Coutinho MC, Cortez-Diaz N, Cantinho G, et al. Reduced myocardial 123-iodine metaiobenzylguanidine uptake: a prognostic marker in familial amyloid polyneuropathy. Circ Cardiovasc Imaging 2013;6(5): 627–36.
63. Dorbala S, Vangala D, Semer J, et al. Imaging cardiac amyloidosis: a pilot study using ^{18}F-florbetapir positron emission tomography. Eur J Nucl Med Mol Imaging 2014;41(9):1652–62.
64. Mohtya D, Damy T, Cosnay P, et al. Cardiac amyloidosis: update in diagnosis and management. Arch Cardiovasc Dis 2013;106:528–40.
65. Lachmann HJ, Booth DR, Booth SE, et al. Misdiagnosis of hereditary amyloidosis as AL (primary) amyloidosis. N Engl J Med 2002;346(23): 1786–91.
66. Austin BA, Tang WH, Rodriguez ER, et al. Delayed hyper-enhancement of magnetic resonance imaging provide incremental diagnostic and prognostic utility in suspected cardiac amyloidosis. JACC Cardiovasc Imaging 2009;2(12):1369–77.
67. Di Bella G, Minutoli F, Mazzeo A, et al. MRI of cardiac involvement in transthyretin familial amyloid polyneuropathy. AJR Am J Roentgenol 2010; 195(6):394–9.

Clinical Applications of Myocardial Innervation Imaging

Mark I. Travin, MD

KEYWORDS

• Molecular imaging • *m*IBG • Heart failure • Cardiac arrhythmias • Adrenergic innervation

KEY POINTS

- Adrenergic imaging with iodine 123 *meta*-iodobenzylguanidine (^{123}I-*m*IBG) and analogous PET tracers assesses direct cardiac sympathetic innervation and is potentially useful in managing various cardiac diseases.
- ^{123}I-*m*IBG effectively risk stratifies patients with advanced heart failure (HF) independently of standard parameters, including left ventricular ejection fraction (LVEF) and B-type natriuretic peptide (BNP).
- In HF and primary arrhythmic conditions, ^{123}I-*m*IBG and PET imaging with ^{11}C-meta-hydroxyephedrine (HED) can help identify increased risk for lethal ventricular arrhythmias and show promise for guiding use of an implantable cardiac defibrillator (ICD).
- Adrenergic imaging has potential for guiding end-stage HF management use of cardiac resynchronization therapy (CRT), left ventricular assist devices (LVADs), and transplant.

INTRODUCTION

The autonomic nervous system plays a key role in regulating cardiac function and consists of circulating hormones and directs neural control by sympathetic and parasympathetic innervation. Circulating mediators, including epinephrine, norepinephrine (NE), arginine vasopressin, BNP, and substances of the renin-angiotensin-aldosterone system (RAAS), control cardiac output (CO), vascular tone, and blood volume to maintain perfusion to body organs.[1] Although measurements of these substances can help manage conditions such as HF, they are not specific to the heart and may reflect noncardiac pathologic conditions.[2,3]

Radiotracer analogues of sympathetic innervation mediators such as NE and of parasympathetic mediators such as acetylcholine allow visualization of cardiac autonomic innervation function and can thus help assess pathologic abnormalities. Given the low density of cardiac cholinergic neurons and difficulties designing suitable tracers, human studies of parasympathetic imaging are limited. In contrast, cardiac sympathetic innervation is abundant, and as single-photon computed tomography (SPECT) and PET analogues of NE have been easy to synthesize, human cardiac sympathetic innervation has been well studied, with applications proposed for a variety of cardiac diseases.

CARDIAC SYMPATHETIC INNERVATION

Sympathetic cardiac control is initiated by regulatory centers in the brain that respond to input signals from the brain and body. Output signals travel along descending pathways, synapsing with preganglionic fibers that synapse with paravertebral stellate ganglia innervating the left and right

Division of Nuclear Medicine, Department of Radiology, Montefiore Medical Center, 111 East-210th Street, Bronx, NY 10467-2490, USA
E-mail address: mtravin@montefiore.org

Cardiol Clin 34 (2016) 133–147
http://dx.doi.org/10.1016/j.ccl.2015.06.003
0733-8651/16/$ – see front matter

ventricles. Sympathetic nerves follow the coronary arteries in the subepicardium before penetrating into the myocardium.[4]

Radiotracers that have been used clinically image presynaptic anatomy and function. As in **Fig. 1**, NE is synthesized in presynaptic terminals and stored in vesicles. In response to sympathetic stimuli, NE is released into synaptic spaces and interacts with postsynaptic membrane α, β1, and β2 receptors, leading to increased heart rate (HR), augmented contractility, and enhanced conduction effects.[5] To control and terminate these effects, NE is actively taken back into presynaptic terminals, mostly via the energy-dependent norepinephrine transporter-1 (NET-1) membrane protein, for storage or catabolic disposal.[6] Some free NE is also taken up by nonneuronal postsynaptic cells, probably by passive diffusion (ie, uptake 2).

Radiotracer Analogues of Norepinephrine

The development of autonomic radiotracers has been well described.[7] To develop scintigraphic adrenal imaging, researchers explored modifying iodine (I)-labeled analogues of the adrenergic blocking antiarrhythmic drug bretylium.[8] Wieland and colleagues[9] investigated guanethidine, a false neurotransmitter analogue of NE, and determined that iodine in the meta position, that is, *meta*-iodobenzylguanidine (*m*IBG), was suitable for both adrenomedullary and cardiac imaging. Unlike NE, *m*IBG is not catabolized after presynaptic uptake,

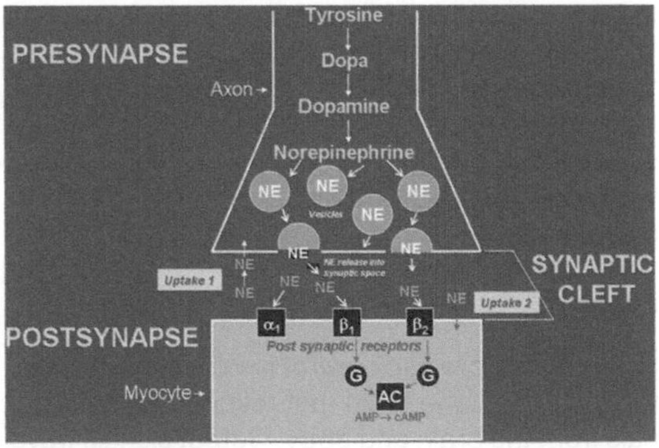

Fig. 1. The sympathetic neuron synapse. In response to a stimulus, vesicles containing NE are released into the synaptic space and interact with postsynaptic receptors. Sympathetic response is controlled by reuptake of NE into the presynaptic terminal via the Uptake-1 norepinephrine transporter. AC, adenyl cyclase; AMP, adenosine monophosphate; cAMP, cyclic adenosine monophosphate; G, G proteins. (*From* Travin MI. Cardiac neuronal imaging at the edge of clinical application. Cardiol Clin 2009;27:312; with permission.)

thus localizing in high concentrations. The first publication of human heart imaging was by Kline and colleagues.[10] In accord with observations of Wieland that in contrast to thallium, which depicts the plumbing of the heart, *m*IBG visualizes wiring of the heart, the potential to assess the pathophysiology of HF and identify patients with autonomic neuropathies that predispose to arrhythmias and sudden cardiac death (SCD) was recognized.[7,11] Current labeling is with ^{123}I, which emits predominantly 159 keV gamma photons, with a half-life of 13.2 hours, well tolerated and easily imaged by SPECT.[11] Used clinically for many years in Europe and Japan, ^{123}I-*m*IBG was approved in 2013 in the United States for cardiac imaging in patients with New York Heart Association (NYHA) class II–III HF and an LVEF 35% or less to help identify patients with lower 1- and 2-year mortality risks.

Various PET analogues of NE have also been studied.[12] Compared with ^{123}I-*m*IBG, these have better physical properties for imaging and also have biologic advantages. The most widely studied PET tracer is ^{11}C-HED, which has higher NET-1 selectivity than ^{123}I-*m*IBG resulting in better differentiation between innervated and denervated myocardium, potentially advantageous in evaluating neuronal heterogeneity in hibernating myocardium.[13] Other less well-studied PET tracers include ^{11}C-epinephrine and ^{11}C-phenylephrine. Nevertheless, as the need for a nearby cyclotron makes ^{11}C-tracers impractical for most practitioners, ^{18}F compounds, such as ^{18}F-LMI-1195 (fluorobenzylguanidine) are under investigation.[14]

CLINICAL IMAGING WITH IODINE 123 *META*-IODOBENZYLGUANIDINE

Patient Preparation and Imaging Techniques

Patient preparation and imaging techniques are summarized in **Box 1**, and readers are referred to various references for more detail.[15–18] ^{123}I-*m*IBG is imaged with a standard Anger camera using a low-energy collimator, although some advocate a medium-energy collimator, as high-energy (>400 keV) ^{123}I photon emissions, especially those at 529 keV, penetrate collimator septa.[19] As parameters vary among different low-energy collimators, a calibration factor derived from a phantom for individual camera-collimator systems has been proposed.[20] There are reports of cardiac ^{123}I-*m*IBG imaging using a solid-state camera, but differences from Anger cameras in terms of quantitative image values need to be determined.[21,22] Acquisition and processing of ^{123}I-*m*IBG images use customary perfusion imaging techniques. Although clinical utility of SPECT imaging is uncertain, tomographic acquisitions are

Box 1
Cardiac ^{123}I-*m*IBG imaging technique

- Patient preparation
  - Continue standard HF medications, for example, β-blockers, angiotensin converting enzyme inhibitors, angiotensin receptor blockers, aldosterone antagonists.
  - Hold for 24 hours or more medications and substances that potentially interfere with NE uptake.
    - Tricyclic antidepressants
    - Antipsychotics
    - Sympathomimetics
    - Some antihypertensives (especially reserpine, labetolol)
    - Opioids and cocaine
    - Foods containing vanillin and catecholamine-like compounds (eg, chocolate, blue cheese)
  - Consider preadministration of a thyroid-blocking agent.
    - Individually balance risk (potential allergic reaction) versus benefit (thyroid radiation exposure)
- Tracer administration
  - Have patients lie quietly for 5 minutes.
  - Administer 10 mCi (370 MBq) slowly over 1 to 2 minutes followed by saline flush.
  - Radiation exposure is approximately 5 mSv.
- Imaging
  - Hardware
    - Standard Anger camera, 20% energy window around main 159-keV peak
    - Low-energy high-resolution collimator is customary
  - Procedure
    - Planar (anterior): early (~15–25 minutes after tracer administration) and late (~4 hours after tracer administration) 10-minute supine acquisitions with 128 × 128 or 256 × 256 matrix
    - SPECT ^{123}I-*m*IBG: Early and late, immediately following planar images; 64 projections at 30 seconds each, supine, with 64 × 64 matrix
    - SPECT perfusion: standard rest SPECT imaging (technetium Tc 99m sestamibi or technetium Tc 99m tetrofosmin) on a different day

Data from Refs.[15–18]

commonly performed immediately after planar imaging. Although most studies report processing with filtered back projection, iterative reconstruction techniques are being explored with deconvolution of septal penetration (DSP) used to compensate for the aforementioned higher-energy ^{123}I photon emissions.[23]

Image Interpretation

^{123}I-*m*IBG image interpretation consists of quantitation of global cardiac tracer uptake in reference to background, that is, the heart to mediastinum ratio (H/M); retention of tracer between early and late images, that is, washout (WO) or washout rate (WR); and regional uptake on SPECT images often in reference to perfusion images, summarized in **Box 2**. The best methods for all techniques remain under discussion.[15]

H/M is customarily assessed from anterior planar images, but there are reports of H/M derivation from SPECT acquisition images with small field of view cameras, either Anger or solid-state systems.[24,25] Typically, only the late H/M shows prognostic statistical significance in multivariate analyses.[18] Although several techniques for creating regions of interest (ROIs) have been reported, the current approach favors measuring heart counts via an ROI around the epicardial border and valve plane. An H/M less than 1.6 (2 SD less than the mean) is

Box 2
Cardiac ^{123}I-*m*IBG image interpretation

- Heart to mediastinum ratio
  - Assesses global cardiac ^{123}I-*m*IBG uptake in reference to background
    - Mean counts per pixel in the myocardium divided by mean counts per pixel in mediastinum.
    - Current approach favors measuring cardiac counts via a region of interest around epicardial border and valve plane, excluding liver and lung as much as possible.
    - Mediastinal counts are derived from a 7 $\times$ 7 pixel box in the upper mediastinum below lung apices.
    - Normal values range from 1.9 to 2.8, mean 2.2 $\pm$ 0.3. H/M less than 1.6 (2 SD less than mean) indicates increased risk.
- Washout rate
  - Assess ability to retain tracer
  - Various techniques reports
  - Higher value associated with increased risk
- SPECT
  - Can be scored similar to perfusion imaging with adjustment for globally decreased uptake
  - Regional heterogeneity may help arrhythmic risk stratification

Data from Refs.[15–18]

considered to indicate increased patient risk,[17] although risk increases in a continuous manner as the H/M decreases.[26,27] **Fig. 2** shows examples of normal and abnormal cardiac ^{123}I-*m*IBG uptake.

The WR not only assesses the ability of the myocardium to retain the tracer but may also reflect competition for the NET-1 receptor by circulating NE.[28] A normal WR is reported as 10% $\pm$ 9%, with 27% or more associated with increased mortality risk.[29,30]

Regional assessment of ^{123}I-*m*IBG using SPECT PET imaging can assess heterogeneous sympathetic innervation and may be advantageous for arrhythmic risk stratification.[31,32] A summed score greater than 26 has been associated with increased risk.[33]

CLINICAL APPLICATIONS OF IMAGING WITH IODINE 123 *META*-IODOBENZYLGUANIDINE AND OTHER SYMPATHETIC INNERVATION TRACERS

Myocardial innervation imaging has potential benefits in numerous clinical situations, including HF

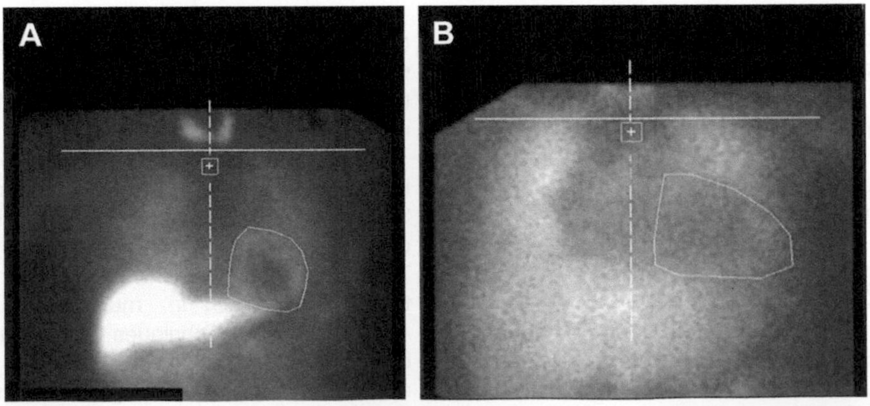

Fig. 2. Examples of planar ^{123}I-*m*IBG images for determination of H/M in patients with systolic heart failure. In (*A*) the H/M was 1.68 consistent with lower risk, and in (*B*) the H/M was 1.17 consistent with increased cardiac risk.

and associated arrhythmias, post–cardiac transplant, primary arrhythmic diseases, myocardial ischemia, diabetes mellitus (DM), and monitoring toxic effects of chemotherapy. Given widespread prevalence, high mortality, and close association with neurohormonal and sympathetic perturbations, HF has been most studied with ^{123}I-*m*IBG imaging.

Iodine 123 meta-Iodobenzylguanidine Imaging to Assess Heart Failure

HF affects approximately 5 million Americans, expected to increase to greater than 8 million by 2030.[34] Annual mortality is 40% to 60%, with a cost greater than $30 billion. Cardiac autonomic abnormalities contribute much to poor outcome. Increased sympathetic tone initially compensates for low CO, but the response often becomes excessive and is then maladaptive with deleterious activation of the RAAS and release of vasoactive substances that contribute to hypertrophy, remodeling, and apoptosis. Further injury and dysfunction often result in a downward clinical spiral toward end-stage HF and death.

Potential utility of ^{123}I-*m*IBG imaging in HF was first reported by Schofer and colleagues[35] who found decreasing tracer uptake as disease worsened. A key study by Merlet and colleagues[36] of NYHA class II–III patients with HF with LVEF less than 45% found an H/M less than 1.2 to be independently associated with 6- and 12-month survivals of 60% and 40%, respectively, versus no deaths when the H/M was 1.2 or more. Nakata and colleagues[26] showed H/M to be related in a continuous fashion to survival. In a meta-analysis of 1755 patients, Verberne and colleagues[37] found an abnormal WR to have a pooled hazard ratio of 1.72 (*P* = .006) for cardiac death and 1.08 (*P*<.001) for cardiac events (cardiac death, myocardial infarction [MI], transplant, HF hospitalization), with the 3 best studies reporting a hazard ratio for late H/M of 1.82 (*P* = .015) for cardiac death and 1.98 (*P*<.001) for cardiac events. A 290-patient study pooling previously collected data from 6 European sites of patients with LVEF 35% or less found that the cardiac event rate increased in a continuous manner as H/M decreased, ranging from less than 5% when H/M was 2.18 or more to more than 50% when H/M was 1.45 or less.[38]

The landmark international AdreView Myocardial Imaging for Risk Evaluation in Heart Failure (ADMIRE-HF) study of 961 patients with NYHA class II–III HF and LVEF 35% or less reported that, an H/M less than 1.6 increased the 17-month occurrence of cardiac events (worsening NYHA class, life-threatening arrhythmias, and cardiac death) from 15% to 37%, with H/M independently predictive relative to numerous variables, including LVEF and BNP, with results shown in **Fig. 3**.[18] Most striking was the extremely high, that is, greater than 99%, negative predictive value for cardiac death. For patients who had H/M 1.6 or more (20% of HF cohort), there were only 2 cardiac deaths, one an arrhythmic death in a patient with an H/M of 1.6 and the other from progressive HF (**Fig. 4**).[39] Among patients with BNP greater than or equal to 100 ng/dL, none with H/M 1.6 or more suffered cardiac death. Thus, among patients with advanced HF and high clinical risk, ^{123}I-*m*IBG imaging identifies a subgroup that is at extremely low risk at least for approximately 2 years. In a subanalysis of ADMIRE-HF data, Ketchum and colleagues[27] reported that H/M added incremental risk stratification power to the

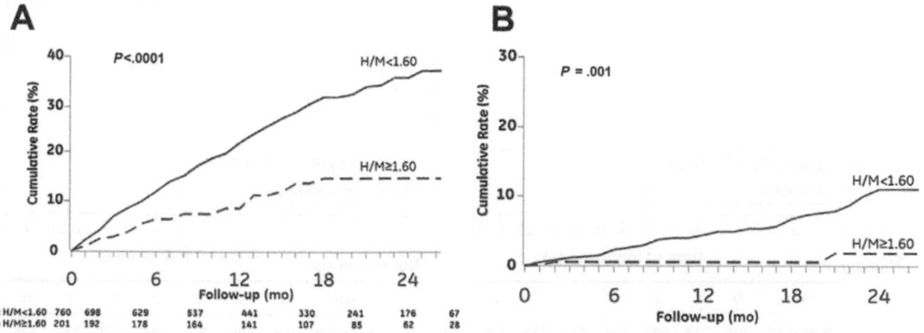

Fig. 3. Cumulative event curves comparing subjects with H/M less than 1.60 versus greater than or equal to 1.60. (*A*) Composite primary end point events including HF progression (increase in NYHA functional class), potentially life-threatening arrhythmic events, and cardiac death. (*B*) Cardiac death in relation to H/M, showing an extremely low 24-month (only 2 of 192 patients) death occurrence for patients with H/M 1.6 or more. (*From* Jacobson AF, Senior R, Cerqueira MD, et al. Myocardial iodine-123 meta-iodobenzylguanidine imaging and cardiac events in heart failure. Results of the prospective ADMIRE-HF (AdreView Myocardial Imaging for Risk Evaluation in Heart Failure) study. J Am Coll Cardiol 2010;55:2216; with permission.)

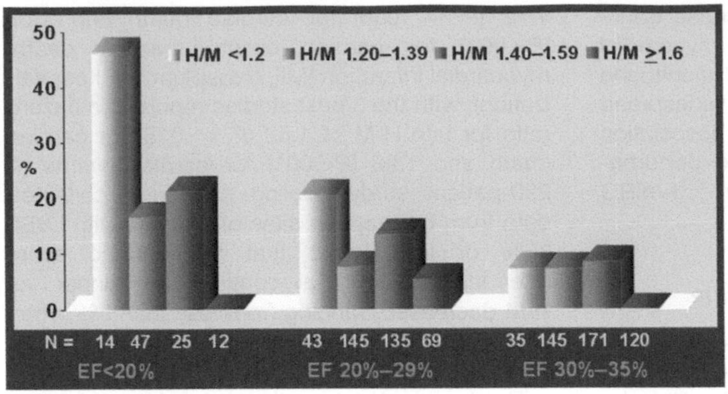

Fig. 4. Relationship of left ventricular ejection fraction (EF) and H/M to 2-year cardiac mortality in the ADMIRE-HF study. (*From* Chirumamilla A, Travin MI. Cardiac applications of ^{123}I-mIBG imaging. Semin Nucl Med 2011;41:380; with permission.)

Seattle Heart Failure Model algorithm of routinely collected demographic, imaging, laboratory, and therapeutic parameters, with 14.9% of subjects who died correctly reclassified as higher risk and 7.9% of patients who survived correctly reclassified as lower risk, a net 22.7% improvement.

Findings similar to ADMIRE-HF were reported by Nakata and colleagues[40] from previously acquired ^{123}I-*m*IBG data of 1322 patients from 6 Japanese centers. As in **Fig. 5**, over approximately 6½ years of follow-up, late HMR (at 1.68) as well as WR (at 43%) well separated patients in terms of all-cause mortality, independent of NYHA class, BNP, LVEF, and age.[40]

Iodine 123 meta-Iodobenzylguanidine Imaging to Manage Patients with Heart Failure

Based on current data, cardiac ^{123}I-*m*IBG imaging is approved in the United States to help identify patients with lower 1- and 2-year mortality risks, as indicated by an H/M greater than or equal to 1.6.[41] Although use of ^{123}I-*m*IBG or PET imaging to direct management, including medical therapy, ICD implantation, CRT, an LVAD, and cardiac transplantation, has not been established, much potential exists in this regard.

Medical Therapy

H/M consistently improves in response to guidelines-directed HF management.[42] Gerson and colleagues[43] showed improved cardiac ^{123}I-*m*IBG uptake after carvedilol therapy, particularly when baseline H/M was less than 1.40. Improved symptoms, functional class, cardiac function, and H/M were reported by various investigators after treatment with metoprolol, angiotensin converting enzyme inhibitors/angiotensin receptor blockers, spironolactone, and amiodarone.[44–48] Nevertheless, innervation imaging is unlikely to

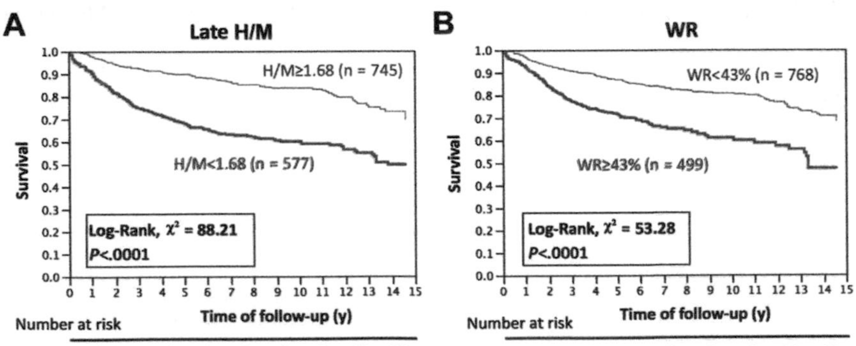

Number at risk

Year	0	1	2	3	5	7	10
H/M≥1.68	745	729	689	634	438	288	179
H/M<1.68	577	526	466	403	290	190	123

Number at risk

Year	0	1	2	3	5	7	10
WR<43%	768	746	700	643	450	330	228
WR≥43%	499	465	415	359	257	129	60

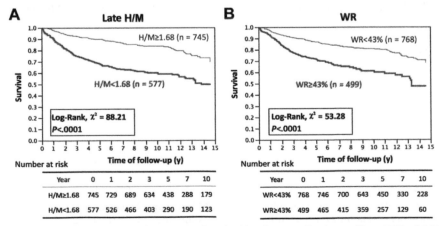

Fig. 5. Kaplan-Meier event-free curves of 2 groups classified by the cutoff values of late H/M of 1.68 (*A*) and WR of 43% (*B*), showing significantly worse survival rates of patients with late H/M <1.68 or WR <43% (*in red*) than their counterparts (*in blue*). (*Reprinted from* Nakata T, Nakajima K, Yamashina S, et al. A pooled analysis of multicenter cohort studies of I-123-mIBG cardiac sympathetic innervation imaging for assessment of long-term prognosis in chronic heart failure. JACC Cardiovascular Imaging 2013;6:776; with permission.)

be used for directing conventional medical therapies as benefit to risk/cost ratios are high. However, Matsui and colleagues[49] reported an H/M decline to be associated with increased mortality, suggesting that ^{123}I-*m*IBG can indicate when medical therapy is insufficient and thus when invasive, high-risk, expensive device therapies should be considered.

Implantable Cardiac Defibrillator

Given reported associations of ^{123}I-*m*IBG image abnormalities with a predisposition to ventricular arrhythmias,[50] attention has been paid to using ^{123}I-*m*IBG to guide ICD implantation.[51] Guidelines recommend LVEF 35% or less as the key parameter for determining ICD need in patients with NYHA class II–III HF.[52] However, this approach is widely understood to be deficient, as most patients with a costly ICD do not receive therapeutic discharges and there are potential serious complications.[53–55] Clinicians often do not follow guidelines indicating that better patient selection methods are essential.[56] As cardiac autonomic innervation more closely relates to the underlying mechanisms of ventricular arrhythmias than LVEF, imaging with ^{123}I-*m*IBG or a PET tracer should help guide ICD use.[57]

Among the first in this regard was Arora and colleagues[58] who reported that, in 17 patients with an ICD, a lower H/M (<1.54) was associated with more frequent ICD discharges (**Fig. 6**). Subsequently, Nagahara and colleagues[59] showed that late H/M correlated with appropriate ICD discharges and SCD and was additive to BNP and LVEF. Studies by Kasama and colleagues[60] and Tamaki and colleagues[61] found WO to be associated with SCD, with the latter study showing statistical independence from HR variability, QT dispersion, and signal-averaged electrocardiogram. In ADMIRE-HF, arrhythmic events (ArEs) and SCD during the 2-year follow-up were rare in patients with H/M 1.6 or greater.[18]

^{123}I-*m*IBG imaging may also identify patients with LVEFs greater than or equal to 35% not meeting ICD implantation criteria but who nevertheless are at risk of ArEs. In fact, the absolute majority of people who suffer fatal ArEs have higher LVEFs and often minimal to no evidence of risk.[62] In an ADMIRE-HF subanalysis, H/M continued to effectively risk stratify patients whose LVEFs at a core laboratory were measured at greater than 35%.[63] Similarly, in patients with LVEF from 36% to more than 50%, Nakata and colleagues[40] reported increased mortality for patients with an H/M less than 1.68.

Despite these robust planar imaging data, many investigators believe that tomographic imaging should be superior for prediction of ArEs given its ability to detect regional abnormalities that would predispose to action potential and impulse conduction heterogeneity. A recent 636-patient meta-analysis study by Verschure and colleagues[64] found that arrhythmic risk assessment with planar imaging was limited. A few small studies have shown potential strength of tomographic imaging for arrhythmic risk stratification. In 50 post-MI patients, Bax and colleagues[31] found an association between inducibility of sustained ventricular arrhythmias and the summed ^{123}I-*m*IBG defect score. In 116 patients with HF receiving ICD implantation, Boogers and

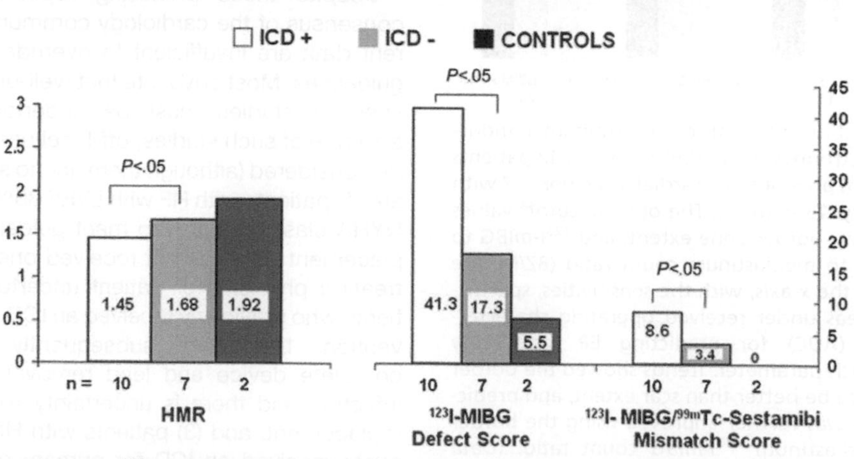

Fig. 6. Planar and SPECT ^{123}I-mIBG results in relation to the occurrence of implantable ICD discharges in 17 patients with ICDs and 2 control patients without heart disease. Compared with patients who did not have an ICD discharge (ICD–), patients with a discharge (ICD+) had a lower mean H/M, a higher mean ^{123}I-*m*IBG defect score, and a higher mean ^{123}I-mIBG/perfusion tracer mismatch score. Tc, technetium. (*From* Travin MI. Cardiac neuronal imaging at the edge of clinical application. Cardiol Clin 2009;27:318; with permission.)

colleagues[33] found that an ^{123}I-*m*IBG SPECT defect score more than a prospectively selected median value of 26 independently predicted future ICD discharges (*P*<.001). Arora and colleagues[58] found that patients with ICD discharges had more extensive tomographic ^{123}I-*m*IBG defects and more extensive autonomic/perfusion mismatches (see **Fig. 6**). A 27-patient study by Marshall and colleagues[65] also found that both summed innervation and innervation/perfusion mismatch scores predicted ArEs.

A potential focus for tomographic ^{123}I-*m*IBG is border zone regions containing mixtures of scar and viable tissue that increase susceptibility to arrhythmias.[66] In particular, in patients with scar from prior MI or another pathologic process, such border zones may become fully or partially denervated as sympathetic fibers are more easily damaged and dysfunctional longer than are cardiomyocytes. Zhou and colleagues[67] fount that a border zone ^{123}I-*m*IBG to mediastinum count cut-off ratio of 2.2 was better predictive of electrophysiologic inducibility than both scar and border zone extent (**Fig. 7**). Klein and colleagues[68] reported on 15 patients with ischemic cardiomyopathy referred for electrophysiologic ventricular tachycardia (VT) ablation, showing that successful ablation sites were often located in ^{123}I-*m*IBG denervation border areas outside of voltage-mapped scar.

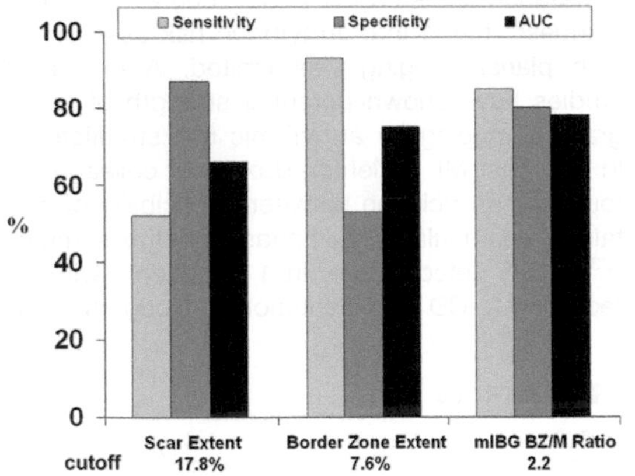

Fig. 7. Prediction of ventricular arrhythmia inducibility on electrophysiologic (EP) testing in 42 patients with scar from previous myocardial infarction, 27 with EP inducibility, 15 without. The optimal cutoff values for scar extent, border zone extent, and ^{123}I-*m*IBG to border zone to mediastinum count ratio (BZ/M) are indicated on the *x*-axis, with the sensitivities, specificities, and areas under received operating characteristic curves (AUC) for predicting EP inducibility shown for each parameter. Trends showed the border zone extent to be better than scar extent, and predictive accuracy was further improved using the border zone to mediastinum ^{123}I-*m*IBG count ratio. (*Data from* Zhou Y, Zhou W, Folks RD, et al. I-123 mIBG and Tc-99m myocardial SPECT imaging to predict inducibility of ventricular arrhythmia on electrophysiology testing: a retrospective analysis. J Nucl Cardiol 2014;21:913–20.)

Unfortunately, there are problems using SPECT for fine assessment of regional adrenergic abnormalities. In many cases, tracer uptake is minimal and sometimes barely appreciated. Image interpretation is often impaired by overlying lung and liver activity. A potential solution may be use of newer solid-state cadmium-zinc-telluride detector cameras with enhanced collimation that have superior count detection and improved spatial and energy resolution compared with standard Anger cameras. Using a Discovery NM 530c imaging system (GE Healthcare, Haifa, Israel), Gimelli and colleagues[21] reported that 85% of patients had good or better ^{123}I-*m*IBG images with 97% and 98% intraobserver and interobserver agreement, respectively.

Further evidence of tomographic imaging helping to identifying risk of lethal arrhythmias was provided by Fallavollita and colleagues[69] using ^{11}C-HED. The higher resolution of PET improved defect detection in a porcine model.[13] As in **Fig. 8**, the Prediction of Arrhythmic Events with Positron Emission Tomography (PARAPET) study of 200 patients with ischemic cardiomyopathy reported that, over 4 years, sudden cardiac arrest (arrhythmic death or ICD shock for VT >240 per minute or ventricular fibrillation) increased in relation to the severity/extent of ^{11}C-HED tomographic abnormalities independent of BNP, clinical symptoms, or LVEF.[69]

Despite these promising reports, it is the consensus of the cardiology community that current data are insufficient to override established guidelines. Most advocate that well-designed prospective studies must be undertaken. In the absence of such studies, off-label uses that might be considered (although there are no specific data) are (1) patients with HF with LVEF 35% or less and NYHA class II or III who meet guidelines for ICD placement but have not received one because of treating physician or patient uncertainty, (2) patients who previously received an ICD for SCD prevention but who subsequently underwent complete device and lead removal because of infection and there is uncertainty regarding ICD replacement, and (3) patients with HF who previously received an ICD for primary prevention of SCD when their LVEF was 35% or less, have had no clinically relevant ventricular arrhythmias since implant, have had improvement of LVEF, but require generator replacement. Development of

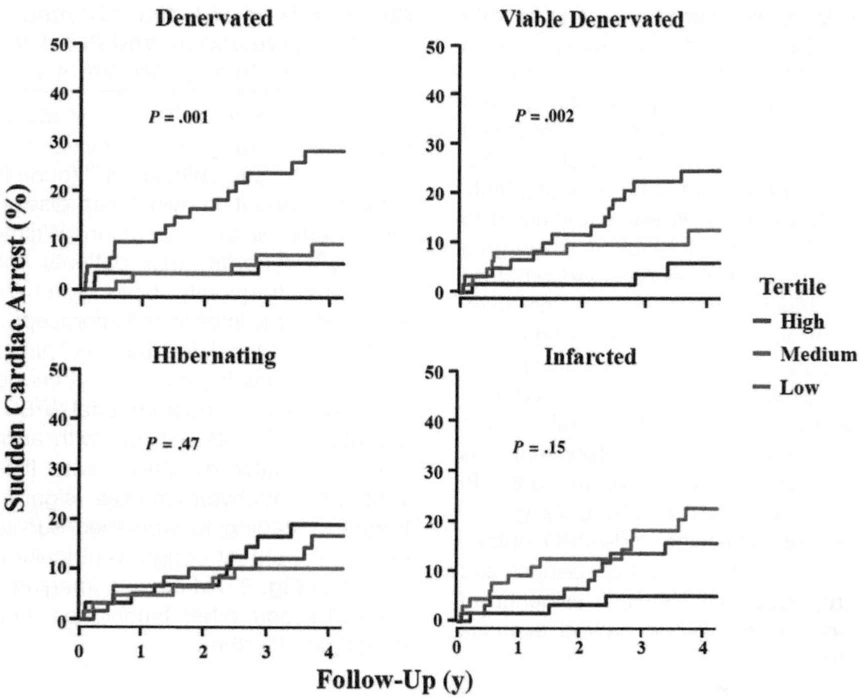

Fig. 8. PET parameters and sudden cardiac arrest. Kaplan-Meier curves showing the incidence of sudden cardiac arrest for tertiles of PET-defined myocardial substrates (median follow-up 4.1 years). As continuous variables, the total volume of denervated, as well as viable denervated, myocardium predicted sudden cardiac arrest. Neither infarct volume nor hibernating myocardium was significant as continuous variable. (*From* Fallavollita JA, Heavey BM, Luisi AJ Jr, et al. Regional myocardial sympathetic denervation predicts the risk of sudden cardiac arrest in ischemic cardiomyopathy. J Am Coll Cardiol 2014;63:145; with permission.)

registries has been suggested to assess practical clinical utility, but at the moment financial considerations are a major challenge.

End-Stage Heart Failure: Cardiac Resynchronization Therapy, Left Ventricular Assist Device, Transplant

Patients with class IV HF have an extremely poor prognosis despite optimal medical therapy and are candidates for advanced therapies, including CRT, implantation of an LVAD, and if not sufficient then cardiac transplant. ^{123}I-*m*IBG imaging shows potential utility for guiding these therapies.

CRT improves outcome in selected patients, but one-fourth to one-third who meet current indications do not respond. D'Orio Nishioka and colleagues[70] reported that an H/M greater than 1.36 predicted CRT response better than echocardiographic dimensions, LVEF, age, and NYHA class, with a sensitivity of 75% and specificity of 71%. Tanaka and colleagues[71] saw that H/M combined with dyssynchrony on echocardiography separated CRT responders from nonresponders. Low H/M may indicate a severely damaged ventricle unable to remodel despite CRT, or excessively damaged, scarred myocytes unresponsive to pacer stimuli.

^{123}I-*m*IBG imaging could conceivably guide LVAD therapy initiation, but the author is unaware of reports at this time. Small studies have shown improvement in tracer uptake in response to LVAD therapy. After 3 months of HeartMate (Thoratec Corporation, Pleasanton, CA, USA) therapy in 12 patients with end-stage HF, Drakos and colleagues[72] found that an H/M increase correlated with improvements in other HF markers. George and colleagues[73] studied 14 patients with a HeartMate II LVAD and after about 200 days saw a 54.7% increase in H/M, trending higher in 10 patients who underwent LVAD explantation. Potentially, ^{123}I-*m*IBG imaging could help identify patients amenable to explantation rather than permanent device therapy or transplant.

In many patients with end-stage HF, the only hope for improved life quality and survival is transplantation, but donor shortages require prioritization. ^{123}I-*m*IBG could potentially assist with patient selection. Cohen-Solal and colleagues[74] found that H/M predicted death or need for transplant better than LVEF in patients with class II–III HF but was not better than peak exercise oxygen consumption (V_{O_2}). In contrast, in patients with advanced HF, Gerson and colleagues[75] found that only H/M predicted transplant independently of peak V_{O_2} and other variables. Previously cited work by Verschure and colleagues[64] reported that late H/M, LVEF, age, and baseline LVEF were independent predictors of future transplant.

There are data on using adrenergic imaging to help manage patients after transplant. Although a transplanted heart is initially denervated with loss of proper ventricular function and coronary blood flow control, there is partial progressive sympathetic reinnervation that can be imaged. At about 7 years posttransplant, DiCarli and colleagues[76] saw increased ^{11}C-HED uptake in the left anterior descending artery territory that was associated with an improved flow response to cold pressor stimuli. Estorch and colleagues[77] found that lack of increasing ^{123}I-*m*IBG uptake was associated with vasculopathy. Bengel and colleagues[78] reported that ^{11}C-HED evidence of reinnervation correlated with improved exercise hemodynamics.

Potential Uses of Iodine 123 meta-iodobenzylguanidine and PET Adrenergic Imaging for Primary Arrhythmias

There are numerous reports of abnormal adrenergic image findings in primary ventricular arrhythmias. Mitrani and colleagues[79] found that patients with VT without known heart disease had ^{123}I-*m*IBG regional dysinnervation. Wichter and colleagues[80] reported that patients with Brugada syndrome frequently have adrenergic defects localized to the inferior and inferoseptal walls, suggesting that a local dominance of parasympathetic tone there may increase arrhythmogenesis. Paul and colleagues[81] reported focal SPECT ^{123}I-*m*IBG defects in 59% of patients with arrhythmogenic right ventricular dysplasia, with life-threatening ventricular tachyarrhythmias significantly more frequent, leading to worsened survival independent of the extent of right ventricular dysfunction, shown in **Fig. 9**. Adrenergic imaging provides insights beyond other techniques and should be investigated further.

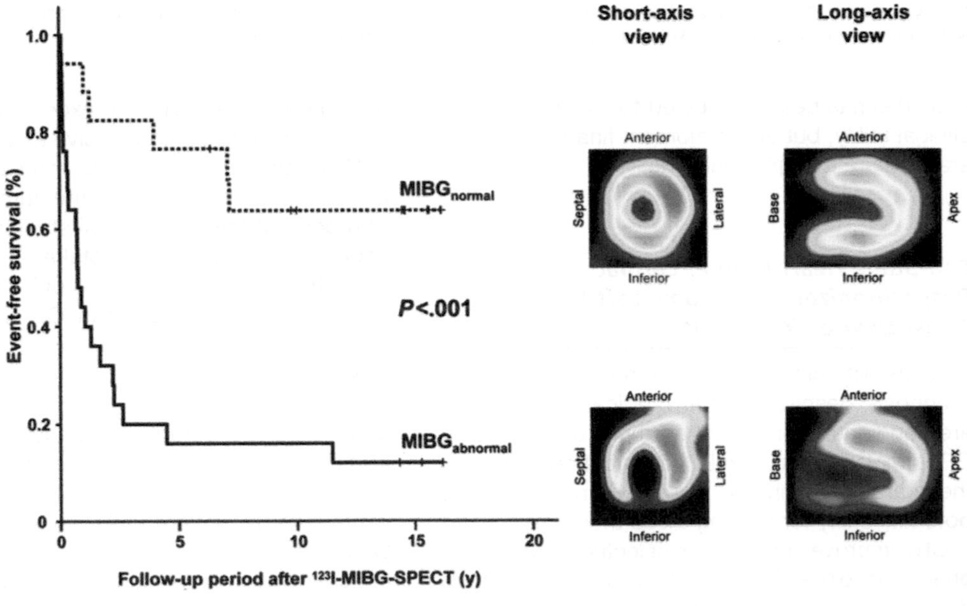

Event-free survivors at time	0 y	5 y	10 y	15 y of follow-up
$MIBG_{normal}$, *n*	17	13	9	5
$MIBG_{abnormal}$, *n*	25	4	4	2

Fig. 9. Event-free survival (ie, sustained VT) during years of follow-up of study population for normal ($MIBG_{normal}$) versus abnormal ($MIBG_{abnormal}$) ^{123}I-*m*IBG uptake. At right are typical ^{123}I-*m*IBG images. (*From* Paul M, Wichter T, Kies P, et al. Cardiac sympathetic dysfunction in genotyped patients with arrhythmogenic right ventricular cardiomyopathy and risk of recurrent ventricular tachyarrhythmias. J Nucl Med 2011;52:1563; with permission.)

Potential Uses of Adrenergic Imaging to Assess Ischemia

Although cardiomyocytes are affected by myocardial ischemia, adrenergic innervation is affected more so because of increased sensitivity to oxygen deprivation.[82] As sympathetic nerves follow the course of coronary arteries, infarction affects not only the vascular distribution at risk but also the distal adrenergic innervation.[32,82] Infarction can result in both denervation (from fibrotic replacement of tissue) and dysinnervation (ie, dysfunction). Ischemic adrenergic dysinnervation persists longer than myocyte impairment. About 1 to 2 weeks after infarction, although perfusion abnormalities reflect final myocyte damage, adrenergic defects represent the larger area that had been threatened.[83,84] ^{123}I-*m*IBG imaging also shows potential as ischemic memory imaging tool.[85] As adrenergic imaging has much potential for assessing ischemia and infarction, more investigations are warranted.

Adrenergic Imaging to Assess Myocardial Effects of Diabetes Mellitus

DM is associated with autonomic neuropathy. Cardiac imaging with ^{123}I-*m*IBG or ^{11}C-HED shows abnormalities even in the absence of clinically manifest neuropathy.[86] In a study by Hattori and colleagues,[87] ^{123}I-*m*IBG SPECT defects were seen in 80% of 31 patients with type II DM, most often involving the inferior wall and adjacent regions. Image findings of cardiac autonomic neuropathy have been associated with a worsened clinical situation. Sacre and colleagues[88] found regional ^{123}I-*m*IBG defects to correlate with diastolic abnormalities on tissue Doppler echocardiography. Nagamachi and colleagues[89] reported that for diabetic patients, a late H/M less than 1.7 was independently associated with worsened 7-year survival.

SUMMARY

There is vast potential for clinical applications of cardiac adrenergic imaging with ^{123}I-*m*IBG and analogous PET tracers. The technique examines underlying cardiac physiology and pathophysiology in ways that other imaging or clinical techniques cannot. Studies report consistent, robust ability to detect high risk in a variety of clinical scenarios, most notably HF and associated ventricular arrhythmias, following heart transplant, in the setting of primary ventricular arrhythmias, for patients with ischemic heart disease, and in diabetic patients. However, as with all medical testing in the current era and for imaging procedures in particular, it has become essential not only to show high diagnostic and risk stratification power but also to demonstrate that there is improved patient outcome beyond other methods. As per Shaw and colleagues,[90] the value of any form of cardiovascular imaging depends on the findings leading to "appropriate and targeted therapies that improve symptom burden and long-term outcomes…[that] are not offset by high upfront procedural and induced costs, [and the clinical benefit] must significantly outweigh any untoward risks associated with imaging…." Imaging myocardial innervation should be able to meet this standard, but clear demonstration is still required.

REFERENCES

1. Bell DR. Control mechanisms in circulatory function. In: Rhoades RA, Bell DR, editors. Medical physiology: principles of clinical medicine. 4th edition. Philadelphia: Lippincott, Williams & Wilkins; 2013. p. 317–20.
2. Anand IS, Fisher LD, Chiang YT, et al, Val-HeFT Investigators. Changes in brain natriuretic peptide and norepinephrine over time and mortality and morbidity in the Valsartan Heart Failure Trial (Val-HeFT). Circulation 2003;107:1278–83.
3. Goldstein DS, Eisenhofer G, Kopin IJ. Sources and significance of plasma levels of catechols and their metabolites in humans. J Pharmacol Exp Ther 2003;305:800–11.
4. Kapa S, Somers VK. Cardiovascular manifestations of autonomic disorders. In: Libby P, Bonow RO, Mann DL, et al, editors. Braunwald's heart disease: a textbook of cardiovascular medicine. 8th edition. Philadelphia: Saunders Elsevier; 2008. p. 2171–83.
5. Travin MI. Cardiac neuronal imaging at the edge of clinical application. Cardiol Clin 2009;27:311–27.
6. Sisson JC, Wieland DM. Radiolabeled meta-iodobenzylguanidine pharmacology: pharmacology and clinical studies. Am J Physiol Imaging 1986;1:96–103.
7. Raffel DM, Wieland DM. Development of mIBG as a cardiac innervation imaging agent. JACC Cardiovasc Imaging 2010;3:111–6.
8. Counsell RE, Yu T, Ranade VV, et al. Radioiodinated bretylium analogs for myocardial scanning. J Nucl Med 1974;15:991–6.
9. Wieland DM, Mangner TJ, Inbasekaran MN, et al. Adrenal medulla imaging agents: a structure distribution relationship study of radiolabeled aralkylguandines. J Med Chem 1984;27:149–55.
10. Kline RC, Swanson DP, Wieland DM, et al. Myocardial imaging in man with I-123 meta-iodobenzylguanidine. J Nucl Med 1981;22:129–32.
11. Sisson J, Shapiro B, Meyers L, et al. Metaiodobenzylguanidine to map scintigraphically the

adrenergic nervous system in man. J Nucl Med 1987;28:1625–36.
12. Bengel FM, Schwaiger M. Assessment of cardiac sympathetic neuronal function using PET imaging. J Nucl Cardiol 2004;11:603–16.
13. Luisi AJ, Suzuki G, deKemp R, et al. Regional ^{11}C-hydroxyephedrine retention in hibernating myocardium: chronic inhomogeneity of sympathetic innervation in the absence of infarction. J Nucl Med 2005;46:1368–74.
14. Sinusas AJ, Lazewatsky J, Brunetti J, et al. Biodistribution and radiation dosimetry of LMI1195: first-in-human study of a novel 18F-labeled tracer for imaging myocardial innervation. J Nucl Med 2014;55:1–7.
15. Flotats A, Carrió I, Agostini D, et al. Proposal for standardization of ^{123}I-metaiodobenzylguanidine (MIBG) cardiac sympathetic imaging by the EANM Cardiovascular Committee and the European Council of Nuclear Cardiology. Eur J Nucl Med Mol Imaging 2010;37:1802–12.
16. Travin MI. Cardiac autonomic imaging with SPECT tracers. J Nucl Cardiol 2013;20:128–43.
17. Jacobson AF, Lombard J, Banerjee G, et al. ^{123}I-*m*IBG scintigraphy to predict risk for adverse cardiac outcomes in heart failure patients: design of two prospective multicenter international trials. J Nucl Cardiol 2009;16:113–21.
18. Jacobson AF, Senior R, Cerqueira MD, et al. Myocardial iodine-123 meta-iodobenzylguanidine imaging and cardiac events in heart failure. Results of the prospective ADMIRE-HF (AdreView Myocardial Imaging for Risk Evaluation in Heart Failure) study. J Am Coll Cardiol 2010;55:2212–21.
19. Verberne HJ, Feenstra C, de Jong WM, et al. Influence of collimator choice and simulated clinical conditions on ^{123}I-MIBG heart/mediastinum ratios: a phantom study. Eur J Nucl Med Mol Imaging 2005; 32:1100–7.
20. Nakajima K, Okuda K, Matsuo S, et al. Standardization of metaiodobenzylguanidine heart to mediastinum ratio using a calibration phantom: effects of correction on normal databases and a multicentre study. Eur J Nucl Med Mol Imaging 2012; 39:113–9.
21. Gimelli A, Liga R, Giorgetti A, et al. Assessment of myocardial adrenergic innervation with a solid-state dedicated cardiac cadmium-zinc-telluride camera: first clinical experience. Eur Heart J Cardiovasc Imaging 2014;15:575–85.
22. Bellevre D, Manrique A, Baavour R, et al. First determination of the heart-to-mediastinum ratio in I-123-MIBG cardiac adrenergic CZT imaging in patients with heart failure. A D-SPECT versus A-SPECT prospective study. J Nucl Med 2014;55(Suppl 1):1725.
23. Jacobson AF, Chen J, Verdes L, et al. Impact of age on myocardial uptake of ^{123}I-*m*IBG in older subjects without coronary heart disease. J Nucl Cardiol 2013; 20:406–14.
24. Chen JI, Folks RD, Verdes L, et al. Quantitative I-123 mIBG SPECT in differentiating abnormal and normal mIBG myocardial uptake. J Nucl Cardiol 2012;19:92–9.
25. Strydhorst J, Wells RG, Ruddy T. Phantom validation of 123-I-mIBG imaging with a dedicated solid state SPECT camera. J Nucl Med 2014;55(Suppl 1):1689.
26. Nakata T, Miyamoto K, Doi A, et al. Cardiac death prediction and impaired cardiac sympathetic innervation assessed by MIBG in patients with failing and nonfailing hearts. J Nucl Cardiol 1998;5:579–90.
27. Ketchum ES, Jacobson AF, Caldwell JH, et al. Selective improvement in Seattle Heart Failure Model risk stratification using iodine-123 meta-iodobenzylguanidine imaging. J Nucl Cardiol 2012;19:1007–16.
28. Chen GP, Tabibiazar R, Branch KR, et al. Cardiac receptor physiology and imaging: an update. J Nucl Cardiol 2005;12:714–30.
29. Somsen GA, Verberne HJ, Fleury E, et al. Normal values and within-subject variability of cardiac I-123 MIBG scintigraphy in healthy individuals: implications for clinical studies. J Nucl Cardiol 2004;11: 126–33.
30. Ogita H, Shimonagata T, Fukunami M, et al. Prognostic significance of cardiac ^{123}I metaiodobenzylguanidine imaging for mortality and morbidity in patients with chronic heart failure: a prospective study. Heart 2001;86:656–60.
31. Bax JJ, Kraft O, Buxton AE, et al. ^{123}I-*m*IBG scintigraphy to predict inducibility of ventricular arrhythmias on cardiac electrophysiology testing: a prospective multicenter pilot study. Circ Cardiovasc Imaging 2008;1:131–40.
32. Minardo JD, Tuli MM, Mock BH, et al. Scintigraphic and electrophysiologic evidence of canine myocardial sympathetic denervation and reinnervation produced by myocardial infarction or phenol application. Circulation 1988;78:1008–19.
33. Boogers MJ, Borleffs CJ, Henneman MM, et al. Cardiac sympathetic denervation assessed with 123-iodine metaiodobenzylguanidine imaging predicts ventricular arrhythmias in implantable cardioverter-defibrillator patients. J Am Coll Cardiol 2010;55: 2769–77.
34. Go AS, Mozaffarian D, Roger VL, et al, on behalf of the American Heart Association Statistics Committee and Stroke Statistics Subcommittee. Heart disease and stroke statistics – 2014 update: a report from the American Heart Association. Circulation 2014;129:e28–292.
35. Schofer J, Spielmann R, Schuchert A, et al. Iodine-123 meta-iodobenzylguanidine scintigraphy: a noninvasive method to demonstrate myocardial adrenergic nervous system disintegrity in patients with idiopathic dilated cardiomyopathy. J Am Coll Cardiol 1988;12:1252–8.

36. Merlet P, Valette H, Dubois-Randé J, et al. Prognostic value of cardiac metaiodobenzylguanidine in patients with heart failure. J Nucl Med 1992;33: 471–7.
37. Verberne HJ, Brewster LM, Somsen GA, et al. Prognostic value of myocardial 123I-metaiodobenzylguanidine (MIBG) parameters in patients with heart failure: a systematic review. Eur Heart J 2008;29: 1147–59.
38. Agostini D, Verberne HJ, Burchert W, et al. I-123-*m*IBG myocardial imaging for assessment of risk for a major cardiac event in heart failure patients: insights from a retrospective European multicenter study. Eur J Nucl Med Mol Imaging 2008;35:535–46.
39. Chirumamilla A, Travin MI. Cardiac applications of ^{123}I-mIBG imaging. Semin Nucl Med 2011;41: 374–87.
40. Nakata T, Nakajima K, Yamashina S, et al. A pooled analysis of multicenter cohort studies of I-123-mIBG cardiac sympathetic innervation imaging for assessment of long-term prognosis in chronic heart failure. JACC Cardiovasc Imaging 2013;6:772–84.
41. FDA [package insert]. Available at: http://medlibrary.org/lib/rx/meds/adreview-1/. Accessed March 2, 2015.
42. Treglia G, Stefanelli I, Giordano BA. Clinical usefulness of myocardial innervation imaging using iodine-123-meta-iodobenzylguanidine scintigraphy in evaluating the effectiveness of pharmacological treatments in patients with heart failure: an overview. Eur Rev Med Pharmacol Sci 2013;17:56–8.
43. Gerson MC, Craft LL, McGuire N, et al. Carvedilol improves left ventricular function in heart failure with idiopathic dilated cardiomyopathy and a wide range of sympathetic nervous system function as measured by iodine 123 metaiodobenzylguanidine. J Nucl Cardiol 2002;9:608–15.
44. Toyama T, Aihara Y, Iwasaki T, et al. Cardiac sympathetic activity estimated by 123I-MIBG myocardial imaging in patients with dilated cardiomyopathy after β-blocker or angiotensin-converting enzyme inhibitor therapy. J Nucl Med 1999;40:217–23.
45. Somsen GA, Vlies BV, de Milliano PA, et al. Increased myocardial [123-I]-metaiodobenzylguanidine uptake after enalapril treatment in patients with chronic heart failure. Heart 1996;76:218–22.
46. Kasama S, Toyama T, Kumakura H. Effects of candesartan on cardiac sympathetic nerve activity in patients with congestive heart failure and preserved LVEF. J Am Coll Cardiol 2005;45:661–7.
47. Kasama S, Toyama T, Kumakura H, et al. Effect of spironolactone on cardiac sympathetic nerve activity and left ventricular remodeling in patients with dilated cardiomyopathy. J Am Coll Cardiol 2003; 41:574–81.
48. Toyama T, Hoshizaki H, Seki R, et al. Efficacy of amiodarone treatment on cardiac symptom, function and sympathetic nerve activity in patients with dilated cardiomyopathy: comparison with beta-blocker therapy. J Nucl Cardiol 2004;11:134–41.
49. Matsui T, Tsutamoto T, Maeda K, et al. Prognostic value of repeated ^{123}I-metaiodobenzylguanidine imaging in patients with dilated cardiomyopathy with congestive heart failure before and after optimized treatments – comparison with neurohumoral factors. Circ J 2002;66:537–43.
50. Klein T, Dilsizian V, Chen W, et al. The potential role of iodine-123 *meta*iodobenzylguanidine imaging for identifying sustained ventricular tachycardia in patients with cardiomyopathy. Curr Cardiol Rep 2013; 15:359–67.
51. Gerson MC, Abdallah M, Muth JN, et al. Will imaging assist in the selection of patients with heart failure for an ICD? JACC Cardiovasc Imaging 2010;3:101–10.
52. Jessup M, Abraham WT, Casey DE, et al, writing on behalf of the 2005 Guideline Update for the Diagnosis and Management of Chronic Heart Failure in the Adult Writing Committee. 2009 Focused update: ACCF/AHA guidelines for the diagnosis and management of heart failure in adults: a report of the American College of Cardiology/American Heart Association Task Force on Practice Guidelines. J Am Coll Cardiol 2009;53:1343–82.
53. Buxton AE, Lee KL, Hafley GE, et al. Limitations of ejection fraction for prediction of sudden death risk in patients with coronary artery disease: lessons from the MUSTT study. J Am Coll Cardiol 2007;50:1150–7.
54. Myerburg RJ. Implantable cardioverter-defibrillators after myocardial infarction. N Engl J Med 2008;359: 2245–53.
55. Lee DS, Krahn AD, Healey JS, et al. Evaluation of early complications related to de novo cardioverter defibrillator implantation insights from the Ontario ICD database. J Am Coll Cardiol 2010;55:774–82.
56. Al-Khatib SM, Hellkamp A, Curtis J, et al. Non-evidence-based ICD implantations in the United States. JAMA 2011;305:43–9.
57. Tomaselli GF, Zipes DP. What causes sudden death in heart failure? Circ Res 2004;95:754–63.
58. Arora R, Ferrick KJ, Nakata T, et al. I-123 MIBG imaging and heart rate variability analysis to predict the needs for an implantable cardioverter defibrillator. J Nucl Cardiol 2003;10:121–31.
59. Nagahara D, Nakata T, Hashimoto A, et al. Predicting the need for an implantable cardioverter defibrillator using cardiac metaiodobenzylguanidine activity together with plasma natriuretic peptide concentration or left ventricular function. J Nucl Med 2008;49:225–33.
60. Kasama S, Toyama T, Sumino H, et al. Prognostic value of serial cardiac 123I-MIBG imaging in patients with stabilized chronic heart failure and reduced left ventricular ejection fraction. J Nucl Med 2008;49:907–14.

61. Tamaki S, Yamada T, Okuyama Y, et al. Cardiac iodine-123 metaiodobenzylguanidine imaging predicts sudden cardiac death independently of left ventricular ejection fraction in patients with chronic heart failure and left ventricular systolic dysfunction: results from a comparative study with signal-averaged electrocardiogram, heart rate variability, and QT dispersion. J Am Coll Cardiol 2009;53:426–35.
62. Stecker EC, Vickers C, Waltz J, et al. Population-based analysis of sudden cardiac death with and without left ventricular systolic dysfunction: two-year findings from the Oregon Sudden Unexpected Death Study. J Am Coll Cardiol 2006;47:1161–6.
63. Shah AM, Bourgoun M, Narula J, et al. Influence of ejection fraction on the prognostic value of sympathetic innervation imaging with iodine-123 MIBG in heart failure. JACC Cardiovasc Imaging 2012;5:1139–46.
64. Verschure DO, Veltman CE, Manrique A, et al. For what endpoint does myocardial ^{123}I-MIBG scintigraphy have the greatest prognostic value in patients with chronic heart failure? Results of a pooled individual patient data meta-analysis. Eur Heart J Cardiovasc Imaging 2014;15:996–1003.
65. Marshall A, Cheetham A, George RS, et al. Cardiac iodine-123 metaiodobenzylguanidine imaging predicts ventricular arrhythmia in heart failure patients receiving an implantable cardioverter-defibrillator for primary prevention. Heart 2012;98:1359–65.
66. Roes SD, Borleffs XJ, van der Geest RJ, et al. Infarct tissue heterogeneity assessed with contrast-enhanced MRI predicts spontaneous ventricular arrhythmia in patients with ischemic cardiomyopathy and implantable cardioverter-defibrillator. Circ Cardiovasc Imaging 2009;2:183–90.
67. Zhou Y, Zhou W, Folks RD, et al. I-123 mIBG and Tc-99m myocardial SPECT imaging to predict inducibility of ventricular arrhythmia on electrophysiology testing: a retrospective analysis. J Nucl Cardiol 2014;21:913–20.
68. Klein T, Abdulghani MS, Asoglu R, et al. Three-dimensional 123I-meta-iodobenzylguanidine (123I mIBG) cardiac innervation maps to guide ablation of ventricular tachycardia - a novel paradigm introducing innervation imaging in ablation therapy. Circulation 2014;130:A17789.
69. Fallavollita JA, Heavey BM, Luisi AJ Jr, et al. Regional myocardial sympathetic denervation predicts the risk of sudden cardiac arrest in ischemic cardiomyopathy. J Am Coll Cardiol 2014;63:141–9.
70. D'Orio Nishioka SA, Filho MM, Soares Brandão SC, et al. Cardiac sympathetic activity pre and post resynchronization therapy evaluated by ^{123}I-MIBG myocardial scintigraphy. J Nucl Cardiol 2007;14:852–9.
71. Tanaka H, Tatsumi K, Fujiwara S, et al. Effect of left ventricular dyssynchrony on cardiac sympathetic activity in heart failure patients with wide QRS duration. Circ J 2012;76:382–9.
72. Drakos SG, Athanasoulis T, Malliaras KG, et al. Myocardial sympathetic innervation and long-term left ventricular mechanical unloading. JACC Cardiovasc Imaging 2010;3:64–70.
73. George RS, Birks EJ, Cheetham A, et al. The effect of long-term left ventricular assist device support on myocardial sympathetic activity in patients with non-ischaemic dilated cardiomyopathy. Eur J Heart Fail 2013;15:1035–43.
74. Cohen-Solal A, Esanu Y, Logeart D, et al. Cardiac metaiodobenzylguanidine uptake in patients with moderate chronic heart failure: relationship with peak oxygen uptake and prognosis. J Am Coll Cardiol 1999;33:759–66.
75. Gerson MC, McGuire N, Wagoner LE. Sympathetic nervous system function as measured by I-123 metaiodobenzylguanidine predicts transplant-free survival in heart failure patients with idiopathic dilated cardiomyopathy. J Card Fail 2003;9:384–91.
76. Di Carli MF, Tobes MC, Mangner T, et al. Effects of cardiac sympathetic innervation on coronary blood flow. N Engl J Med 1997;336:1208–15.
77. Estorch M, Campreciós M, Flotats A, et al. Sympathetic reinnervation of cardiac allografts evaluated by ^{123}I-MIBG imaging. J Nucl Med 1999;40:911–6.
78. Bengel FM, Ueberfuhr P, Schiepel N, et al. Effect of sympathetic reinnervation on cardiac performance after heart transplantation. N Engl J Med 2001;345:731–8.
79. Mitrani RD, Klein LS, Miles WM, et al. Regional cardiac sympathetic denervation in patients with ventricular tachycardia in the absence of coronary artery disease. J Am Coll Cardiol 1993;22:1344–53.
80. Wichter T, Matheja P, Eckardt L, et al. Cardiac autonomic dysfunction in Brugada syndrome. Circulation 2002;105:702–6.
81. Paul M, Wichter T, Kies P, et al. Cardiac sympathetic dysfunction in genotyped patients with arrhythmogenic right ventricular cardiomyopathy and risk of recurrent ventricular tachyarrhythmias. J Nucl Med 2011;52:1559–65.
82. Henneman MM, Bengel FM, Bax JJ. Will innervation imaging predict ventricular arrhythmias in ischaemic cardiomyopathy? Eur J Nucl Med Mol Imaging 2006;33:862–5.
83. Matsunari I, Schricke U, Bengel FM, et al. Extent of cardiac sympathetic neuronal damage is determined by the area of ischemia in patients with acute coronary syndromes. Circulation 2000;101:2579–85.

84. Simões MV, Barthel P, Matsunari I, et al. Presence of sympathetically denervated but viable myocardium and its electrophysiologic correlates after early revascularised, acute myocardial infarction. Eur Heart J 2004;25:551–7.

85. Inobe Y, Kugiyama K, Miyagi H, et al. Long-lasting abnormalities in cardiac sympathetic nervous system in patients with coronary spastic angina: quantitative analysis with iodine 123 metaiodobenzylguanidine myocardial scintigraphy. Am Heart J 1997;134:112–8.

86. Langer A, Freeman MR, Josse RG, et al. Metaiodobenzylguanidine imaging in diabetes mellitus: assessment of cardiac sympathetic denervation and its relation to autonomic dysfunction and silent myocardial ischemia. J Am Coll Cardiol 1995;25:610–8.

87. Hattori N, Tamaki N, Hayashi T, et al. Regional abnormality of iodine-123-MIBG in diabetic hearts. J Nucl Med 1996;37:1985–90.

88. Sacre JW, Franjic B, Jellis CL, et al. Association of cardiac autonomic neuropathy with subclinical myocardial dysfunction in type 2 diabetes. JACC Cardiovasc Imaging 2010;3:1207–15.

89. Nagamachi S, Fujita S, Nishii R, et al. Prognostic value of cardiac I-123 metaiodobenzylguanidine imaging in patients with non-insulin-dependent diabetes mellitus. J Nucl Cardiol 2006;13:34–42.

90. Shaw LJ, Min JK, Hachamovitch R, et al. Cardiovascular imaging research at the crossroads. JACC Cardiovasc Imaging 2010;3:316–24.

Radionuclide Imaging of Cardiovascular Infection

Fozia Zahir Ahmed, MBChB, MRCP[a,1], Jackie James, MBChB, MSc, MD, FRCP[b,1], Matthew J. Memmott, MSci, MSc[b], Parthiban Arumugam, MBBS, MSc, FRCP[b,*]

KEYWORDS

• Cardiovascular infection • Pacemaker infection • Infective endocarditis • Radionuclide imaging • [^{18}F] FDG-PET/CT

KEY POINTS

- There is growing evidence to support the role of fludeoxyglucose F 18 ([^{18}F] FDG) PET/computed tomographic (CT) imaging in patients with suspected cardiovascular prosthetic and device infections.
- Diagnosis of cardiac implantable electronic device (CIED)-generator pocket infection (GPI) is challenging because of nonspecific clinical presentations, and [^{18}F] FDG-PET/CT may be most valuable in this group because of its high negative predictive value.
- [^{18}F]-FDG PET/CT could be a problem-solving tool in patients with suspected valve infective endocarditis (IE) (particularly prosthetic valves), with positive blood cultures but negative echocardiogram, and also in the detection of distant septic emboli.
- Evidence is emerging regarding the potential utility of hybrid radionuclide imaging in suspected vascular graft infection.

INTRODUCTION

Cardiovascular infection can be broadly split into 2 main groups: nonvalvular infections, which are usually associated with a CIED or prosthetic material, and valvular infections, which can affect both native and prosthetic valves. Despite this arbitrary classification, both types of infection are associated with significant morbidity and mortality. Furthermore, delays in diagnosing infection in difficult cases may delay appropriate treatment, further complicating the clinical course. The American Heart Association (AHA) has published guidelines for the investigation and management of cardiovascular infections.[1] These guidelines highlight the role of echocardiography and microbiological culture to confirm diagnosis. More recently, PET/CT has been used for infection imaging in patients with both low and high probability of CIED infection, with high sensitivity and specificity. However, the utility of radionuclide imaging to function as a stand-alone noninvasive diagnostic imaging test in patients with suspected endocarditis has been less frequently examined. In this article, the authors summarize the recent advances in radionuclide imaging for the evaluation of patients with suspected cardiovascular infections.

GENERAL PRINCIPLES

The basic principle underlying radionuclide imaging is administration of a tracer that targets the

Conflicts of interest: none.

[a] Department of Cardiology, Manchester Heart Centre, Central Manchester University Hospitals NHS Foundation Trust, Oxford Road, Manchester M13 9WL, UK; [b] Department of Nuclear Medicine, Central Manchester University Hospitals NHS Foundation Trust, Oxford Road, Manchester M13 9WL, UK
[1] F.Z. Ahmed and J. James contributed equally to the article.
* Corresponding author. Nuclear Medicine Centre, Central Manchester University Hospitals NHS Foundation Trust, Manchester M13 9WL, UK.
E-mail address: parthiban.arumugam@cmft.nhs.uk

Cardiol Clin 34 (2016) 149–165
http://dx.doi.org/10.1016/j.ccl.2015.06.004

function of a particular organ or a particular metabolic process. The tracer is labeled with a radionuclide, and it is the gamma emissions, from the radionuclide as it decays, that are detected by the gamma camera or the PET camera.

Until the mid-1990s, radionuclide imaging provided two-dimensional (2D) functional images of 3-dimensional (3D) structures without the degree of anatomic information afforded by other forms of imaging such as CT and MRI. With the development of hybrid imaging technology, the addition of CT to the gamma camera or PET camera gantry allowed the fusion of functional information with anatomy. This development represented a major breakthrough, allowing accurate 3D localization of tracer distribution.

HISTORICAL PERSPECTIVE

Attempts were made to use radionuclide imaging for detection of endocarditis over 50 years ago; however, these early studies suffered from the limitations of planar (2D) imaging and also the unfavorable imaging characteristics of the then available radionuclide, ^{67}Ga citrate. The radiation dose to the patient was high and imaging continued for 3 or more days after intravenous tracer injection.

The emergence of techniques to radiolabel autologous leukocytes in the 1970s[2,3] constituted a major breakthrough in imaging of infection and inflammation. The radionuclide, either ^{99m}Tc or ^{111}In, bound to a lipophilic chelate, crosses the phospholipid leukocyte cell membrane. Following reinjection of the radiolabeled cells, the leukocyte migration pathway and incorporation of leukocytes into areas of infection or inflammation can be mapped. Both remain in use for leukocyte labeling, and this technique is widely available.

PET/CT offers several advantages over gamma camera imaging including increased sensitivity, increased image resolution, accurate attenuation correction, and accurate quantification, hence autologous leukocyte labeling with a positron-emitting radionuclide presents an attractive alternative to ^{99m}Tc or ^{111}In labeling.[4,5] The short physical half-life of PET tracers is, however, problematic, being insufficient to encompass the time course of labeled leukocyte migration into infection sites.

GENERAL PRINCIPLES OF FLUDEOXYGLUCOSE F 18-PET/COMPUTED TOMOGRAPHIC IMAGING

The positron-emitting radionuclide, [^{18}F] FDG, has been widely used in oncologic imaging for over a decade, and in recent years, it has been proposed for imaging of infection and inflammation.[6–12] The tracer [^{18}F] FDG is taken up by metabolically active cells via glucose transporters, primarily GLUT 1 and also GLUT 4, which is insulin sensitive and present in myocardium and skeletal muscle. Once inside the cell, [^{18}F] FDG is phosphorylated by hexokinase to [^{18}F]-2′-FDG-6-phosphate and remains intracellular without undergoing further metabolism.

Activated neutrophils, monocytes, macrophages, and lymphocytes express high levels of glucose transporters especially GLUT 1 and GLUT 3, hence [^{18}F] FDG uptake by these cells and migration to sites of infection is to be expected. The technique has high sensitivity, but [^{18}F] FDG avidity is also shown by active thrombi, soft atherosclerotic plaques, vasculitis, inflammation, and many primary and secondary malignancies (**Fig. 1**).[6–13] In addition, many tissues, including the myocardium, show high and sometimes heterogeneous physiologic [^{18}F] FDG activity, therefore clinical correlation and consideration of other imaging is required when interpreting [^{18}F] FDG images to avoid significant decrease in specificity.

Dual time point imaging, in which the acquisition is repeated after sufficient delay to allow for reduction in normal physiologic uptake, may be of value in differentiating normal physiologic or inflammatory [^{18}F] FDG activity from pathologic increased accumulation.[14–17] High physiologic myocardial activity may be problematic when using the technique for detection of endocarditis, valve infection, or intracardiac lead infection (LI); however, dietary manipulation has been reported to reduce physiologic uptake.[15,18,19] In the authors' experience, use of a carbohydrate-restricted diet for 24 hours before the standard 4- to 6-hour fast required for [^{18}F] FDG studies (**Box 1**) significantly decreases physiologic myocardial activity and permits adequate visualization of abnormal myocardial activity (see **Fig. 1**; **Figs. 2** and **3**).[20]

There is now a body of published literature detailing the use of [^{18}F] FDG in suspected cardiovascular-related infection, including both case reports and retrospective studies. A summary of radionuclides in current use for imaging of infection and inflammation is provided in **Table 1**. Advantages and disadvantages of the radionuclides are detailed in **Table 2**. [^{18}F] FDG-PET/CT is the authors' preferred option in suspected CIED infection and endocarditis, and accordingly, a more detailed protocol for this radionuclide is presented in **Table 3** and a proposed algorithm is presented in **Fig. 4**.

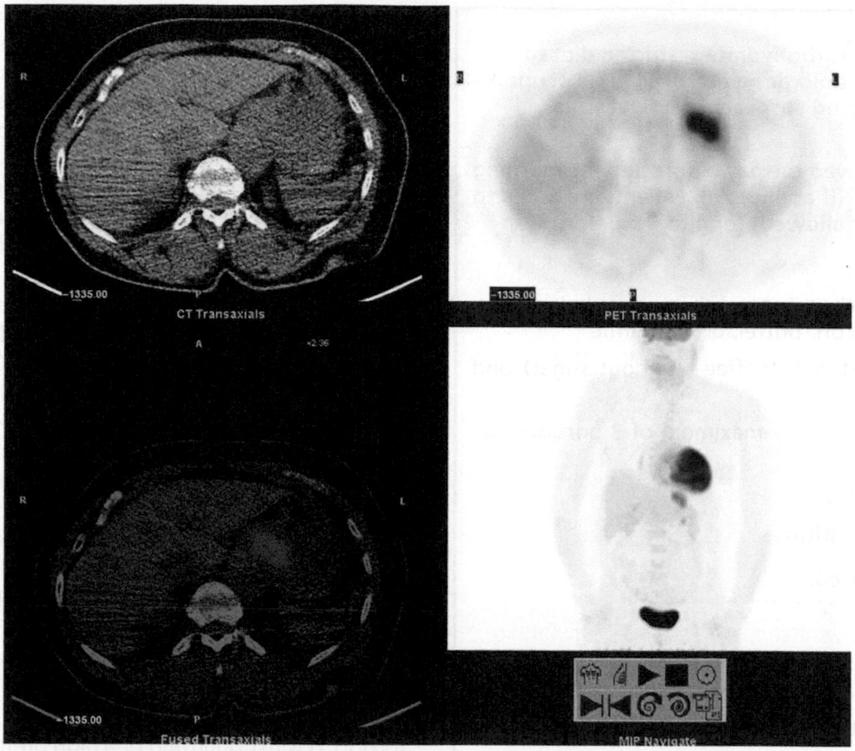

Fig. 1. Incidental identification of malignant polyp in the cardia of the stomach. Patient presented with swelling and tenderness in the region of the device. An incidental finding of high activity in the cardia of the stomach was noted. A malignant gastric polyp was found on subsequent oesphogastroduodenoscopy. Patient did not follow carbohydrate-restricted diet, and high physiologic myocardial uptake is noted. All images are corrected for attenuation. MIP, maximum intensity projection.

FLUDEOXYGLUCOSE F 18-PET/COMPUTED TOMOGRAPHY FOR CARDIAC IMPLANTABLE ELECTRONIC DEVICE INFECTION

Owing to expanding clinical indications, increasing numbers of patients are being treated with CIEDs. Despite improved surgical techniques and the use of prophylactic antimicrobial therapy, the rate of CIED-related infection is also increasing. Between 2004 and 2006, there was a 57% increase in the rate of CIED infection, while during the same period, CIED implantation rates rose by only 12%.[21]

Infection is a serious complication of CIED implantation. Clinical manifestations range from surgical site infection and local symptoms in the region of the generator pocket to fulminant endocarditis, usually affecting the right heart valves. The AHA and the North American Society for Pacing and Electrophysiology recommend complete system removal in all patients with definite CIED infection, regardless of whether it is limited to the pocket, involves the transvenous leads, or is associated with valvular endocarditis or sepsis.[1] The assessment of CIED infection using [^{18}F] FDG is a recent development, and there has been significant variation in the [^{18}F] FDG scanning protocols that have been reported in the literature. The optimal scan protocol remains to be defined, and most published data focus on the utility of PET/CT to diagnose CIED-related infections. These studies are relatively few in number and consist of small patient cohorts.

Enthusiasm for evaluating the role of [^{18}F] FDG in CIED infection has, for the most part, been driven by recent proof-of-concept studies that have shown [^{18}F] FDG-PET/CT to have high sensitivity and specificity for the diagnosis of CIED-GPI. There have been 4 published studies evaluating the role of [^{18}F] FDG-PET/CT in cases of CIED-GPI.[22,23,25,27] One further preliminary study evaluated the role of [^{18}F] FDG-PET/CT to identify LIs and guide decision to extract the CIED.[24]

Although the utility of [^{18}F] FDG-PET/CT in CIED infection is very much in its infancy, the available evidence indicates considerable promise for future use in routine clinical practice. Published studies agree that both the clinical presentation and the diagnostic accuracy of [^{18}F] FDG-PET/CT varies

Box 1
Suggested carbohydrate-restricted diet to reduce physiologic myocardial [^{18}F] FDG uptake when imaging suspected cardiovascular infection

To be followed the day before and the morning of the scan (if applicable). Patients are asked to fast (water allowed) for 4 to 6 h before scan

Permitted:

- Plain chicken, meat, fish, meat-only sausages, eggs, bacon, butter, or margarine
- Liquids (tea or coffee—without sugar) and water
- Dairy products—maximum of 3 portions per day
- Vegetables
- Sugar substitutes

Not permitted:

- Bread
- Cereals
- Pasta
- Soup with pasta
- Potatoes
- Rice
- Crackers
- Beans
- Peanut butter
- Jam
- Nuts
- Fruit juice
- Sweets—mints, cough drops
- Chewing gum
- Alcohol

depending on the site of infection (ie, generator pocket vs intravascular leads and intracardiac portions of the device) (**Table 4**).

REVIEW OF PUBLISHED LITERATURE

The first study to evaluate the diagnostic utility of [^{18}F] FDG-PET/CT to identify cases of CIED-GPI and LI was published in 2011. Bensimhon and colleagues[25] examined 21 cases of suspected CIED infection and 14 noninfected controls with devices implanted for long term. All patients underwent whole-body [^{18}F] FDG-PET/CT examination. The 21 cases of suspected CIED infection had individuals with (1) unexplained or persistent recurrent fever greater than 38°C (n = 17), (2) chronic inflammatory syndrome with elevated levels of C-reactive protein (n = 15), (3) positive result of blood cultures (n = 11), and/or (4) clinical suspicion of GPI (n = 5). Importantly, the vast majority of these subjects had fever and/or abnormal levels of blood markers for infection, while a smaller number of patients had only local signs in the region of the generator pocket. Infection was confirmed in 10 of 21 cases, either from bacteriologic culture after CIED extraction or during follow-up according to modified Duke criteria. In cases of suspected infection, visual analysis of [^{18}F] FDG uptake at an individual patient level identified 8 patients with true-positive results, 11 with true-negative results, and 2 with false-negative results. There were no false-positive results in the control group. Accordingly, sensitivity and specificity of [^{18}F] FDG-PET/CT to diagnose infection on a per patient basis was 80% and 100% for GPI and/or LI.

Sarrazin and colleagues[22] undertook the largest study to date of patients with confirmed or high probability of CIED infection and substantiated the high diagnostic accuracy of [^{18}F] FDG-PET/CT to diagnose CIED-GPI. A total of 42 patients (group 1) with confirmed or a high pretest probability of CIED infection (clinical features of pocket infections [n = 26], device erosion [n = 6], lead endocarditis [n = 7], and persistent or recurrent bacteremia without another obvious source [n = 3]) underwent PET/CT examination. A further group of patients (group 2, n = 12) with recent CIED implantation (4 to 8 weeks postimplantation) but no features of infection served as acute-phase controls to evaluate [^{18}F] FDG activity in the setting of recent postoperative inflammation. Group 3 was composed of patients with CIEDs implanted for long term (implanted $\geq$6 months) and no indication of infection (n = 12). All patients underwent [^{18}F] FDG-PET/CT examination. In addition to a qualitative visual score, a semiquantitative ratio (SQR) comparing the maximum [^{18}F] FDG uptake in the region of interest, generally the device pocket, with the mean uptake in normal tissue (lung parenchyma on the non-attenuation corrected [NAC] PET images) was also calculated. Of 42 patients, 35 were treated for confirmed CIED infection; of these 24 underwent CIED extraction. SQR was statistically significantly higher in group 1 than in groups 2 and 3. These investigators defined an SQR cutoff greater than 1.87 as being both sensitive and specific for diagnosing the presence of infection. Above this value, 100% specificity was achieved for the diagnosis of infection. This study established that [^{18}F] FDG-PET/CT was useful in differentiating between CIED infection and recent postimplant changes. Furthermore, none of the

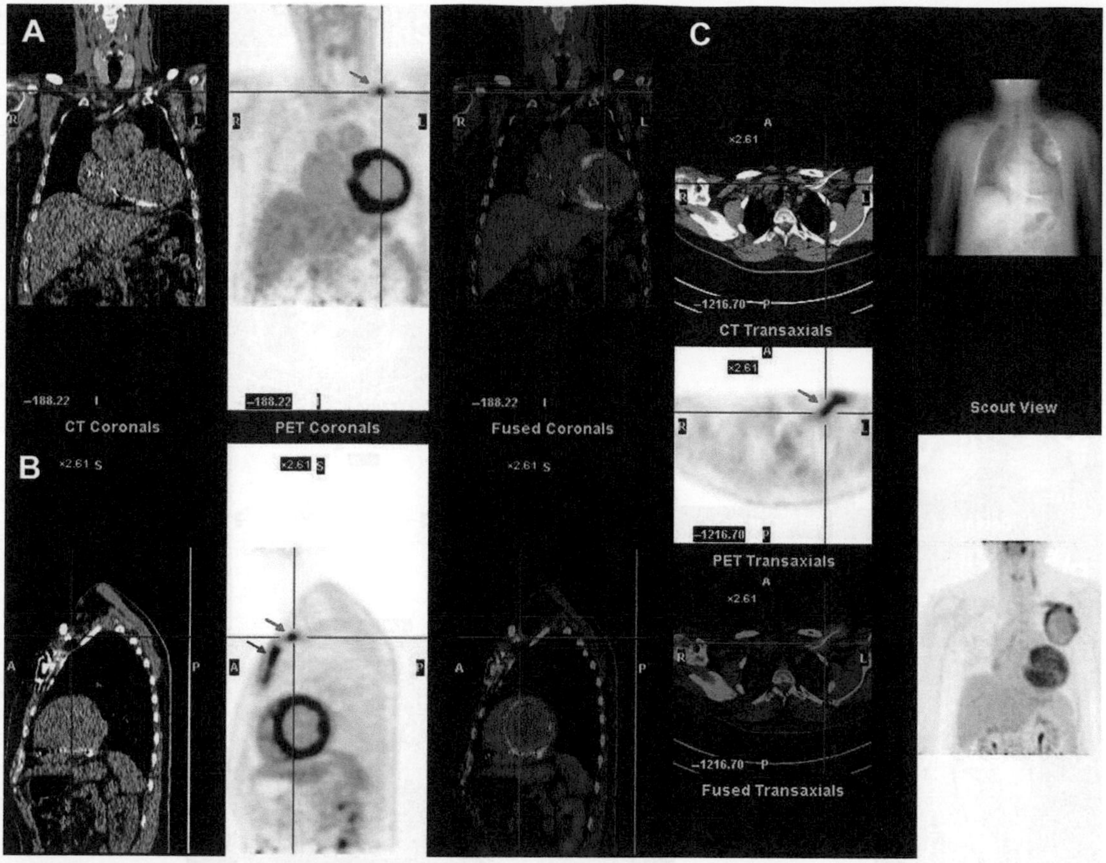

Fig. 2. Positive result of scan in a patient presenting with pain in the region of the generator pocket. Increased [18F] FDG uptake around the CIED within the pocket (*red arrow*) and along the proximal portion of the leads (*yellow arrows*) was demonstrated on coronal (*A*), sagittal (*B*), and axial views (*C*). Patient did not follow carbohydrate-restricted diet, and high physiologic myocardial uptake is noted. All images are corrected for attenuation.

12 controls with CIED implanted for long term had an SQR above 1.00, indicating a strong negative predictive value of [18F] FDG-PET/CT.

In a pilot study, Cautela and colleagues[23] examined the utility of [18F] FDG-PET/CT to diagnose CIED infection, and also specifically evaluated the diagnostic yield for CIED-associated IE (CIED-IE) and pocket infections. Of 21 patients evaluated, 15 had evidence of CIED-GPI and 1 patient had superficial skin infection; 13 patients had definite or probable endocarditis. The sensitivity and specificity for diagnosis of skin infection or CIED-GPI was 87% and 100%, respectively. On NAC images, using an SQR (defined as the ratio of the maximal count rate in the region of the generator pocket to the contralateral prepectoral region) of greater than 1.06, both sensitivity and specificity reached 100%. On the contrary, accuracy for CIED-IE was significantly lower (sensitivity and specificity of 30.8% and 62.5%, respectively). These results suggested that [18F] FDG-PET/CT had a high diagnostic accuracy for skin infection and CIED-GPI, whereas the diagnostic accuracy in cases of CIED-IE fell well below what would be desired of a diagnostic test. It is relevant that a significant proportion of these patients had received treatment with antimicrobials before PET/CT examination; this has been reported to be associated with attenuated [18F] FDG uptake in other conditions and false-negative results in patients with confirmed CIED infection.[24,26] In addition, physiologic myocardial [18F] FDG uptake needs to be considered as a confounding factor when interpreting the low sensitivities and specificities reported for the diagnosis of CIED-IE.

CIED infection can occur anywhere along the course of the device; from the generator pocket and endovascular portions to the intracardiac portions of the lead and the endocardium (**Figs. 5** and **6**). Patients with CIED-GPI usually report local symptoms and/or signs in the region of the generator pocket. Individuals with CIED-IE are typically

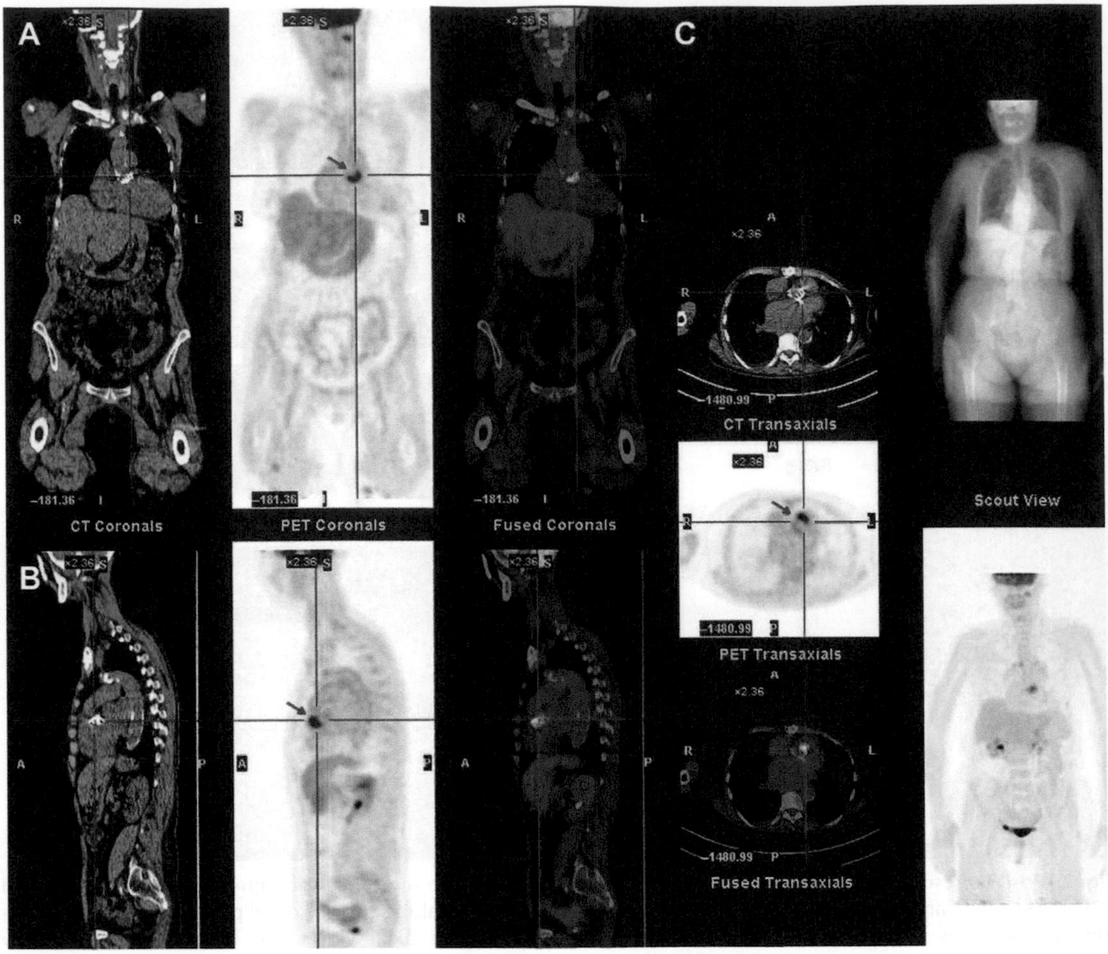

Fig. 3. Positive [^{18}F] FDG-PET/CT in a patient with a metallic aortic valve infective endocarditis. Increased [^{18}F] FDG activity was observed in the region of the aortic valve prosthesis (*red arrow*) in the coronal (*A*), sagittal (*B*) and transaxial (*C*) slices, consistent with infective endocarditis. Patient followed a restricted carbohydrate diet; note the reduced physiologic uptake in the myocardium. All images are corrected for attenuation.

systemically unwell with raised levels of inflammatory markers and/or evidence of vegetations on transthoracic or transesophageal echocardiography. In comparison, individuals with isolated LIs (ie, infection usually, but not exclusively, limited to the pacing lead) often present with pyrexia and/or bacteremia (without another identifiable source). In cases of isolated pacing LI, there may be a paucity of local symptoms in the region of the pocket. Furthermore, unless there is involvement of the intracardiac portion of the lead, the echocardiogram may also be unremarkable. To investigate the utility of [^{18}F] FDG-PET/CT in these patients, Ploux and colleagues[27] examined 10 patients with pyrexia of unknown origin and an implanted device. The decision to extract was based on the presence of increased [^{18}F] FDG uptake along the pacing lead. Six patients had abnormal uptake and therefore underwent complete CIED extraction. A pathogen was recovered in all 6 cases. The remaining 4 cases, with no abnormal uptake along the pacing leads, did not undergo system extraction and were successfully managed with a conservative strategy.

All the aforementioned studies have, for the most part, evaluated the utility of [^{18}F] FDG in cases with a high pretest probability of CIED infection. Fulminant signs of infection with obvious inflammatory changes are observed in the vast majority of cases of CIED-GPI, and in these patients, device extraction is immediately indicated without the need for additional tests. In other instances, a persistent bacteremia or pyrexia of unknown origin in patients with a CIED may prompt investigation to exclude CIED-related or ectopic infection (**Fig. 7**).

Table 1
Overview of radionuclides currently used in the evaluation of cardiovascular-related infection

Modality	Radionuclide	Emission Energy	Physical Half-Life	Typical Administered Activity	Patient Radiation Dose	No. of Visits	Imaging Time Points	Duration (min)
PET/CT	[^{18}F] FDG	511 keV	110 min	Up to 400 MBq[a]	0.02 mSv/MBq ([^{18}F] FDG) + 2–4 mSv (CT)[c]	1	60 or 90 & 180 min	20–25
Gamma camera SPECT/CT + planar[b]	^{99m}Tc-HMPAO autologous leukocytes	140 keV	6 h	200 MBq	2 mSv (^{99m}Tc) + 1–4 mSv (CT)	2	30 min 2–4 h 24 h	20–30 40–60
	^{111}In (oxine or chloride) autologous leukocytes	245 & 171 keV	67 h	20 MBq	9 mSv (^{111}In) + 1–4 mSv (CT)	2–3	30 min 4 h 24 & 48 h	20–30 40–60

Abbreviations: HMPAO, hexamethylpropyleneamine oxime; SPECT, single-photon emission computed tomography.

[a] Careful implementation of advances in hardware and reconstruction methods, namely, time of flight reconstruction, in current generation PET/CT systems, allow either reduction in administered activity or imaging time per bed position while maintaining image quality and quantitative accuracy. In the authors' institution, they have adopted a combination of the 2 with administered [^{18}F] FDG activity reduced to 3.5 MBq/kg and up to a maximum of 280 MBq. Imaging time per bed position is adjusted according to patient weight, but for most patients, it has been reduced to 2 minutes per bed position.[43,44]

[b] ^{67}Ga citrate has not been included because of reduced prevalence of use in clinical practice.

[c] CT examination radiation dose depends on the number and extent of the low-dose CT scan. The above figure is based on 1 to 2 half-body studies, from orbits to midthigh, performed at 90 and 180 minutes.

Table 2
Advantages and disadvantages of radionuclides in current use for the evaluation of suspected cardiovascular-related infection

Modality	Advantages	Disadvantages
[^{18}F] FDG	• Single appointment • Excellent image resolution • Whole-body imaging allows detection of ectopic foci; see **Fig. 7** • Accurate anatomic localization • Accurate attenuation correction • Accurate quantification	• Moderate radiation dose • Physiologic myocardial, bone marrow, renal, and bowel activity may hamper interpretation • Fasting & dietary manipulation required • High cost • Variable availability • Prior antibiotic therapy may reduce sensitivity • Potential false-positive results caused by early postsurgical scans and certain surgical glues
^{99m}Tc-HMPAO autologous leukocytes	• Multi-time-point imaging feasible • Low radiation dose	• Multiple appointments over 1–2 d • Labor intensive • Risk associated with blood handling • Physiologic hepatic, splenic, renal, and bone marrow activity may hamper interpretation • Hepatobiliary excretion/labeling instability can be problematic • Long image acquisition times if > single SPECT/CT field of view required • High cost • Prior antibiotic therapy may reduce sensitivity
^{111}In autologous leukocytes	• Multi-time-point imaging feasible • Imaging up to 48 h useful if low leukocyte migration/chronic sepsis	• Multiple appointments over 1–3 d • High radiation dose • Labor intensive • Risk associated with blood handling • Physiologic hepatic, splenic, and bone marrow activity may hamper interpretation • Long image acquisition times if > single SPECT/CT field of view required • High cost • Not readily available • Prior antibiotic therapy may reduce sensitivity
^{67}Ga citrate	• Low cost	• Multiple appointments over 3 or more days • High radiation dose • Poor imaging characteristics • Long image acquisition times for both planar and SPECT/CT • Not readily available • Physiologic bowel and bone marrow activity may hamper interpretation • Prior antibiotic therapy may reduce sensitivity

Abbreviation: HMPAO, hexamethylpropyleneamine oxime.

Device extraction is not immediately indicated in patients who present with nonspecific symptoms in the region of the generator pocket in the absence of bloodstream infection. However, some studies suggest that infection is present in a significant proportion of patients who present with local symptoms.[28] Diagnosis of CIED-GPI is challenging in this group of patients, and the authors think that this is the area where a sensitive and specific imaging modality may be most valuable.

Table 3
Suggested [18F] FDG-PECT/CT study protocol for investigation of suspected cardiovascular-related infection

Patient Preparation Before the scan	Nondiabetic patients: • Carbohydrate-restricted diet to be followed on the day before and morning of the scan (see **Table 1**). • 6-h fast Diabetic patients: • No specific diet. • Insulin dependent: 4-h fast. Need to ensure a minimum of 4-h insulin-free period before tracer injection • Oral hypoglycemic or diet controlled: 6-h fast All patients: • Allowed plain water freely; advised 500 mL in the 2 h before appointment • Avoid excessive exercise, caffeine, alcohol, and nicotine for 24 h before appointment
Patient Preparation On arrival	• Check blood sugar; allowed range 3.5–12.0 mmol/L (63–216 mg/dL) • Detailed clinical history particularly pertaining to device implantation, previous revision, and extraction • Site cannula in arm or hand opposite to CIED site
Scan Protocol	• Scan limits: orbits to diaphragm, or skull base to proximal thighs if suspected ectopic source of infection, at 90 min after injection • Ensure MAR-enabled technique (when available) • Repeat imaging at 180 min postinjection; acquisition time increased to 5 min per bed position
Reporting	• Review both nonattenuation- and attenuation-corrected PET images for areas of increased metabolic activity in relation to the device and/or leads or in ectopic sites • Quantification as per local protocols • Review CT data for incidental findings

Abbreviation: MAR, metallic artifact reduction.

Ahmed and colleagues[24] sought to specifically evaluate the diagnostic utility of [18F] FDG PET CT in cases with a lower pretest probability of CIED-GPI at initial presentation. A total of 46 patients with suspected CIED-GPI were divided according to specific clinical criteria into either possible (n = 26) or definite (n = 20) CIED-GPI; 40 control subjects had CIEDs implanted for long term and no indication of infection. All patients underwent [18F] FDG-PET/CT assessment and standard clinical management independent of PET/CT findings. Patients with CIED-GPI who required extraction (n = 32) had significantly higher uptake in the region of the pocket, relative to blood pool activity, compared with patents who were managed conservatively (n = 14) (**Fig. 8**) and control subjects (n = 40). Furthermore the SQR, as per Sarrazin and colleagues,[22] was also significantly increased in extracted cases compared with nonextracted cases and controls. The investigators concluded that [18F] FDG-PET/CT had a high diagnostic accuracy in differentiating CIED-GPI (defined by need for extraction) from noninfected devices with sensitivity and specificity of 97% and 98%, respectively. Further large-scale studies are necessary to establish the use of [18F] FDG-PET/CT in this particular group of patients.

INFECTIVE ENDOCARDITIS (SINGLE-PHOTON EMISSION COMPUTED TOMOGRAPHY/ COMPUTED TOMOGRAPHY AND PET/ COMPUTED TOMOGRAPHY)

The incidence of IE has remained stable for the past 50 years with an incidence of 2 to 4 per 100,000.[5] IE is suspected in patients with fever of unknown origin when associated with a heart murmur or heart failure and/or evidence of septic emboli. This fact is true of acute IE, but in a subacute or chronic presentation, there may be a paucity of clinical features, particularly in the elderly and in immunocompromised patients, rendering assessment less straightforward. Diagnosis is essentially clinical and based on the modified Duke criteria (positive result of blood cultures with typical IE microorganisms and echocardiographic findings) with a sensitivity of 80%.[5] Result of blood culture can be negative in patients

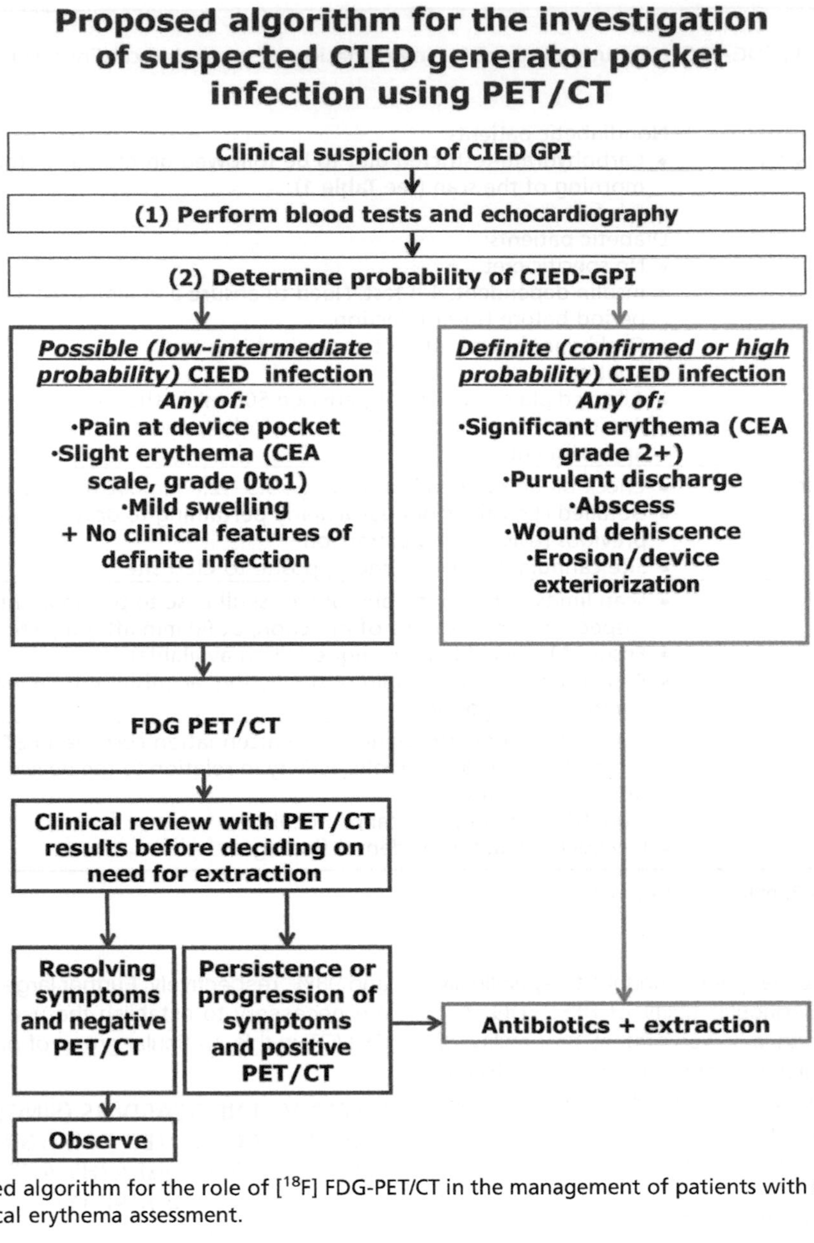

Fig. 4. Proposed algorithm for the role of [^{18}F] FDG-PET/CT in the management of patients with suspected CIED-GPI. CEA, clinical erythema assessment.

pretreated with antibiotics or when the organisms are difficult to culture. Similarly, the echocardiogram can yield negative result in the early stages, when the vegetations may be small or have embolized. Conversely, falsely positive lesions may be reported in the presence of significant valve degeneration, mechanical valves, thrombus, or cardiac tumors.

Radionuclide imaging could be useful when there is a high clinical suspicion of IE but blood cultures remain negative for a pathogen and echocardiogram is inconclusive particularly in the setting of prosthetic valves and when looking for ectopic infective sites or distant septic emboli. Most of the current published literature surrounding the role of radionuclide imaging with both labeled white cells and [^{18}F] FDG-PET is limited to case series or case reports.

Erba and colleagues[29] evaluated the role of ^{99m}Tc-labeled hexamethylpropyleneamine oxime (HMPAO) single-photon emission computed tomography (SPECT)/CT imaging in 131 patients with suspected or definite endocarditis based on modified Duke criteria. Of the 131 patients, 51 had confirmed IE (comparable number of native, bioprosthetic, and metallic valves); 46 of 51 (23

Table 4
Summary of contemporaneous studies evaluating the utility of [^{18}F] FDG-PET/CT in cases of CIED-related infection

Study	N (Controls)	Site	Analysis	Quoted Sensitivity and Specificity
Bensimhon et al[25]	21 (14)	Pocket & leads	Visual	80% and 100%
		Leads	Quantitative	—
Sarazzin et al[22]	42 (24)	Pocket & leads	Visual (NAC)	89% and 86%
			Quantitative (NAC)	Specificity of 100%
Cautela et al[23]	21 (0)	Pocket	Visual	87% and 100% (Pocket)
		CIED-IE		31% and 63% (CIED-IE)
			Quantitative (AC)	93% and 83% (Pocket)
			Quantitative (NAC)	100% and 100% (Pocket)
Ploux et al[27]	10 (40)	Leads	Visual	100% and 93%
Ahmed et al[24]	46 (40)	Pocket	Visual	—
			Quantitative (NAC)	97% and 98%

Abbreviations: AC, attenuation corrected; NAC, non-attenuation corrected.

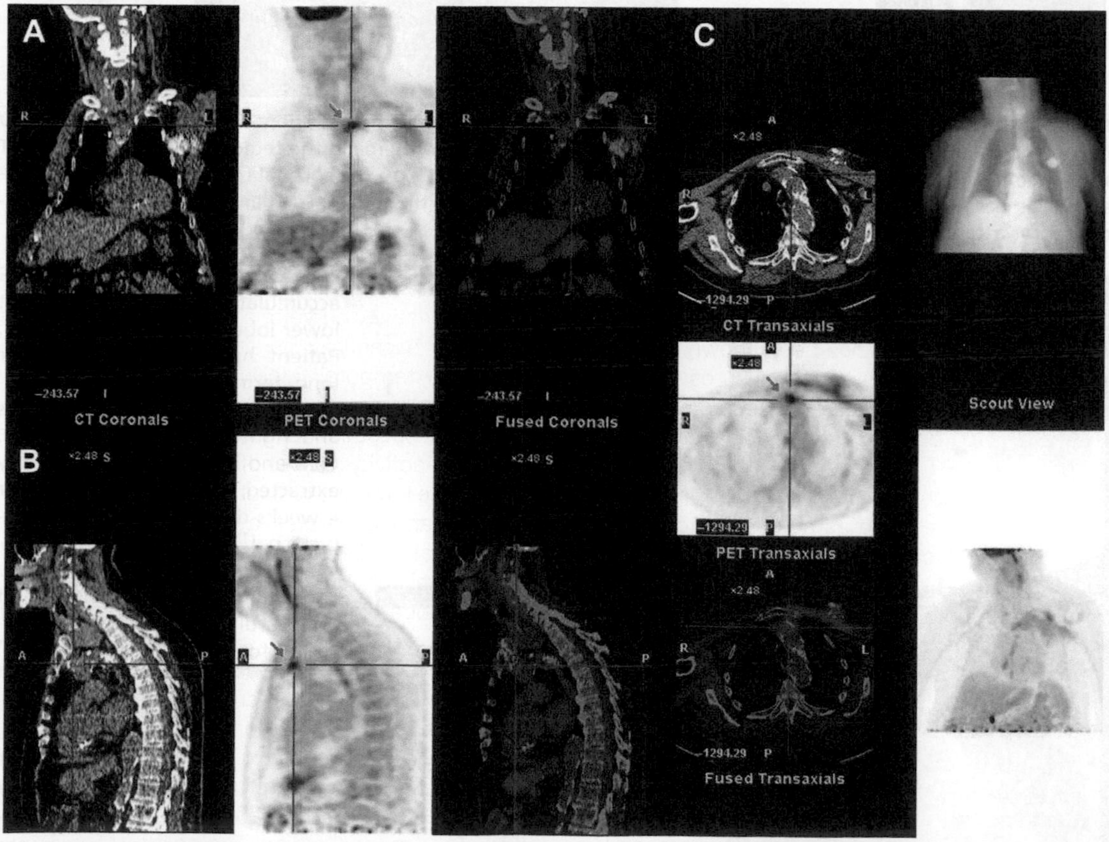

Fig. 5. Positive [^{18}F] FDG-PET/CT study indicating lead involvement. Patient presented with localized erythema in the region of the generator pocket and an elevated C-reactive protein. Increased [^{18}F] FDG activity is observed on the transvenous portion of the pacing lead (*yellow arrow*), indicating lead involvement, on coronal (*A*), sagittal (*B*), and transaxial views (*C*). Less-intense uptake was also observed around the pocket. All images are corrected for attenuation.

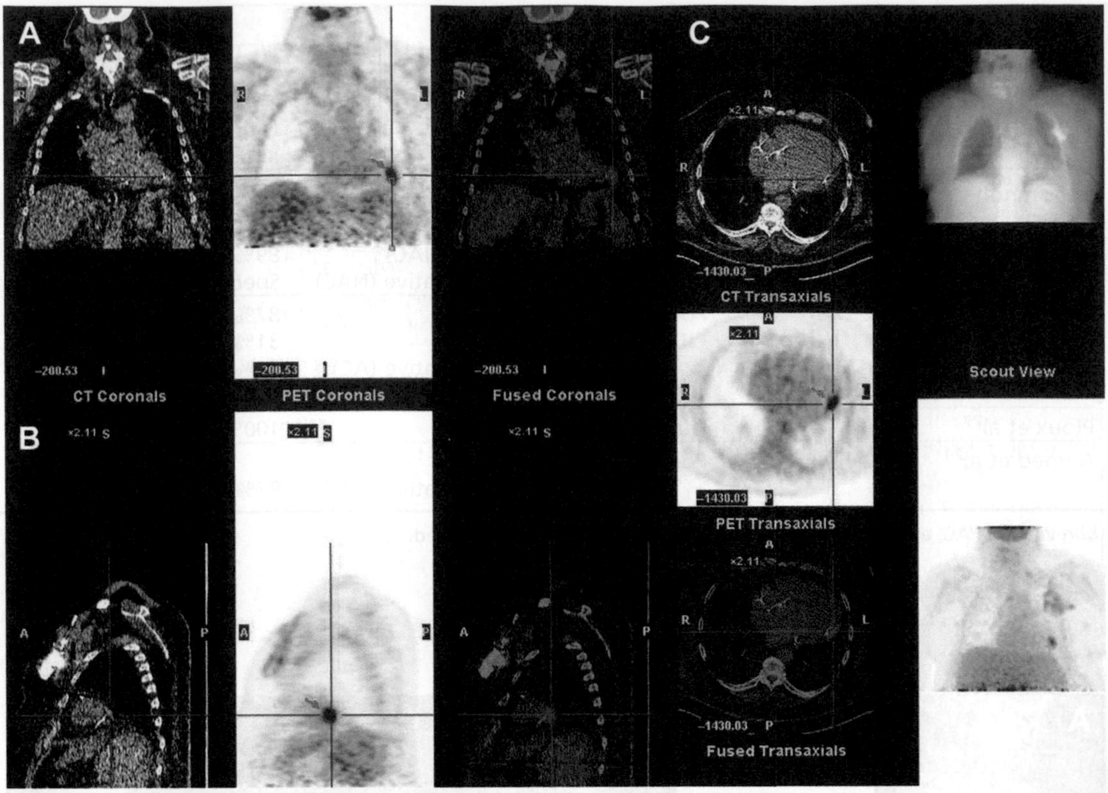

Fig. 6. Positive [^{18}F] FDG-PET/CT study indicating intracardiac lead involvement. Patient had left prepectoral CIED implanted in 2005, with a box change in 2013, and presented with erythema in the region of the pocket. PET/CT study demonstrates increased activity around the device (*yellow arrow*) on the coronal (*A*), sagittal (*B*) and transaxial (*C*) slices, and a further focus of high uptake in association with the left ventricular lead. All images are corrected for attenuation.

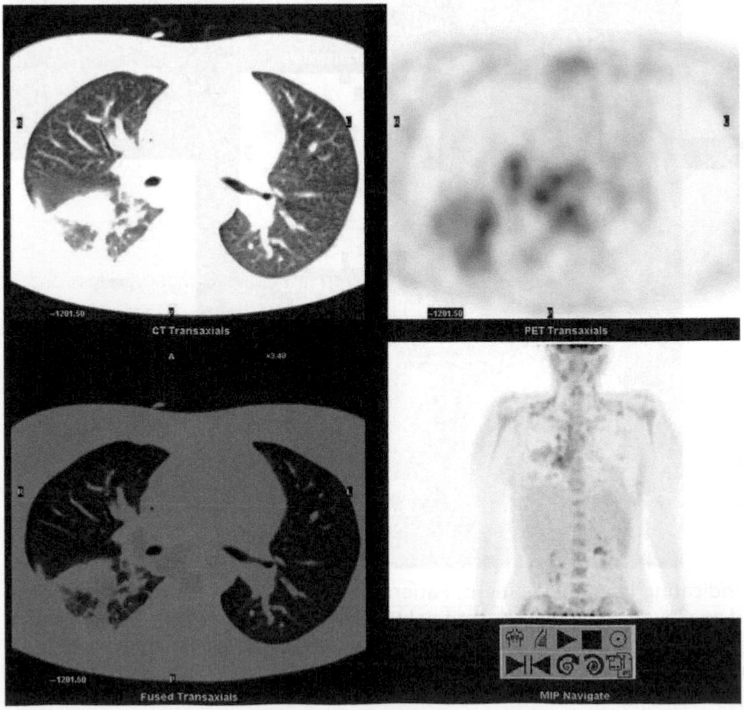

Fig. 7. Ectopic foci of [^{18}F] FDG accumulation in the region of right lower lobe collapse/consolidation. Patient had CIED implanted for long term (11 years) and developed tricuspid valve endocarditis and right ventricular vegetation. CIED and leads were subsequently extracted, but fever persisted for 4 weeks despite intravenous antibiotics. [^{18}F] FDG-PET/CT scan revealed right lower lobe collapse/consolidation with no evidence of endocarditis. All images are corrected for attenuation.

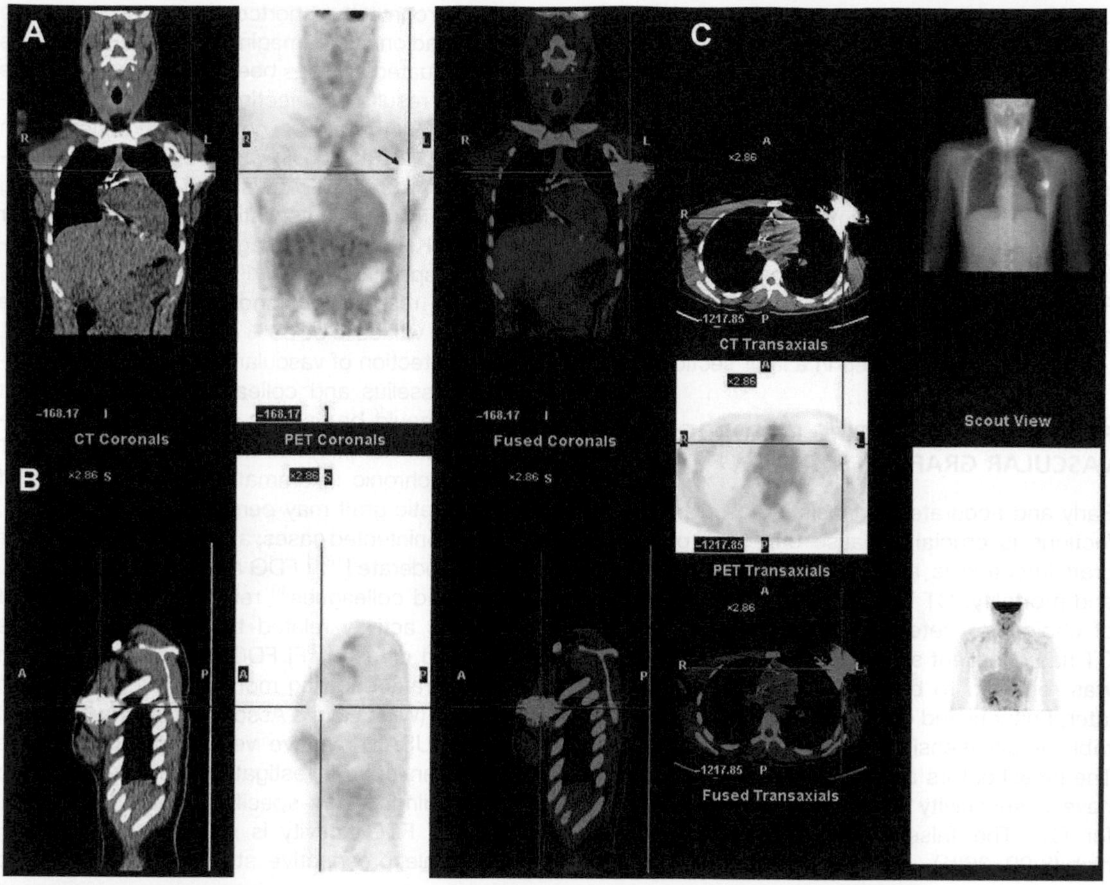

Fig. 8. Negative scan in a patient with a chronically implanted device presenting with pain in region of the generator pocket. No increased uptake was visualized along the course of the CIED on the coronal (*A*), sagittal (*B*) or transaxial (*C*) slices. The patient was managed conservatively and remained well on follow-up (14 months) with no features of infection. Arrow points to the site of the generator in the pre-pectoral pocket, which is clear of increased [^{18}F] FDG activity. All images are corrected for attenuation.

valve only and 23 valve and extracardiac infection) were identified on radionuclide imaging including 11 patients who had a negative result of echocardiogram and 17 patients with negative result of blood cultures. The 5 false-negative study results were attributed to small vegetations in the presence of *Enterococcus* (n = 4) or *Candida* (n = 1) sp, all of which were in patients who were receiving high-dose antibiotic therapy. There were no false-positive scan results for valvular endocarditis. The investigators recommended use of white cell imaging as a second-line imaging modality in clinically challenging cases in detecting valvular endocarditis and highlighted the ability of SPECT/CT to accurately localize ectopic infection. Despite impressive results albeit from a single-center study, this technique remains underused because of the perceived limitations of this modality.

Millar and colleagues,[30] in a review article, discuss in detail the potential role of [^{18}F] FDG-PET/CT in patients with suspected IE. A further review article by Erba and colleagues[5] elegantly highlights the role of [^{18}F] FDG-PET/CT in IE. It is beyond the scope of this article to detail individual case reports, hence the authors recommend further reading of the 2 review articles citied above. It can be concluded that [^{18}F] FDG-PET/CT may have a role as a problem-solving tool (1) in patients with suspected valve IE, particularly in prosthetic valves; (2) where there is a high clinical suspicion with positive results of blood cultures, but negative result of echocardiogram; and (3) in the detection of complications related to IE, namely, distant septic emboli.

In a recent article[31] poor sensitivity (39%) of [^{18}F] FDG-PET/CT imaging in IE was reported. It was suggested that use of advanced imaging technology and low carbohydrate diets could improve sensitivity, because variable uptake within the left ventricular myocardium renders the distinction between physiologic and pathologic uptake difficult. While blood glucose level is thought to have a nonlinear relationship to myocardial uptake, fasting time and age do not seem to have an influence.[32] In the authors' own experience and in that of others,[19,20,33] a low carbohydrate diet (see **Box 1**) seems to reduce physiologic myocardial uptake. A further limitation as identified by several investigators[5,30] relates to metallic artifacts affecting the attenuation-corrected (AC) PET images, but this could potentially be overcome by using metallic artifact reduction (MAR) techniques, as discussed in a later section.

RADIONUCLIDE IMAGING IN AORTIC VASCULAR GRAFT INFECTIONS

Early and accurate diagnosis of vascular graft infections is crucial because untreated prosthetic graft infection is associated with high morbidity and mortality. CT has been the imaging modality of choice for detecting graft infection. Although CT has excellent specificity (100%), its sensitivity was reported to be only 55%.[34] Over a decade later, Fukuchi and colleagues[35] published comparable results (sensitivity 64% and specificity 86%). The investigators also reported [^{18}F] FDG-PET to have a sensitivity of 91%, compared with 64% for CT. The false-positive rate, however, was high (8/22, 36%).

To overcome the shortcomings of stand-alone CT and radionuclide imaging, hybrid imaging has been evaluated and has been shown to have more favorable results in detecting vascular graft infection (**Fig. 9**). Erba and colleagues[36] quote high sensitivity (82%–100%) and specificity (85%–100%) for ^{99m}Tc-HMPAO-labeled white cells using SPECT/CT in patients with suspected vascular infection. Keidar and colleagues[37] report the sensitivity and specificity of [^{18}F] FDG-PET/CT to be 93% and 91%, respectively, and positive and negative predictive values to be 88% and 96%, respectively, for the detection of vascular graft infections. However, Wasselius and colleagues[38] underline that caution should be used in the evaluation of suspected vascular infection using [^{18}F] FDG-PET/CT because chronic inflammation on the surface of the synthetic graft may persist long after implant, even in noninfected cases, and may result in diffuse low to moderate [^{18}F] FDG activity along the graft. Kieder and colleagues[39] retrospectively reviewed metabolic activity related to 107 vascular grafts and found diffuse [^{18}F] FDG activity in 92%, with Dacron grafts showing more intense activity than Gore-Tex (W. L. Gore & Associations, Inc. Flagstaff, Arizona. USA) or native vein grafts. One of the above-mentioned investigators recently reiterated these findings,[40] but specifically noted that focal high [^{18}F] FDG activity is suspicious for sepsis. Large-scale prospective studies are required to

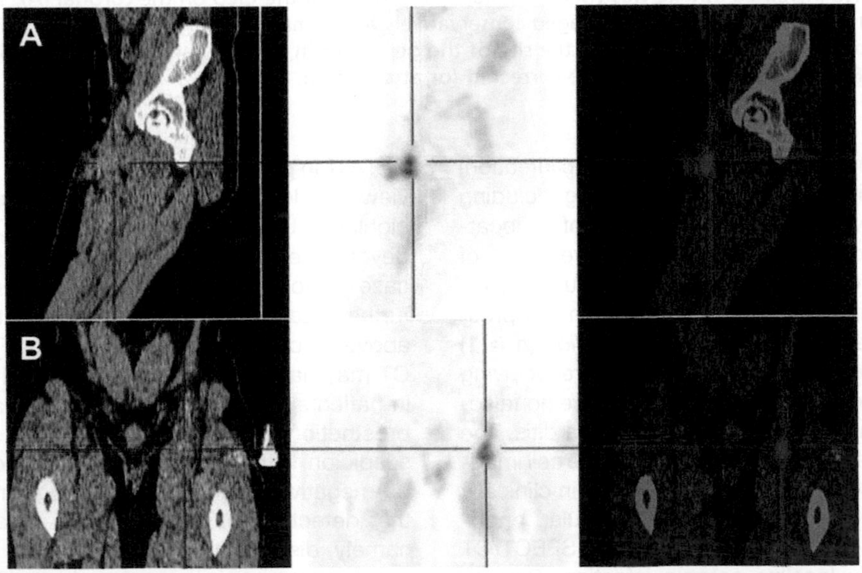

Fig. 9. [^{18}F] FDG-PET/CT study consistent with femoral vascular graft infection. A 42-year-old man with history of left common femoral and sapenofemoral artery pseudoaneursym repair and left common femoral artery graft 3 years previously. Patient presented with 2-day history of subcutaneous serous collection and pain in left groin. Sagittal (*A*) and coronal (*B*) [^{18}F] FDG-PET/CT images demonstrate increased metabolic activity in the soft tissue in the left groin, extending anteriorly in the skin and subcutaneous tissues, and also extending proximally in the graft consistent with sepsis. All images are corrected for attenuation.

further delineate the risk of false-positive results of scans in this population.

TECHNICAL CONSIDERATIONS AND PRACTICAL GUIDE FOR INTERPRETATION

While it is good practice when reporting PET/CT to review the NAC PET images, the use of NAC data in published studies[22,23] reflects the concern and challenges of accurate quantification around metallic devices, which lead to high- and low-density artifacts on the CT data. The resultant streak artifacts have the potential to propagate through to the CT-based attenuation correction, causing inaccuracies in quantification of uptake in relation to the metallic device and/or leads on the AC PET images. To prevent this, MAR algorithms can be used on the CT reconstruction to suppress the high-density regions (**Fig. 10**).[41,42]

Phantom work undertaken using a body torso phantom with CIED plus leads attached has shown that this algorithm[42] consistently underestimates the [^{18}F] FDG uptake in the areas of both low- and high-density streak artifact surrounding the CIED on the CT and that the leads show uptake similar to background. As a consequence, when using this particular MAR algorithm, no false-positive results are expected and any increase in [^{18}F] FDG uptake surrounding the device or leads can be attributed to a true increase in uptake rather than to artifact.[41] Marginal increases in [^{18}F] FDG uptake immediately adjacent to the device may, however,

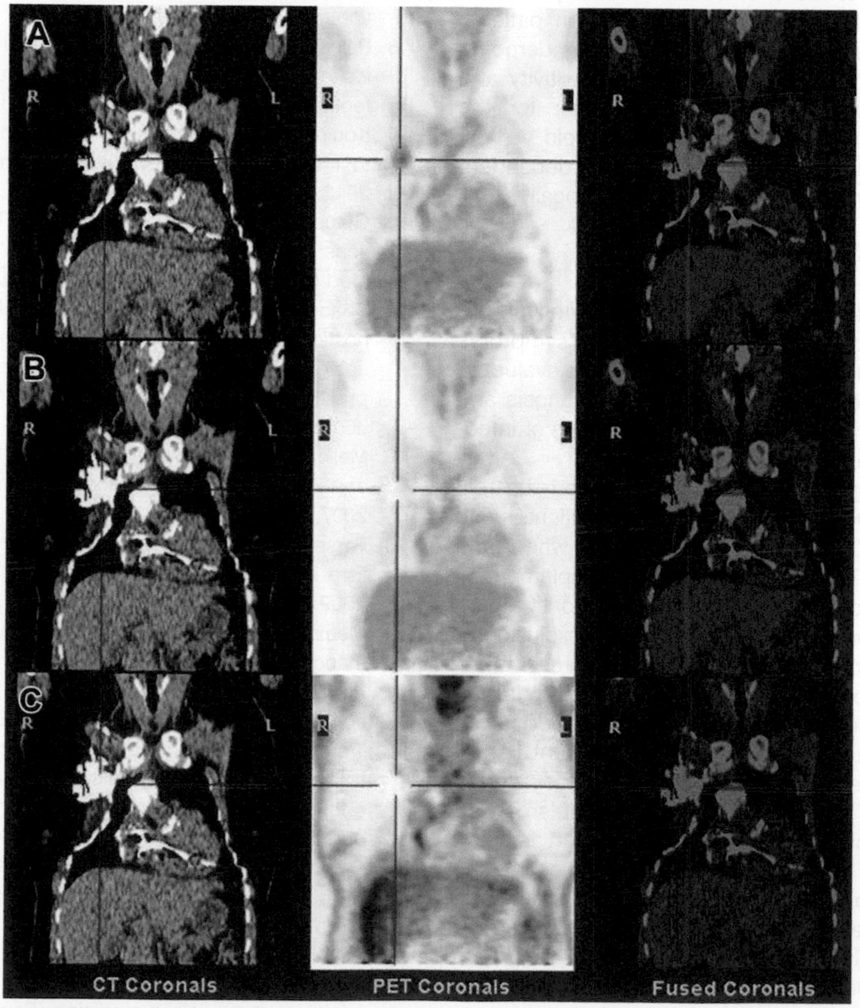

Fig. 10. [^{18}F] FDG-PET/CT study demonstrating the effect of metallic artefact reduction (MAR) techniques. Patient presented with pain in the region of the generator pocket. Previous history of a surgically corrected Tetralogy of Fallot. First CIED implanted in 1975, with several subsequent revisions. Current CIED had been in situ for 4 years. A negative, AC [^{18}F]-FDG PET/CT scan with MAR algorithm enabled (*B*), but positive with MAR algorithm disabled (*A*). NAC images confirm negative study (*C*).

be difficult to detect because of underestimation of uptake in this region.

For reporting, the authors recommend visual inspection of the AC and NAC PET data; assessment of the maximal standardized uptake value (SUV_{max}), calculated as the activity concentration normalized to the patient body weight and injected activity, in relation to the device pocket and along the course of all leads; and comparison of these values to the average SUV (SUV_{mean}) within mediastinal and hepatic blood pool. The authors also find calculation of an SQR, as per Sarrazin and colleagues,[22] which compares maximum uptake around the device or leads on the NAC PET data with the mean uptake within right and left lung parenchyma, to be useful.

The authors have compared the accuracy of several published methods[22,23,25] of quantification, using both AC and NAC data, in patients with suspected CIED infection undergoing [^{18}F] FDG-PET/CT examination.[14] Sensitivity and specificity were found to be superior for the above-mentioned parameters. Threshold values, however, will be system and protocol dependent and therefore need to be established locally.

SUMMARY

Patients with suspected valvular or nonvalvular cardiac infection who present with local symptoms in the absence of bacteremia should be evaluated for the presence of infection. Early diagnosis and treatment is essential to prevent seeding of infection to endovascular structures.

There is growing evidence to support the role of [^{18}F] FDG-PET/CT imaging in patients with suspected CIED-GPI. In this respect, when [^{18}F] FDG-PET/CT has been used as a complementary diagnostic tool, it has consistently demonstrated a high negative predictive value for the exclusion of an infective process, both during initial presentation and during long-term follow-up. Further study is indicated to assess not only involvement of endocardial structures but also the response to treatment. Large-scale prospective studies that base the decision to treat on the [^{18}F] FDG-PET/CT results, implementing dietary manipulation and state-of-the-art imaging technology, are needed, however, to confirm the true utility of [^{18}F] FDG-PET/CT as a stand-alone diagnostic test. Evidence is also emerging regarding the potential utility of hybrid radionuclide imaging in suspected vascular graft infection.

REFERENCES

1. Baddour LM, Epstein AE, Erickson CC, et al. Update on cardiovascular implantable electronic device infections and their management: a scientific statement from the American Heart Association. Circulation 2010;121(3):458–77.
2. Segal AW, Thakur ML, Arnot RN, et al. Indium-111-labelled leucocytes for localization of abscesses. Lancet 1976;13:1056–8.
3. Thakur ML, Lavender JP, Arnot RN, et al. Indium-111-labelled autologous leukocytes in man. J Nucl Med 1977;18(10):1014–21.
4. Forstrom LA, Mullan BP, Hung JC, et al. 18F-FDG labelling of human leukocytes. Nucl Med Commun 2000;21:691–4.
5. Erba PA, Sollini M, Lazzeri E, et al. FDG-PET in cardiac infections. Semin Nucl Med 2013;43(5):377–95.
6. Keidar Z, Nitecki S. FDG-PET in prosthetic graft infections. Semin Nucl Med 2013;43:396–402.
7. Jamar F, Buscombe J, Chiti A, et al. EANM/SNMMI guideline for 18F-FDG use in inflammation and infection. J Nucl Med 2013;54(4):647–58.
8. Palestro CJ, Love C, Miller TT. Infection and musculoskeletal conditions: imaging of musculoskeletal infections. Clin Rheumatol 2006;20(6):1197–218.
9. Kouijzer IJ, Bleaker-Rovers CP, Oyen WJG. FDG-PET in fever of unknown origin. Semin Nucl Med 2013;43:333–9.
10. Glaudemans AW, Signore A. FDG-PET/CT in infections: the imaging method of choice? Eur J Nucl Med Mol Imaging 2010;37(10):1986–91.
11. Spacek M, Belohlavek O, Votrubova J, et al. Diagnostics of "non-acute" vascular prosthesis infection using 18F-FDG PET/CT: our experience with 96 prostheses. Eur J Nucl Med Mol Imaging 2009; 36(5):850–8.
12. Meller J, Sahlmann CO, Scheel AK. 18F-FDG PET and PET/CT in fever of unknown origin. J Nucl Med 2007;48(1):35–45.
13. Farsad M, Pernter P, Triani A, et al. Thromboembolism in pulmonary artery sarcoma. Clin Nucl Med 2009;34:239–40.
14. Memmott M, James J, Ahmed F, et al. The performance of quantitation methods in the evaluation of cardiac implantable electronic device (CIED) infection: a technical review. J Nucl Cardiol 2015, in press.
15. Treglia G, Bertagna F. Factors influencing the sensitivity of 18F-FDG PET/CT in the detection of infective endocarditis. Eur J Nucl Med Mol Imaging 2013; 40(7):1112–3.
16. Caldarella C, Leccisotti L, Treglia G, et al. Which is the optimal acquisition time for FDG PET/CT imaging in patients with infective endocarditis? J Nucl Cardiol 2013;20(2):307–9.
17. O'Doherty M, Barrington SF, Klein JL. Opportunistic infection and nuclear medicine. Semin Nucl Med 2009;39(2):88–102.
18. Balink H, Hut E, Pol T, et al. Suppression of 18F-FDG myocardial uptake using a fat-allowed, carbohydrate-restricted diet. J Nucl Med Technol 2011;39:185–9.

19. Williams G, Kolodny GM. Suppression of myocardial 18F-FDG uptake by preparing patients with a high-fat, low-carbohydrate diet. Am J Roentgenol 2008; 109:W151–6.
20. James J, Memmott MJ, Ahmed FA. Impact of dietary carbohydrate restriction prior to 18F-FDG PET/CT for suspected cardiac implantable electronic device (CIED) infection and endocarditis. Nuc Med Comms 2015;36(5):A37.
21. Voigt A, Shalaby A, Saba S. Rising rates of cardiac rhythm management device infections in the united states: 1996 through 2003. J Am Coll Cardiol 2006; 48:590–1.
22. Sarrazin JF, Philippon F, Tessier M, et al. Usefulness of fluorine-18 positron emission tomography/computed tomography for identification of cardiovascular implantable electronic device infections. J Am Coll Cardiol 2012;59(18):1616–25.
23. Cautela J, Alessandrini S, Cammilleri S, et al. Diagnostic yield of FDG positron-emission tomography/computed tomography in patients with CEID infection: a pilot study. Europace 2013;15(2):252–7.
24. Ahmed FZ, James J, Cunnington C, et al. Early diagnosis of cardiac implantable electronic device generator pocket infection using 18F-FDG-PET/CT. Eur Heart J Cardiovasc Imaging 2015;16(5):521–30.
25. Bensimhon L, Lavergne T, Hugonnet F, et al. Whole body [(18) F]fluorodeoxyglucose positron emission tomography imaging for the diagnosis of pacemaker or implantable cardioverter defibrillator infection: a preliminary prospective study. Clin Microbiol Infect 2011;17(6):836–44.
26. Amin R, Charron M, Grinblat L, et al. Cystic fibrosis: detecting changes in airway inflammation with FDG PET/CT. Radiology 2012;264:868–75. And Ahmed, et al 2015.
27. Ploux S, Riviere A, Amraoui S, et al. Positron emission tomography in patients with suspected pacing system infections may play a critical role in difficult cases. Heart Rhythm 2011;8(9):1478–81.
28. Klug D, Balde M, Pavin D, et al. Risk factors related to infections of implanted pacemakers and cardioverter-defibrillators. Circulation 2007;116:1349–55.
29. Erba A, Conti U, Lazzeri E, et al. Added value of 99mTc-HMPAO-labeled leukocyte SPECT/CT in the characterization and management of patients with infectious endocarditis. J Nucl Med 2012;53(8):1235–43.
30. Millar BC, Prendergast BD, Alavi A, et al. 18FDG-positron emission tomography (PET) has a role to play in the diagnosis and therapy of infective endocarditis and cardiac device infection. Int J Cardiol 2013;167(5):1724–36.
31. Kouijzer IJ, Vos FJ, Janssen MJ, et al. The value of 18F-FDG PET/CT in diagnosing infectious endocarditis. Eur J Nucl Med Mol Imaging 2013;40(7):1102–7.
32. de Groot M, Meeuwis AP, Kok PJ, et al. Influence of blood glucose level, age and fasting period on non-pathological FDG uptake in heart and gut. Eur J Nucl Med Mol Imaging 2005;32(1):98–101.
33. Lum D, Wandell S, Ko J, et al. Positron emission tomography of thoracic malignancies: reduction of myocardial fluorodeoxyglucose uptake artifacts with a carbohydrate restricted diet. Clin Positron Imaging 2000;3:155.
34. Fiorani P, Speziale F, Rizzo L, et al. Detection of aortic graft infection with leukocytes labelled with technetium 99m-hexametazime. J Vasc Surg 1993; 17(1):87–96.
35. Fukuchi K, Ishida Y, Higashi M, et al. Detection of aortic graft infection by fluorodeoxyglucose positron emission tomography: comparison with computed tomographic findings. J Vasc Surg 2005;42(5): 919–25.
36. Erba PA, Leo G, Sollini M, et al. Radiolabelled leucocyte scintigraphy versus conventional radiological imaging for the management of late, low-grade vascular prosthesis infections. Eur J Nucl Med Mol Imaging 2014;41:357–68.
37. Keidar Z, Engel A, Hoffman A, et al. Prosthetic vascular graft infection: the role of 18F-FDG PET/CT. J Nucl Med 2007;48(8):1230–6.
38. Wasselius J, Malmstedt J, Kalin B, et al. High 18F-FDG uptake in synthetic aortic vascular grafts on PET/CT in symptomatic and asymptomatic patients. J Nucl Med 2008;49(10):1601–5.
39. Kieder Z, Pirmisashvili N, Leiderman M, et al. 18F-FDG uptake in noninfected prosthetic vascular grafts: incidence, patterns, and changes over time. J Nucl Med 2014;55(3):392–5.
40. Isreal O. Vascular graft infection. Presented as part of the Categorical Seminar: radionuclide imaging inflammation and infection: State of the art and future directions. SNMMI Annual Meeting. St Louis (MO), June 7–11, 2014.
41. Ahmed FZ, James J, Tout D, et al. Metal artefact reduction algorithms prevent false positive results when assessing patients for cardiac implantable electronic device infection. J Nucl Cardiol 2014;22:219–20.
42. Abdoli M, De Jong JR, Pruim J, et al. Clough-Tocher interpolation of virtual sinogram in a Delaunay triangulated grid for metal artifact reduction of PET/CT images. IEEE Nucl Sci Symp Conf Rec 2012;3197–201.
43. Armstrong IS, James J. Reduced-dose (18F)-FDG PETCT scanning with current generation PETCT systems.Available at: http://www.radmagazine.co.uk/ScientificPDFs/December%202014%20-%20Reduced-dose%20PETCT%20scanning%20with%20current%20generation%20PETCT%20systems.pdf.
44. Armstrong IS, James JM, Williams HA, et al. The assessment of time-of-flight on image quality and quantification with reduced administered activity and scan times in FDG PET. Nucl Med Commun 2015;36(7):728–37.

Novel Applications of Radionuclide Imaging in Peripheral Vascular Disease

Mitchel R. Stacy, PhD[a,*], Albert J. Sinusas, MD[a,b]

KEYWORDS

- Peripheral vascular disease • Molecular imaging • PET • SPECT • Perfusion • Angiogenesis
- Atherosclerosis

KEY POINTS

- Peripheral vascular disease is a prevalent atherosclerotic condition affecting the lower extremities that is associated with significant limb health complications and health care costs.
- Current imaging techniques all have limitations with regard to noninvasive assessment of peripheral vascular disease pathophysiology and treatment responses.
- Radionuclide-based imaging may provide novel opportunities for noninvasive assessment of peripheral vascular disease by allowing the evaluation of various physiologic indices, such as skeletal muscle perfusion, angiogenesis, atherosclerosis, and metabolism.

INTRODUCTION

Peripheral vascular disease (PVD) is a highly prevalent and progressive atherosclerotic disease of the lower extremities that is associated with claudication, nonhealing ulcers, major amputations, and death.[1] In addition to lower extremity complications, PVD is also associated with high rates of myocardial infarction and stroke.[2] In a study of Medicare patients, annual costs for PVD-related treatment totaled $4.37 billion.[3]

Because of the onset of atherosclerosis-induced tissue ischemia and necrosis, many patients with PVD require lower extremity revascularization using endovascular procedures or surgical bypass.[4] Nonsurgical options have traditionally been limited to endovascular procedures that have resulted in high rates of stenosis, but recent developments in drug-eluting balloons[5] and stents,[6,7] which possess antiproliferative agents, have increased the opportunities for novel therapeutics. In addition to endovascular procedures, systemic treatments such as drugs that reduce antiplatelet and cholesterol levels, as well as renin-angiotensin system inhibitors, have been applied for the treatment of patients with PVD who are not candidates for revascularization because of multiple diffuse stenosis or arterial calcification.[8] Gene-based therapies using growth factors such as vascular endothelial growth factor (VEGF),[9] fibroblast growth factor,[10] hepatocyte growth factor,[11] and hypoxia inducible factor 1[12] have also gained attention in recent years. In addition, cell-based therapies for PVD have been assessed using endothelial progenitor cells,[13] bone marrow mononuclear cells,[14] and mesenchymal stem cells[15] and have shown relative benefits. Overall, although

Funding sources: This work was supported in part by American Heart Association grant 14CRP20480404 to Dr M.R. Stacy and NIH grant T32 HL098069 to Dr A.J. Sinusas.
Disclosures: Dr A.J. Sinusas receives financial support and NC100692 from GE Healthcare.
[a] Department of Internal Medicine, Yale University School of Medicine, PO Box 208017, Dana-3, New Haven, CT 06520, USA; [b] Department of Diagnostic Radiology, Yale University School of Medicine, PO Box 208042, New Haven, CT 06520, USA
* Corresponding author.
E-mail address: mitchel.stacy@yale.edu

Cardiol Clin 34 (2016) 167–177
http://dx.doi.org/10.1016/j.ccl.2015.06.005
0733-8651/16/$ – see front matter

early application of both gene-based and cell-based therapies has produced some positive results, there are many inconsistencies that still remain with regard to proper dose size, frequency of therapeutics, and combination therapies incorporating multiple forms of growth factors or cells. Development of standardized end points to evaluate clinical outcomes should facilitate understanding of the clinical potential for these therapies. In particular, the use of noninvasive imaging techniques capable of evaluating physiologic responses to novel therapeutic interventions could enhance the field and provide tools that complement standard clinical and anatomic indices, which may lack the ability to fully assess underlying physiologic changes responsible for positive clinical outcomes.

STANDARD IMAGING MODALITIES FOR EVALUATING PERIPHERAL VASCULAR DISEASE

Common clinical methods for detecting the response to medical treatment in the setting of PVD have been the ankle-brachial pressure index (ABI), duplex ultrasonography, and magnetic resonance (MR) or computed tomography (CT) angiographic parameters; however, each of these techniques has relative limitations for the evaluation of PVD.[1] For example, ABI (ie, the pressure differential between upper and lower extremity arteries) is only efficient for evaluating large-vessel obstructions and has decreased sensitivity in the setting of microvascular disease.[16] In addition, ABI values can be exaggerated in the setting of medical calcification, further weakening their clinical utility.[16] Duplex ultrasonography, although an inexpensive, widely available, and fast imaging technique, only permits evaluation of blood flow in major vessels and is not useful for the estimation of collateral vessel flow.[1] CT and MR angiography can characterize vessel morphology and allow identification of significant stenosis or occlusion, thereby directing targeted revascularization procedures. However, both CT and MR angiography are limited by the lack of standard quantitative tools to assess the physiologic consequences associated with vessel stenosis and occlusion.[17] Additional MR approaches exist for evaluation of lower extremity tissue perfusion and oxygenation, but commonly require exercise, pharmacologic, or reactive hyperemia protocols to produce quantifiable changes in image signal intensity.[18,19] Other techniques that have been used in more severe cases of PVD, such as critical limb ischemia (CLI), have included ankle and toe systolic pressures. However, ankle pressures, like ABIs, are subject to error in the setting of arterial calcification, and toe pressures are not always reliable for predicting amputation risk. Transcutaneous oxygen pressure ($TcPo_2$) is considered to be a more reliable prognostic tool in the setting of CLI, because it provides functional information related to tissue perfusion and viability; however, $TcPo_2$ also has limitations because of the ability to only measure superficial tissue viability.[20]

Lower extremity imaging using radionuclide-based approaches, such as positron emission tomography (PET) and single-photon emission CT (SPECT), may allow not only the physiologic assessment of PVD but may also permit evaluation of molecular events associated with disease progression or treatment response. PET and SPECT use targeted radionuclides capable of high-sensitivity detection of biological processes such as angiogenesis, atherosclerosis, and metabolism (**Table 1**).[1] PET systems offer higher sensitivity than SPECT for targeted molecular imaging and also expose patients to lower levels of ionizing radiation through the use of isotopes with short half-lives. However, SPECT systems are more readily available, less expensive, and permit simultaneous imaging of multiple isotopes. Despite the high sensitivity of PET and SPECT for molecular imaging, both possess low spatial resolution compared with CT and MR systems. Because of this limitation, hybrid imaging systems (PET/CT, SPECT/CT, PET/MR) have emerged that allow the pairing of high-sensitivity physiologic images with high-resolution anatomic images, permitting improved quantification of radionuclide uptake within anatomic regions of interest and allowing for attenuation correction and correction for partial volume effects.[21] This article discusses recent trends in radionuclide imaging of PVD and highlights novel applications that may allow serial evaluation of the progression and treatment of PVD.

RADIONUCLIDE IMAGING OF SKELETAL MUSCLE PERFUSION AND BLOOD FLOW

Because of ongoing exposure to, and severity of, skeletal muscle ischemia and hypoxia within the lower extremities, some of the earliest attempts at evaluating PVD with radionuclide approaches evaluated skeletal muscle blood flow and perfusion using intramuscular[22–24] and intra-arterial[25–27] injections of radionuclides. However, in the 1980s thallium-201 (^{201}Tl) emerged as the predominant radionuclide for planar imaging in patients with PVD because of its high first-pass extraction and the ability to inject ^{201}Tl intravenously under conditions of rest[28] or stress.[29] Early studies established the clinical utility of ^{201}Tl

Table 1
Molecular imaging targets for evaluation of PVD

Physiologic Target	Radionuclide	Application
Perfusion/blood flow	^{201}Tl	Porcine,[32] clinical[28–31,82]
	^{99m}Tc-sestamibi	Clinical[34,35,37]
	^{99m}Tc-tetrofosmin	Clinical[1,38,39]
	^{15}O-water	Canine,[43] clinical[40,42,83]
	$C^{15}O_2$	Clinical[84]
	$^{15}O_2$	Clinical[83,84]
	^{13}N-ammonia	Mouse[44]
Angiogenesis	^{99m}Tc-NC100692	Mouse[47,52,85,86]
	^{111}In-VEGF$_{121}$	Rabbit[48]
	^{125}I-c (RGD(I)yV)	Mouse[51]
	^{76}Br-nanoprobe	Mouse[46]
	^{68}Ga-NOTA-RGD	Mouse[50]
	^{64}Cu-DOTA-VEGF$_{121}$	Mouse[49]
	^{64}Cu-DOTA-CANF-comb	Mouse[53]
	^{64}Cu-NOTA-TRC105	Mouse[45,54]
Atherosclerosis	^{18}F-FDG	Clinical[55–58]
	^{18}F-NaF	Clinical[61–64]
	^{11}C-acetate	Clinical[65]
	^{18}F-galacto-RGD	Mouse,[68] clinical[87]
	^{64}Cu-DOTA-CANF	Rabbit[67]
	^{99m}Tc-PBMC	Clinical[66]
Metabolism	^{18}F-FDG	Clinical[69]

Abbreviations: CANF, C-type atrial natriuretic factor; PBMC, peripheral blood mononuclear cell.

scintigraphy and SPECT for detecting perfusion abnormalities in patients with PVD,[28,30] and they also showed high sensitivity for detecting impaired perfusion in the lower extremities of asymptomatic patients.[31] Recent preclinical work by our research team also showed the feasibility of ^{201}Tl SPECT imaging for tracking serial changes in lower extremity perfusion within specific muscle groups in association with ischemia-induced arteriogenesis and angiogenesis, further indicating the clinical utility of ^{201}Tl.[32]

Despite the established value of ^{201}Tl for evaluating patients with PVD, technetium-99m (^{99m}Tc)-labeled tracers have recently emerged as the SPECT perfusion agents of clinical choice because of the shorter half-life, higher-energy gamma rays, and minimal redistribution that characterizes ^{99m}Tc-labeled perfusion agents, thus reducing patient exposure to ionizing radiation and also improving image quality.[33] Planar imaging studies using ^{99m}Tc-sestamibi (MIBI) have shown significant reductions in proximal and distal lower extremity perfusion in asymptomatic patients who presented with early stages of atherosclerosis,[34] and have also revealed impairments in rest and exercise stress perfusion when comparing patients with PVD with controls.[35,36] In addition, Miles and colleagues[35] showed that ^{99m}Tc-MIBI possessed a very high sensitivity (91%) and specificity (94%) for diagnosing PVD, and also showed that ^{99m}Tc-MIBI uptake significantly correlated with angiographic and Doppler findings. Because of the limited redistribution associated with ^{99m}Tc-MIBI, there has been a recent focus on ^{99m}Tc-MIBI lower extremity imaging in patients already undergoing myocardial perfusion imaging for the purposes of identifying potential lower extremity abnormalities in asymptomatic and symptomatic patients.[37] Another ^{99m}Tc-labeled tracer, ^{99m}Tc-tetrofosmin, with no demonstrable redistribution, has also emerged as a tool for assessing lower extremity perfusion, and has shown potential clinical utility in evaluating the response to cell-based and growth factor-based therapies in patients with PVD.[38,39] Our group has established tools for quantifying regional differences in ^{99m}Tc-tetrofosmin uptake in patients with unilateral PVD[1] and have recently transitioned ^{99m}Tc-tetrofosmin SPECT imaging into patients with PVD with CLI to evaluate serial changes in foot perfusion following revascularization procedures (**Fig. 1**).

In addition to radionuclides for SPECT imaging of lower extremity perfusion, PET tracers have also been used for evaluation of skeletal muscle blood flow. One potential benefit that PET may

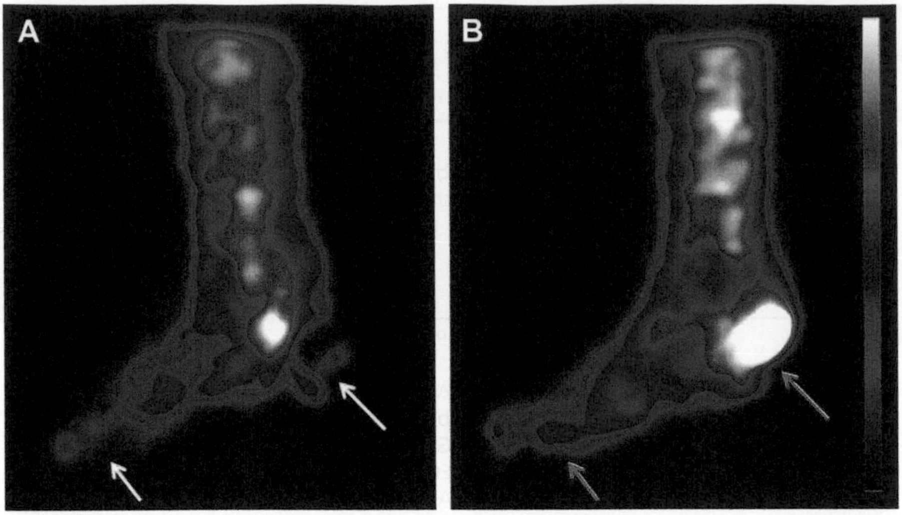

Fig. 1. Sagittal view of ^{99m}Tc-tetrofosmin SPECT imaging in a patient with nonhealing heel ulcer before (*A*) and after (*B*) lower extremity revascularization and wound debridement shows increased tracer uptake in the heel and distal foot. Prerevascularization regions of ischemia are identified by white arrows and improvements in postrevascularization perfusion are denoted by yellow arrows.

offer compared with SPECT in the evaluation of PVD is the ability to quantify absolute muscle blood flow, compared with the standard use of relative uptake values with SPECT. In addition, PET tracers typically possess shorter half-lives, which allows repeated measurements on a patient within the same day.[40] However, a primary limitation of PET, compared with SPECT imaging, is the requirement of exercise or a pharmacologic stressor to induce quantifiable changes in muscle blood flow.[41] An early study by Burchert and colleagues[41] established the clinical utility of PET imaging for evaluation of muscle blood flow in patients with PVD using vasodilator and exercise stress. Further work by Schmidt and colleagues[40] showed the ability of $H_2{}^{15}O$ PET imaging to detect significant impairments in calf muscle flow reserve in patients with PVD compared with healthy subjects, and also found a close correlation between thermodilution-derived and PET-derived flow reserve values. In addition to the utility of PET imaging in the setting of PVD, $H_2{}^{15}O$ PET has also identified the anatomic level of muscle blood flow deficits in the limbs of patients with CLI, suggesting that radionuclide imaging may be a specific indicator of tissue viability and a predictor of future amputation level of the lower extremity.[42]

Preclinical work with $H_2{}^{15}O$ PET imaging has shown a close matching of PET-derived and microsphere-derived measurements of limb blood flow in healthy canines under baseline resting conditions and vasodilator stress.[43] In addition, PET-derived measurements of muscle blood flow have been found to correlate significantly with Doppler flow probe measurements across a variety of physiologic states ($r^2 = 0.92$), further indicating the clinical potential of PET imaging for assessing lower extremity blood flow.[43] In a mouse model of hind limb ischemia, PET imaging of nitrogen-13 (^{13}N) ammonia has been used to evaluate serial changes in tissue perfusion following iliac occlusion and has shown that serial improvements in relative tissue perfusion of the ischemic hind limb closely correlated with the amount of tissue necrosis and fibrosis quantified histologically 30 days following occlusion.[44]

Application of SPECT and PET imaging for serial evaluation of muscle perfusion or blood flow in patients with PVD has yet to reach full potential. Further development of fluorine-18 (^{18}F)–labeled perfusion tracers for PET, which would possess longer half-lives than standard tracers (~110 minutes vs <5 minutes), may assist in expanding the application of PET for assessment of PVD through the combination of myocardial and lower extremity perfusion imaging. In addition, ongoing development of high-sensitivity, high-resolution cadmium zinc telluride SPECT systems should allow the absolute quantification of blood flow in the lower extremities, thereby improving the future potential of SPECT applications in the setting of PVD.

RADIONUCLIDE IMAGING OF SKELETAL MUSCLE ANGIOGENESIS

In addition to imaging of lower extremity perfusion and blood flow, radionuclide-based imaging of angiogenesis has also been established as an effective tool in the evaluation of limb ischemia in preclinical animal models.[44–47] To date, molecular imaging of peripheral angiogenesis with PET and SPECT has relied on radionuclides targeting VEGF receptors and the $\alpha v\beta 3$ integrin, which both play important roles in the angiogenic process. Early work by Lu and colleagues[48] targeted VEGF receptors using indium-111 (^{111}In)–labeled recombinant human $VEGF_{121}$ and showed increased tracer uptake in ischemic hind limbs that peaked 10 days following induction of limb ischemia. More recent work by Willmann and colleagues[49] used in vivo micro-PET imaging and gamma counting of copper-64 (^{64}Cu)–$VEGF_{121}$ for evaluating peripheral angiogenesis and revealed peak tracer uptake at 8 days after femoral artery ligation. In addition, ^{64}Cu-$VEGF_{121}$ showed a significantly higher angiogenic response in mice exposed to an exercise training regimen, suggesting that serial imaging of peripheral angiogenesis may have clinical utility for patients undergoing exercise therapy.

Along with targeting of VEGF receptors, other work has used gallium-68 (^{68}Ga)-labeled,[50] iodine-125 (^{125}I)–labeled,[51] and ^{99m}Tc-labeled[52] RGD peptides (composed of L-arginine, glycine, and L-aspartic acid) for targeting of the $\alpha v\beta 3$ integrin. The RGD peptide moiety allows selective imaging of angiogenesis, because the $\alpha v\beta 3$ integrin is expressed on proliferating endothelial cells and activated macrophages that are involved in the angiogenic process. Early work by Lee and colleagues[51] assessed an ^{125}I-labeled RGD peptide in mice and showed serial changes in radionuclide uptake (via gamma counting) in ischemic limbs that corresponded with postmortem immunohistochemistry evaluation of $\alpha v\beta 3$ integrin expression. Serial in vivo Doppler imaging also revealed improvements in tissue perfusion within the ischemic limb after surgery. Additional work by Hua and colleagues[52] used planar imaging of another radiolabeled RGD tracer, ^{99m}Tc-NC100692 (Maraciclatide, GE Healthcare), to evaluate serial changes in angiogenesis and showed increased radionuclide uptake at 3 and 7 days after induction of limb ischemia that was associated with serial improvements in microvascular density. Further immunofluorescent analysis revealed specificity and colocalization of NC100692 to endothelial cells. Our research team has expanded on this early work with RGD peptides to also validate SPECT/CT image analysis tools for serial regional assessment of angiogenesis in endothelial nitric oxide synthase–deficient mice exposed to limb ischemia and has shown impaired angiogenesis in the distal limbs of these mice compared with wild-type counterparts.[47] Ongoing work in our laboratory is directed at applying ^{99m}Tc-NC100692 SPECT/CT imaging in large animal models of limb ischemia to assess serial changes in angiogenesis and has recently revealed the potential of this tracer for evaluating ischemic hind limb tissue in a porcine model 2 weeks after femoral artery occlusion (**Fig. 2**).

Targeted nanoprobes have also been in recent development for noninvasive assessment of peripheral angiogenesis.[46,53] Specifically, ^{64}Cu-labeled C-type atrial natriuretic factor (CANF)–conjugated comblike nanoprobes have been developed and applied for PET imaging of angiogenesis in mice, showing high sensitivity and specificity for angiogenesis-specific vascular targets.[53] In addition, biodegradable dendritic nanoprobes labeled with either ^{125}I or bromine-76 (^{76}Br) have been developed for PET imaging of the $\alpha v\beta 3$ integrin through the use of polyethylene oxide chains fitted with RGD motifs and have revealed specific uptake in $\alpha v\beta 3$-positive cells as well as in angiogenic tissue within the mouse hind limb.[46]

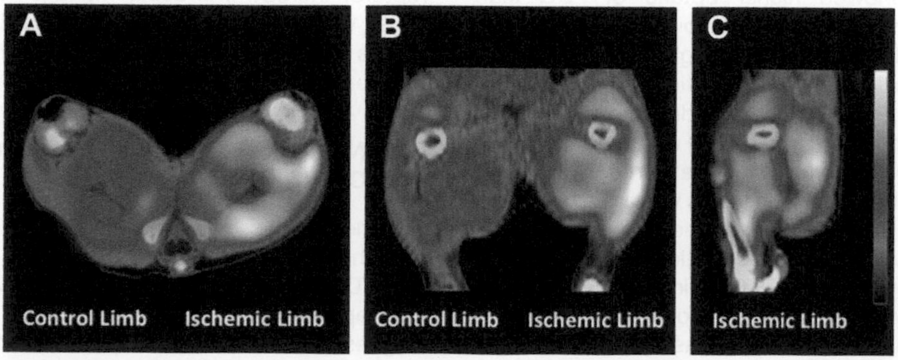

Fig. 2. Transverse (*A*), coronal (*B*), and sagittal (*C*) views of angiogenesis-targeted imaging in a pig model of unilateral hind limb ischemia using ^{99m}Tc-NC100692 SPECT/CT shows marked tracer uptake in ischemic tissue 2 weeks following femoral artery occlusion.

Along with the previously established $\alpha v\beta 3$ and VEGF targets for noninvasive imaging of angiogenesis, ^{64}Cu-NOTA-TRC1005, a CD105 antibody, has recently been developed and validated for evaluating serial changes in angiogenesis following surgically induced limb ischemia.[45,54] In addition to ^{64}Cu-NOTA-TRC1005 showing significantly increased uptake in the setting of hind limb ischemia, this tracer has also shown significantly higher uptake in mice exposed to a combination of limb ischemia and statin therapy, indicating further potential for clinical translation of angiogenesis-targeted imaging in the assessment of medical treatment.[45]

RADIONUCLIDE IMAGING OF ATHEROSCLEROSIS

Another area of radionuclide imaging research that has developed interest is molecular imaging of atherosclerosis. Atherosclerotic plaque progression and stability are regulated by multiple signaling events and cell interactions. Therefore, incorporation of noninvasive imaging tools may offer new insight into plaque evolution and may also assist with monitoring of disease progression and therapeutic responses. To date, the most popular plaque targets have been metabolism and inflammation using PET/CT imaging of ^{18}F-fluorodeoxyglucose (FDG), which is a glucose analogue that is metabolized by resident macrophages, thus providing a noninvasive dual marker of ongoing metabolic activity and inflammation within remodeling plaque.[55–57] Early work by Yun and colleagues[57] showed a strong correlation ($r = 0.99$) between increasing age and increasing FDG uptake in peripheral arteries, and also found an increased prevalence of FDG uptake in peripheral vessels in patients with at least 1 atherogenic risk factor.[58] Further work by Rudd and colleagues[56] revealed that symptomatic, unstable plaques showed higher uptake of FDG than asymptomatic lesions and showed high reproducibility of ^{18}F-FDG-PET/CT imaging for evaluation of plaque burden within the carotid, iliac, and femoral arteries.[55] Recent clinical studies have found significant reductions in ^{18}F-FDG uptake within lower extremity vessels following the increase of plasma high-density lipoprotein levels via atherogenic risk reduction,[59] as well as reduced vascular FDG uptake following high-dose statin therapy.[60] These results suggest that PET/CT imaging of ^{18}F-FDG may provide a sensitive noninvasive tool for tracking atherosclerotic disease progression and therapeutic responses in PVD.

Another radionuclide approach that may allow the evaluation of atherosclerotic plaque progression is PET/CT imaging of ^{18}F-sodium fluoride (^{18}F-NaF). ^{18}F-NaF was originally approved by the US Food and Drug Administration in 1972 as a bone imaging tracer because of the tendency of fluoride ^{18}F to deposit within sites of calcium minerals. Recent work has shown that PET/CT imaging of ^{18}F-NaF may also have value as a noninvasive tool for evaluating active microcalcifications in atherosclerotic plaques (**Fig. 3**).[61–64] In initial atherosclerosis imaging work by Derlin and colleagues,[61] ^{18}F-NaF uptake was highest in the femoral arteries compared with other major peripheral vessels. Further PET/CT imaging studies have since shown a strong correlation between ^{18}F-NaF femoral[64] and carotid[63] artery uptake and atherogenic risk factors, as well as the ability to pair ^{18}F-NaF with ^{18}F-FDG for potential dual analysis of pathophysiologic stages of plaque formation and progression.[62]

Additional radionuclide techniques have also shown feasibility for targeted imaging of atherosclerosis. Derlin and colleagues[65] applied carbon-11 (^{11}C) acetate PET/CT imaging for evaluation of fatty acid synthesis within atherosclerotic plaque of patients and showed increased tracer uptake that was colocalized with regions of arterial calcification. In addition to imaging of fatty acid synthesis, ^{99m}Tc-labeled peripheral blood mononuclear cells have also been used for targeted SPECT/CT imaging of arterial wall inflammation in patients with advanced atherosclerosis and revealed a correlation between tracer uptake and disease severity.[66] Preclinical imaging work in atherosclerosis-induced animal models has also shown the potential for ^{64}Cu-labeled natriuretic peptide in a rabbit model of hypercholesterolemia[67] and ^{18}F-galacto-RGD in evaluating the effect of dietary intervention in hypercholesterolemic mice.[68] The active development of radionuclide-based approaches for evaluation of atherosclerosis should elucidate the various mechanisms regulating plaque progression and vulnerability to rupture, thereby improving management of patients with PVD at high risk for cardiovascular events and allowing the assessment of therapeutic interventions.

POTENTIAL FOR APPLICATION OF NOVEL RADIONUCLIDES

A variety of less-established radionuclide approaches may also have potential for evaluation of PVD and these warrant further investigation and application. Specifically, Pande and colleagues[69] showed impairment of skeletal muscle metabolism in patients with PVD with claudication using ^{18}F-FDG-PET/CT imaging. ^{18}F-FDG has also shown clinical potential for assessing local

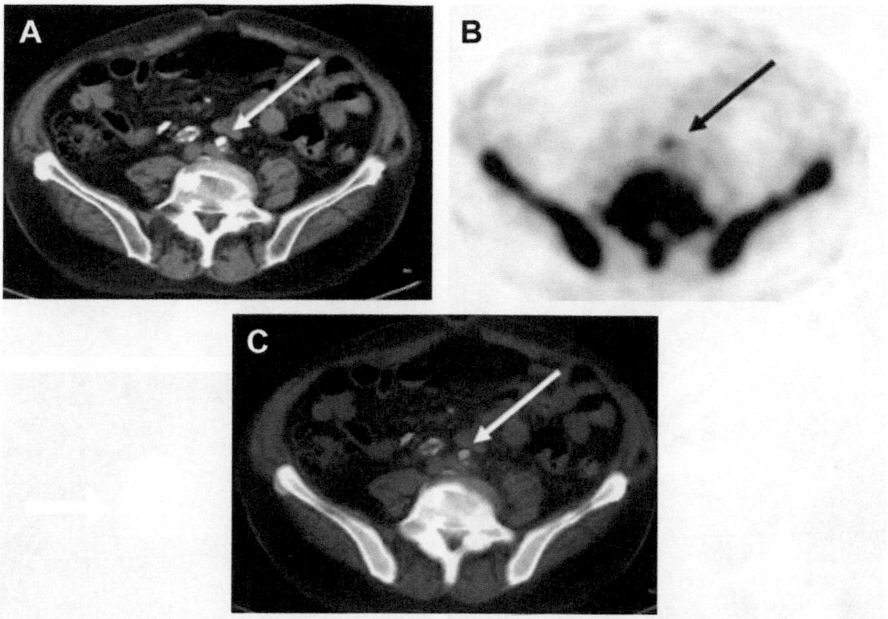

Fig. 3. Targeted imaging of atherosclerosis in the common iliac arteries using CT (*A*), ^{18}F-NaF PET (*B*), and fused ^{18}F-NaF PET/CT imaging (*C*). Fused imaging shows ^{18}F-NaF accumulation in atherosclerotic lesion of iliac artery that is colocalized with calcification. Arrows indicate the region of calcified lesion. (*From* Derlin T, Richter U, Bannas P, et al. Feasibility of 18F-Sodium Fluoride PET/CT for Imaging of Atherosclerotic Plaque. J Nucl Med 2010;51:864.)

infection within fractured peripheral stents and guiding subsequent antibiotic therapy (**Fig. 4**).[70] Both of these studies represent novel applications of ^{18}F-FDG imaging in the evaluation and management of patients with PVD, and warrant future clinical investigations that may further expand on the current role of PET/CT imaging in PVD.

Other radiotracer-based imaging approaches have been developed, but have not yet been applied in the setting of PVD. For example, hypoxia-targeted imaging has been developed and applied for assessment of myocardial ischemia, but application of hypoxia imaging for evaluation of PVD may represent an alternative use, providing an assessment of the balance between tissue blood flow and oxygen utilization.[71] Another noninvasive probe for application in PVD might be the pH (low) insertion peptide, which has been applied for evaluating changing levels in tissue pH and acidosis in the setting of myocardial ischemia and showed sensitivity for detecting tissue exposed to acidic pH levels.[72] In addition, an ^{18}F-labeled PET tracer has recently been developed for assessment of reactive oxygen species and applied in the setting of myocardial inflammation, representing another novel noninvasive approach that may have potential for evaluating stages of atherosclerotic plaque progression or the angiogenic process.[73]

Ongoing development and application of cell-based and gene-based therapies that are being used in clinical trials of patients with PVD should offer additional opportunities for high-sensitivity radionuclide-based approaches for evaluation of PVD.[8,74] The ability to noninvasively evaluate the biodistribution of transplanted cells should be achievable through the use of high-sensitivity PET and SPECT imaging of radiolabeled cells ($\sim 10^4$–10^6 cells/voxel).[75] Multiple clinical trials have already shown the feasibility of tracking effective cell delivery in the myocardium of patients following myocardial infarction.[76–79] However, to date, the short half-lives of PET and SPECT radionuclides has limited the ability to track long-term cell fate in vivo. The development of reporter probes, such as the sodium iodide symporter (NIS), may overcome this limitation by allowing noninvasive detection of viable NIS-transfected cells through retention of isotopes by NIS.[80] NIS has already shown potential for noninvasive assessment of viable cells within infarcted porcine myocardium for 15 weeks following cell transplantation using iodine-123 (^{123}I) SPECT/CT imaging.[81] Future use of radionuclide imaging for serial tracking of cell-based and gene-based therapies is encouraging and should have an expanding role in the evaluation of these novel treatments of PVD.

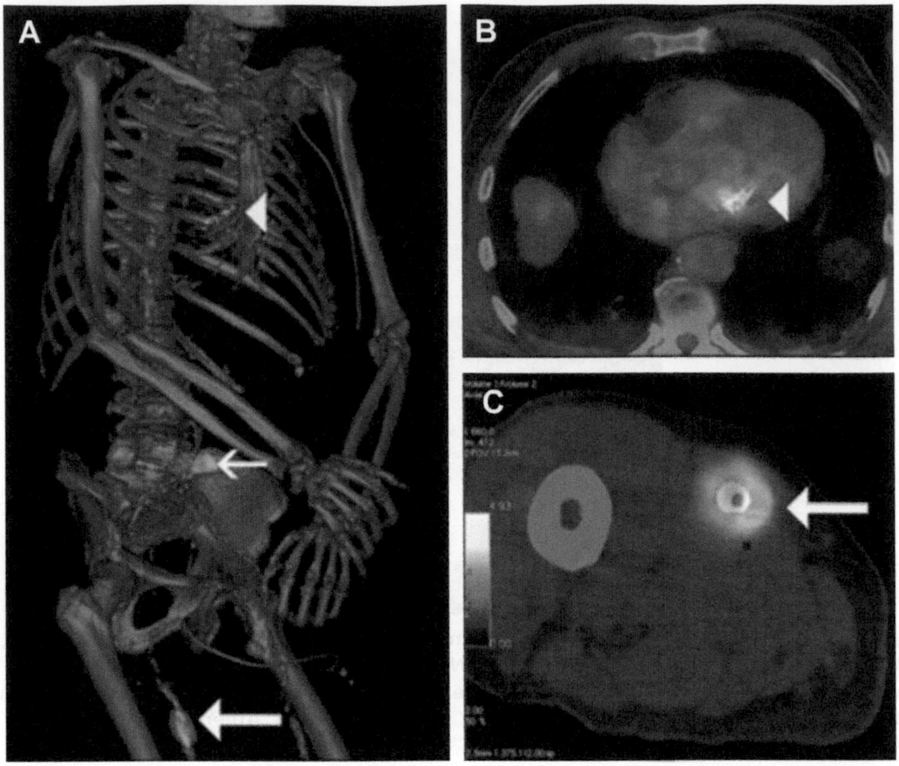

Fig. 4. (*A*) Volume rendering of ^{18}F-FDG-PET/CT shows focal uptake of tracer in regions of mitral valve (*arrowhead*), L4 to L5 discus (*thin arrow*), and right femoral artery stent (*thick arrow*) in a patient found to have mitral endocarditis, peridural abscess, and stent dislocation and fracture. Transverse images further reveal focal ^{18}F-FDG uptake in the infected (*B*) mitral valve and (*C*) femoral artery stent. (*From* Berard X, Pinaquy J-B, Stecken L, et al. Use of 18F-fluorodeoxyglucose positron emission tomography-computed tomography and sonication for detection of infection after peripheral stent fracture. Circulation 2014;129:2439.)

SUMMARY

Radionuclide-based approaches for evaluation of PVD continue to show potential in preclinical animal models as well as patient populations. Ongoing development of targeted PET and SPECT tracers should provide high-sensitivity biomarkers for evaluation of a variety of pathophysiologic processes associated with PVD, and should also offer noninvasive imaging tools to complement the existing anatomic and clinical indices. Continued progress in revascularization procedures and gene-based and cell-based therapies for the management of PVD may further expand the role and potential applications for radionuclide-based imaging approaches in the serial evaluation of medical and/or surgical treatments.

REFERENCES

1. Stacy MR, Zhou W, Sinusas AJ. Radiotracer imaging of peripheral vascular disease. J Nucl Med 2013; 54(12):2104–10.
2. Regensteiner JG, Hiatt WR, Coll JR, et al. The impact of peripheral arterial disease on health-related quality of life in the Peripheral Arterial Disease Awareness, Risk, and Treatment: New Resources for Survival (PARTNERS) Program. Vasc Med 2008;13(1):15–24.
3. Hirsch AT, Hartman L, Town RJ, et al. National health care costs of peripheral arterial disease in the Medicare population. Vasc Med 2008;13(3):209–15.
4. Nasr B, Kaladji A, Vent PA, et al. State-of-the-art treatment of common femoral artery disease. J Cardiovasc Surg 2015;56(2):309–16.
5. Tepe G, Zeller T, Albrecht T, et al. Local delivery of paclitaxel to inhibit restenosis during angioplasty of the leg. N Engl J Med 2008;358(7): 689–99.
6. Lammer J, Bosiers M, Zeller T, et al. First clinical trial of nitinol self-expanding everolimus-eluting stent implantation for peripheral arterial occlusive disease. J Vasc Surg 2011;54(2):394–401.
7. Dake MD, Ansel GM, Jaff MR, et al. Sustained safety and effectiveness of paclitaxel-eluting stents for femoropopliteal lesions: 2-year follow-up from the

Zilver PTX randomized and single-arm clinical studies. J Am Coll Cardiol 2013;61(24):2417–27.
8. Sanada F, Taniyama Y, Kanbara Y, et al. Gene therapy in peripheral artery disease. Expert Opin Biol Ther 2015;15(3):381–90.
9. Isner JM, Pieczek A, Schainfeld R, et al. Clinical evidence of angiogenesis after arterial gene transfer of phVEGF 165 in patient with ischaemic limb. Lancet 1996;348(9024):370–4.
10. Nikol S, Baumgartner I, Van Belle E, et al. Therapeutic angiogenesis with intramuscular NV1FGF improves amputation-free survival in patients with critical limb ischemia. Mol Ther 2008;16(5):972–8.
11. Makino H, Aoki M, Hashiya N, et al. Long-term follow-up evaluation of results from clinical trial using hepatocyte growth factor gene to treat severe peripheral arterial disease. Arterioscler Thromb Vasc Biol 2012;32(10):2503–9.
12. Rajagopalan S, Olin J, Deitcher S, et al. Use of a constitutively active hypoxia-inducible factor-1alpha transgene as a therapeutic strategy in no-option critical limb ischemia patients: phase I dose-escalation experience. Circulation 2007;115(10):1234–43.
13. Kawamoto A, Katayama M, Handa N, et al. Intramuscular transplantation of G-CSF-mobilized CD34(+) cells in patients with critical limb ischemia: a phase I/IIa, multicenter, single-blinded, dose-escalation clinical trial. Stem Cells 2009;27(11):2857–64.
14. Walter DH, Krankenberg H, Balzer JO, et al. Intraarterial administration of bone marrow mononuclear cells in patients with critical limb ischemia: a randomized-start, placebo-controlled pilot trial (PROVASA). Circ Cardiovasc Interv 2011;4(1):26–37.
15. Lasala GP, Silva JA, Gardner PA, et al. Combination stem cell therapy for the treatment of severe limb ischemia: safety and efficacy analysis. Angiology 2010;61(6):551–6.
16. Potier L, Abi Khalil C, Mohammedi K, et al. Use and utility of ankle brachial index in patients with diabetes. Eur J Vasc Endovasc Surg 2011;41(1):110–6.
17. Duran C, Bismuth J. Advanced imaging in limb salvage. Methodist Debakey Cardiovasc J 2012; 8(4):28–32.
18. Pollak AW, Meyer CH, Epstein FH, et al. Arterial spin labeling MR imaging reproducibly measures peak-exercise calf muscle perfusion: a study in patients with peripheral arterial disease and healthy volunteers. JACC Cardiovasc Imaging 2012;5(12):1224–30.
19. Ledermann H-P, Schulte A-C, Heidecker H-G, et al. Blood oxygenation level-dependent magnetic resonance imaging of the skeletal muscle in patients with peripheral arterial occlusive disease. Circulation 2006;113(25):2929–35.
20. Becker F, Robert-Ebadi H, Ricco JB, et al. Chapter I: definitions, epidemiology, clinical presentation and prognosis. Eur J Vasc Endovasc Surg 2011;42(52): S4–12.
21. Stacy MR, Sinusas AJ. Emerging imaging modalities in regenerative medicine. Curr Pathobiol Rep 2015; 3(1):27–36.
22. Kety S. Measurement of regional circulation by the local clearance of radioactive sodium. Am Heart J 1949;38:321–8.
23. Lassen OA, Lindberg J, Munck O. Measurement of blood flow through skeletal muscle by intramuscular injection of xenon-133. Lancet 1964;1(7335):686–9.
24. Cutajar CL, Brown NJ, Marston A. Muscle blood-flow studies by the technetium (99m)Tc clearance technique in normal subjects and in patients with intermittent claudication. Br J Surg 1971;58(7):532–7.
25. Rhodes BA, Greyson ND, Siegel ME, et al. The distribution of radioactive microspheres after intra-arterial injection in the legs of patients with peripheral vascular disease. Am J Roentgenol Radium Ther Nucl Med 1973;118:820–6.
26. Coffmann JD, Mannick JA. A simple objective test for arteriosclerosis obliterations. N Engl J Med 1965;273:1297–301.
27. Sheda H, O'Hara I. Study in peripheral circulation using I-131 and macroaggregated serum albumin. J Exp Med 1970;101:311–4.
28. Hamanaka D, Odori T, Maeda H, et al. A quantitative assessment of scintigraphy of the legs using 201Tl. Eur J Nucl Med 1984;9(1):12–6.
29. Siegel ME, Stewart CA. Thallium-201 peripheral perfusion scans: feasibility of single-dose, single-day, rest and stress study. AJR Am J Roentgenol 1981;136(6):1179–83.
30. Oshima M, Akanabe H, Sakuma S, et al. Quantification of leg muscle perfusion using thallium-201 single photon emission computed tomography. J Nucl Med 1989;30(4):458–65.
31. Duet M, Virally M, Bailliart O, et al. Whole-body (201) Tl scintigraphy can detect exercise lower limb perfusion abnormalities in asymptomatic diabetic patients with normal Doppler pressure indices. Nucl Med Commun 2001;22(9):949–54.
32. Stacy MR, Yu DY, Maxfield MW, et al. Multimodality imaging approach for serial assessment of regional changes in lower extremity arteriogenesis and tissue perfusion in a porcine model of peripheral arterial disease. Circ Cardiovasc Imaging 2014;7(1):92–9.
33. Purushothaman K, Sinusas AJ. Technetium-99m-labeled myocardial perfusion agents: are they better than thallium-201? Cardiol Rev 2001;9(3):160–72.
34. Kuśmierek J, Dąbrowski J, Bienkiewicz M, et al. Radionuclide assessment of lower limb perfusion using (99m)Tc-MIBI in early stages of atherosclerosis. Nucl Med Rev Cent East Eur 2006;9(1):18–23.
35. Miles KA, Barber RW, Wraight EP, et al. Leg muscle scintigraphy with (99)Tc-MIBI in the assessment of peripheral vascular (arterial) disease. Nucl Med Commun 1992;13:593–603.

36. Sayman HB, Urgancioglu I. Muscle perfusion with technetium-MIBI in lower extremity peripheral arterial diseases. J Nucl Med 1991;32(9):1700–3.
37. Soyer H, Uslu I. A patient with peripheral arterial stenosis diagnosed with lower extremity perfusion scintigraphy. Clin Nucl Med 2007;32:458–9.
38. Miyamoto M, Yasutake M, Takano H, et al. Therapeutic angiogenesis by autologous bone marrow cell implantation for refractory chronic peripheral arterial disease using assessment of neovascularization by 99mTc-tetrofosmin (TF) perfusion scintigraphy. Cell Transplant 2004;13(4):429–37.
39. Takagi G, Miyamoto M, Tara S, et al. Controlled-release basic fibroblast growth factor for peripheral artery disease: comparison with autologous bone marrow-derived stem cell transfer. Tissue Eng Part A 2011;17:2787–94.
40. Schmidt MA, Chakrabarti A, Shamim-Uzzaman Q, et al. Calf flow reserve with H(2)(15)O PET as a quantifiable index of lower extremity flow. J Nucl Med 2003;44(6):915–9.
41. Burchert W, Schellong S, van den Hoff J, et al. Oxygen-15-water PET assessment of muscular blood flow in peripheral vascular disease. J Nucl Med 1996;37:93–8.
42. Scremin OU, Figoni SF, Norman K, et al. Preamputation evaluation of lower-limb skeletal muscle perfusion with (15)O H_2O positron emission tomography. Am J Phys Med Rehabil 2010;89(6):473–86.
43. Fischman AJ, Hsu H, Carter EA, et al. Regional measurement of canine skeletal muscle blood flow by positron emission tomography with H_2(15)O. J Appl Physiol (1985) 2002;92(4):1709–16.
44. Peñuelas I, Aranguren XL, Abizanda G, et al. (13)N-ammonia PET as a measurement of hindlimb perfusion in a mouse model of peripheral artery occlusive disease. J Nucl Med 2007;48(7):1216–23.
45. Orbay H, Hong H, Koch JM, et al. Pravastatin stimulates angiogenesis in a murine hindlimb ischemia model: a positron emission tomography imaging study with (64)Cu-NOTA-TRC105. Am J Transl Res 2013;6(1):54–63.
46. Almutairi A, Rossin R, Shokeen M, et al. Biodegradable dendritic positron-emitting nanoprobes for the noninvasive imaging of angiogenesis. Proc Natl Acad Sci U S A 2009;106(3):685–90.
47. Dobrucki LW, Dione DP, Kalinowski L, et al. Serial noninvasive targeted imaging of peripheral angiogenesis: validation and application of a semiautomated quantitative approach. J Nucl Med 2009; 50(8):1356–63.
48. Lu E, Wagner WR, Schellenberger U, et al. Targeted in vivo labeling of receptors for vascular endothelial growth factor: approach to identification of ischemic tissue. Circulation 2003;108(1):97–103.
49. Willmann JK, Chen K, Wang H, et al. Monitoring of the biological response to murine hindlimb ischemia with 64Cu-labeled vascular endothelial growth factor-121 positron emission tomography. Circulation 2008;117(7):915–22.
50. Jeong JM, Hong MK, Chang YS, et al. Preparation of a promising angiogenesis PET imaging agent: (68) Ga-labeled c(RGDyK)-isothiocyanatobenzyl1-1,4,7-triazacyclononane-1,4,7-triacetic acid and feasibility studies in mice. J Nucl Med 2008;49:830–6.
51. Lee K, Jung K, Song S, et al. Radiolabeled RGD uptake and alpha(v) integrin expression is enhanced in ischemic murine hindlimbs. J Nucl Med 2005;46: 472–8.
52. Hua J, Dobrucki LW, Sadeghi MM, et al. Noninvasive imaging of angiogenesis with a (99m)Tc-labeled peptide targeted at alpha(v)beta(3) integrin after murine hindlimb ischemia. Circulation 2005; 111(24):3255–60.
53. Liu Y, Pressly ED, Abendschein DR, et al. Targeting angiogenesis using a C-type atrial natriuretic factor-conjugated nanoprobe and PET. J Nucl Med 2011; 52:1956–63.
54. Orbay H, Zhang Y, Hong H, et al. Positron emission tomography imaging of angiogenesis in a murine hindlimb ischemia model with (64)Cu-labeled TRC105. Mol Pharm 2013;10:2749–56.
55. Rudd JHF, Myers KS, Bansilal S, et al. Atherosclerosis inflammation imaging with 18F-FDG PET: carotid, iliac, and femoral uptake reproducibility, quantification methods, and recommendations. J Nucl Med 2008;49(6):871–8.
56. Rudd JHF, Warburton EA, Fryer TD, et al. Imaging atherosclerotic plaque inflammation with [18F]-fluorodeoxyglucose positron emission tomography. Circulation 2002;105:2708–11.
57. Yun M, Yeh D, Araujo LI, et al. F-18 FDG uptake in the large arteries. A new observation. Clin Nucl Med 2001;26(4):314–9.
58. Yun M, Jang S, Cucchiara A, et al. (18)F FDG uptake in the large arteries: a correlation study with the atherogenic risk factors. Semin Nucl Med 2002;32:70–6.
59. Lee SJ, On YK, Lee EJ, et al. Reversal of vascular 18F-FDG uptake with plasma high-density lipoprotein elevation by atherogenic risk reduction. J Nucl Med 2008;49:1277–82.
60. Ishii H, Nishio M, Takahashi H, et al. Comparison of atorvastatin 5 and 20 mg/d for reducing F-18 fluorodeoxyglucose uptake in atherosclerotic plaques on positron emission tomography/computed tomography: a randomized, investigator-blinded, open-label, 6-month study in Japanese adults scheduled for percutaneous coronary intervention. Clin Ther 2010;32:2337–47.
61. Derlin T, Richter U, Bannas P, et al. Feasibility of (18) F-sodium fluoride PET/CT for imaging of atherosclerosis plaque. J Nucl Med 2010;51:862–5.
62. Derlin T, Toth Z, Papp L, et al. Correlation of inflammation assessed by (18)F-FDG PET, active mineral

deposition assessed by (18)F-fluoride PET, and vascular calcification in atherosclerotic plaque: a dual-tracer PET/CT study. J Nucl Med 2011;52: 1020–7.
63. Derlin T, Wisotzki C, Richter U, et al. In vivo imaging of mineral deposition in carotid plaque using 18F-sodium fluoride PET/CT: correlation with atherogenic risk factors. J Nucl Med 2011;52:362–8.
64. Janssen T, Bannas P, Herrmann J, et al. Association of linear (18)F-sodium fluoride accumulation in femoral arteries as a measure of diffuse calcification with cardiovascular risk factors: a PET/CT study. J Nucl Cardiol 2013;20:569–77.
65. Derlin T, Habermann CR, Lengyel Z, et al. Feasibility of (11)C-acetate PET/CT for imaging of fatty acid synthesis in the atherosclerotic vessel wall. J Nucl Med 2011;52:1848–54.
66. Van der Valk FM, Kroon J, Potters WV, et al. In vivo imaging of enhanced leukocyte accumulation in atherosclerotic lesions in humans. J Am Coll Cardiol 2014;64(10):1019–29.
67. Liu Y, Abendschein D, Woodard GE, et al. Molecular imaging of atherosclerotic plaque with (64)Cu-labeled natriuretic peptide and PET. J Nucl Med 2010;51:85–91.
68. Saraste A, Laitinen I, Weidl E, et al. Diet intervention reduces uptake of avB3 integrin-targeted PET tracer (18)F-galacto-RGD in mouse atherosclerotic plaques. J Nucl Cardiol 2012;19:775–84.
69. Pande RL, Park M-A, Perlstein TS, et al. Impaired skeletal muscle glucose uptake by [18F] fluorodeoxyglucose-positron emission tomography in patients with peripheral artery disease and intermittent claudication. Arterioscler Thromb Vasc Biol 2011;31:190–6.
70. Berard X, Pinaquy J-B, Stecken L, et al. Use of 18F-fluorodeoxyglucose positron emission tomography-computed tomography and sonication for detection of infection after peripheral stent fracture. Circulation 2014;129:2437–9.
71. Sinusas AJ. The potential for myocardial imaging with hypoxia markers. Semin Nucl Med 1999;29(4):330–8.
72. Sosunov EA, Anyukhovsky EP, Sosunov AA, et al. pH (low) insertion peptide (pHLIP) targets ischemic myocardium. Proc Natl Acad Sci U S A 2013; 110(1):82–6.
73. Chu W, Chepetan A, Zhou D, et al. Development of a PET radiotracer for non-invasive imaging of the reactive oxygen species, superoxide, in vivo. Org Biomol Chem 2014;12(25):4421–31.
74. Moazzami K, Moazzami B, Roohi A, et al. Local intramuscular transplantation of autologous mononuclear cells for critical lower limb ischaemia. Cochrane Database Syst Rev 2014;(12):CD008347.
75. Nguyen PK, Riegler J, Wu JC. Stem cell imaging: from bench to bedside. Cell Stem Cell 2014;14:431–44.
76. Kang WJ, Kang HJ, Kim HS, et al. Tissue distribution of 18F-FDG-labeled peripheral hematopoietic stem cells after intracoronary administration in patients with myocardial infarction. J Nucl Med 2006;47: 1295–301.
77. Schachinger V, Aicher A, Dobert N, et al. Pilot trial on determinants of progenitor cell recruitment to the infarcted human myocardium. Circulation 2008; 118(14):1425–32.
78. Hofmann M, Wollert KC, Meyer GP, et al. Monitoring of bone marrow cell homing into the infarcted human myocardium. Circulation 2005;111(17):2198–202.
79. Vrtovec B, Poglajen G, Lezaic L, et al. Comparison of transendocardial and intracoronary CD34+ cell transplantation in patients with nonischemic dilated cardiomyopathy. Circulation 2013;128(Suppl 1):S42–9.
80. Dohan O, De la Vieja A, Paroder V, et al. The sodium/iodide symporter (NIS): characterization, regulation, and medical significance. Endocr Rev 2003;24(1):48–77.
81. Templin C, Zweigerdt R, Schwanke K, et al. Transplantation and tracking of human-induced pluripotent stem cells in a pig model of myocardial infarction: assessment of cell survival, engraftment, and distribution by hybrid single photon emission computed tomography/computed tomography of sodium iodide symporter transgene expression. Circulation 2012;126(4):430–9.
82. Earnshaw JJ, Hardy JG, Hopkinson BR, et al. Non-invasive investigation of lower limb revascularisation using resting thallium peripheral perfusion imaging. Eur J Nucl Med 1986;12(9):443–6.
83. Depairon M, Depresseux J-C, Petermans J, et al. Assessment of flow and oxygen delivery to the lower extremity in arterial insufficiency: a PET-scan study comparison with other methods. Angiology 1991; 42(10):788–95.
84. Depairon M, Zicot M. The quantitation of blood flow/metabolism coupling at rest and after exercise in peripheral arterial insufficiency, using PET and 15-0 labeled tracers. Angiology 1996;47(10):991–9.
85. Mehra VC, Jackson E, Zhang XM, et al. Ceramide-activated phosphatase mediates fatty acid-induced endothelial VEGF resistance and impaired angiogenesis. Am J Pathol 2014;184(5):1562–76.
86. Hedhli N, Dobrucki LW, Kalinowski A, et al. Endothelial-derived neuregulin is an important mediator of ischaemia-induced angiogenesis and arteriogenesis. Cardiovasc Res 2012;93(3):516–24.
87. Beer AJ, Pelisek J, Heider P, et al. PET/CT imaging of integrin alpha(v)beta(3) expression in human carotid atherosclerosis. JACC Cardiovasc Imaging 2014;7(2):178–87.

Translational Coronary Atherosclerosis Imaging with PET

Philip D. Adamson, MBChB*, David E. Newby, DSc, Marc R. Dweck, PhD

KEYWORDS

- Coronary atherosclerosis • ^{18}F-FDG • ^{18}F-NaF • PET • Vulnerable plaque

KEY POINTS

- Acute coronary syndromes typically arise from disruption of an underlying atherosclerotic plaque.
- The characteristic features of these plaques include large necrotic cores with thin fibrous caps, persistent inflammation and active microcalcification.
- Existing imaging technologies can identify anatomical features of vulnerability but not plaque biology.
- PET-CT imaging offers the potential to simultaneously assess plaque morphology and pathophysiology.
- Accurate, prospective identification of the vulnerable plaque may improve patient risk stratification and allow tailored therapeutic approaches.

Ever since 1958, when F. Mason Sones unintentionally performed the first in vivo coronary angiogram, the focus of atherosclerosis imaging has been on determining the presence of coronary plaque and the resultant severity of coronary stenosis. Such an approach has allowed the development of effective revascularization techniques that alleviate symptoms related to coronary insufficiency, and, in some patients with complex disease, improve prognosis. Forty years later, the development of cardiac computed tomography (CT) and quantitative calcium scoring enabled similar information to be obtained in a noninvasive manner and initiated attempts at identifying individuals at risk of future cardiac events from within asymptomatic populations. Unfortunately, it was soon recognized that stenosis severity and macroscopic calcification provide incomplete predictive value for determining the event rate related to an individual plaque.

Concurrent with these developments, several pathologic studies were undertaken on autopsied hearts to describe the characteristic features of culprit plaques—those responsible for acute coronary syndromes and sudden death—in the hope of determining the critical determinants of vulnerability. This approach identified hallmarks, such as a thin fibrous cap, large necrotic core, microcalcification, and positive arterial remodeling, and necessarily emphasized anatomic structure over biological function.[1,2] The advent of high-resolution intracoronary imaging tools, such as intravascular ultrasound (IVUS) and optical coherence tomography (OCT), have since determined that these thin-cap fibroatheromas (TCFA) are common relative to clinical events with a relatively benign natural history whereby most high-risk lesions tend to stabilize over time and other apparently

P.D. Adamson is supported by the New Zealand Heart Foundation (1607). M.R. Dweck and D.E. Newby are supported by the British Heart Foundation (FS/14/78/31020 and CH/09/002) and the Wellcome Trust (WT103782AIA).
Disclosures: The authors declare no conflict of interest.
Centre for Cardiovascular Science, University of Edinburgh, Edinburgh, UK
* Corresponding author. SU305 Chancellor's Building, 47 Little France Crescent, Edinburgh EH16 4TJ, UK.
E-mail address: philip.adamson@ed.ac.uk

Cardiol Clin 34 (2016) 179–186
http://dx.doi.org/10.1016/j.ccl.2015.06.002
0733-8651/16/$ – see front matter

low-risk plaques develop de novo features of vulnerability.[3,4] It is now apparent that a deeper understanding of the pathophysiologic processes that alter this equilibrium is needed and it is in this context that the technique of coronary positron emission tomography (PET) has demonstrated an important potential role.

PET relies on the administration of molecularly targeted radioactive isotopes that exhibit beta decay. The emitted positron travels a short distance, rapidly losing energy until it collides with its antiparticle, the electron. The resultant reaction causes in annihilation of both with 2 photons ejected in approximately opposing directions toward the encircling detector ring. It is an imaging tool that has been in clinical use since the 1960s, predominantly in the field of oncology where it has proved particularly useful for detecting occult metastases and as a surrogate marker of treatment response. As a technique for imaging coronary atherosclerosis, it has faced a variety of challenges that have hampered its uptake in both research and clinical settings. The most important of these have been limited spatial resolution and problems with cardiac motion. Fortunately, the recent development of hybridized PET-CT imaging, gated for cardiac and/or respiratory motion, has allowed coregistration of the PET signal with the high anatomic resolution achieved by CT coronary angiography and substantially improved the ability to localize tracer uptake to individual coronary plaques. Despite this achievement, several important questions remain to be addressed before the true clinical utility of coronary PET-CT imaging can be determined.

WHY IMAGE THE VULNERABLE PLAQUE?

Ideally the information gained about plaque biology from PET-CT imaging would enable prediction of clinical events in a manner sufficiently reliable to allow therapeutic strategies targeting those plaques at most risk and obviate costly and potentially hazardous interventions in those at low risk. Despite currently being a long way from that lofty goal, there are several key roles for these techniques that are more readily realized. The ability to perform serial, prospective, nondestructive imaging allows a better understanding of the dynamic pathophysiologic processes occurring within the plaque. The ability to monitor changes in these processes over time creates the opportunity for PET imaging to be used as a surrogate endpoint for clinical trials. In addition, given that the vulnerable plaque seldom occurs in isolation, it seems plausible that identifying the vulnerable plaque will also aid identification of vulnerable patients. This, in turn, could enable earlier intensification of medical therapies in patients deemed high risk and avoid unnecessary treatments in others.

CHOOSING A PET TRACER

Using PET imaging for determining plaque vulnerability is crucially dependent on selecting an appropriate radiopharmaceutical. Two approaches to developing a PET tracer for coronary imaging can be envisioned: the first makes serendipitous use of an established tracer that binds to a known extracardiac target that may also play a role in plaque vulnerability; the second, developed from first principles, relies on identifying an appropriate target of interest within vulnerable plaque and designing a tracer that binds with sufficient specificity to enable reliable detection. To date, the former has predominated over the latter but, regardless of approach, it is vital that there is a clear understanding of both the exact nature of the tracer-target binding and the importance of the target in determining the natural history of the atherosclerotic lesion. If the purpose of the coronary imaging is simply to determine risk of plaque-related vascular events, then there must be a clear correlation between the presence of a particular target ligand and the risk of such an event. If, however, the purpose is to use the imaging tracer as a surrogate endpoint for an investigation of a novel intervention, then there must additionally be a known causative role of the ligand of interest and these events. ^{18}F-FDG and ^{18}F-NaF are 2 tracers that may potentially fulfill both these objectives and both have been the focus of keen research interest.

18F-FLUORODEOXYGLUCOSE AND THE ROLE OF INFLAMMATION IN PLAQUE VULNERABILITY

Inflammation drives atherosclerosis from its earliest stages. Cellular adhesion molecules promote the migration of immune cells into the plaque where they secrete further inflammatory cytokines creating a self-sustaining cycle. These chemical messengers include proteolytic enzymes that alter the homeostasis of the fibrous cap, increasing the likelihood of cap thinning below the critical threshold of 50 to 65 μm that is associated with rupture.[1,5,6] This process is not localized to a single plaque but reflects a high-risk internal milieu from which arises the concept of pan-coronary vulnerability. Autopsy-based studies have consistently identified the presence of macrophages and other inflammatory cells within culprit lesions whereas biomarker studies report a correlation between systemic markers of inflammation and the incidence of vascular events.[2,7,8] Furthermore, the accelerated development of atherosclerosis in patients with concomitant inflammatory connective tissue and infective diseases supports a causative role for inflammation in plaque rupture.[9]

Preclinical 18F-Fluorodeoxyglucose

^{18}F-FDG is a radiolabeled glucose analogue that concentrates in tissues with high metabolic activity via cellular uptake by the glucose transporter protein (GLUT) system. Within the cell ^{18}F-FDG is converted by hexokinase to ^{18}F-FDG-6-phosphate, which cannot be metabolized further, resulting in its intracellular accumulation. Because malignant cells are more metabolically active than surrounding tissues, ^{18}F-FDG has long been used in oncology for diagnosis, staging, and monitoring treatment response. Within the atherosclerotic plaque, it is believed to correspond with macrophage activity which, as a consequence of their high-energy requirements, predominantly rely on anaerobic metabolism via the glycolytic pathway.[10] Hexokinase activity in activated macrophages is 10-fold greater than in those at rest.[11] Histologic samples from animal models of atherosclerosis have consistently shown tracer localization to regions of macrophage differentiation into foam cells and the subsequent activity of those foams cells as determined by a variety of soluble biomarkers.[12] Wenning and colleagues[13] used ^{18}F-FDG imaging in a recent study that implanted a carotid artery cuff to induce shear stress–mediated atherosclerotic inflammation in dyslipidemic mice in an attempt to reflect more closely the inflammatory process that occurs within human plaques. They identified a clear increase in tracer uptake in the low shear-stress, inflammation-prone, upstream arterial region compared with no change in tracer uptake downstream of the iatrogenic stenosis. Furthermore, the increased tracer uptake in the upstream plaques correlated with increased lesion size and macrophage density compared with the smaller, less inflamed downstream plaques (**Fig. 1**). Finally, the predictive value of tracer uptake was demonstrated in a separate study involving atherosclerotic rabbits that were administered Russell's viper venom, a potent procoagulant, with the intention of inducing plaque-related aortic thrombosis. Baseline ^{18}F-FDG uptake

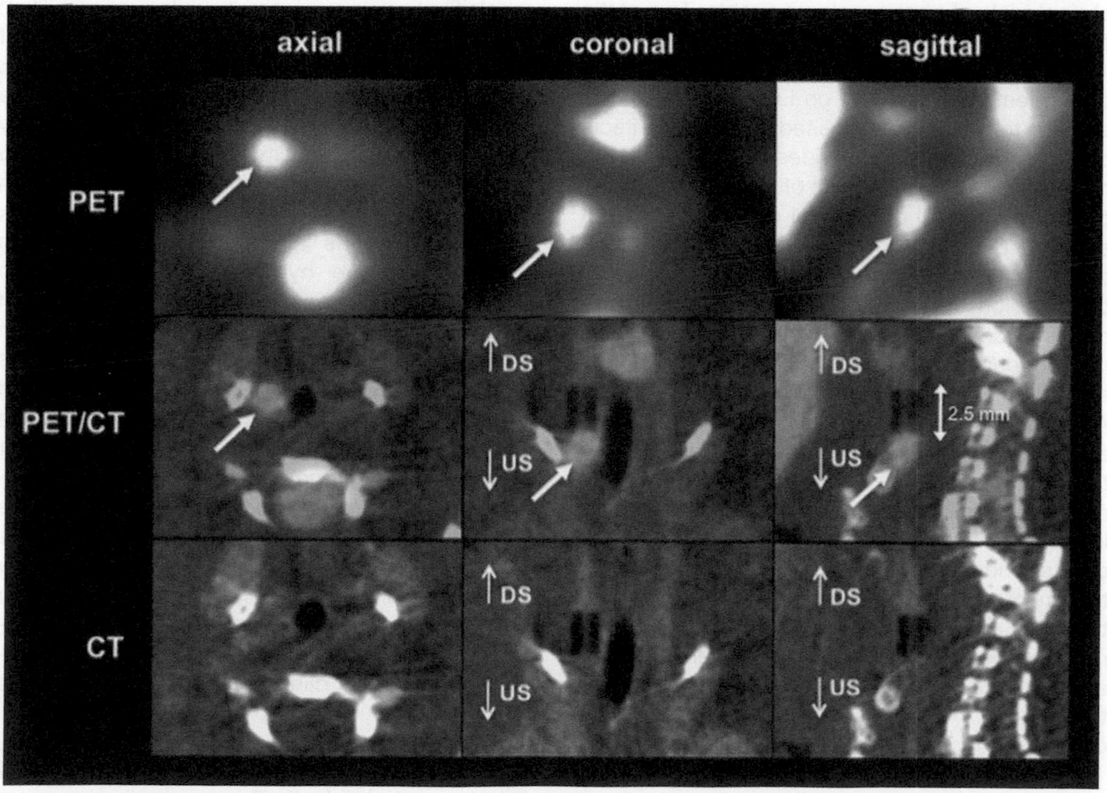

Fig. 1. In vivo ^{18}F-FDG PET/CT 8 weeks after cuff implantation around the right common carotid artery shows increased ^{18}F-FDG uptake in the US plaque (*white arrows*). DS, downstream; US, upstream. (*From* Wenning C, Kloth C, Kuhlmann MT, et al. Serial F-18-FDG PET/CT distinguishes inflamed from stable plaque phenotypes in shear-stress induced murine atherosclerosis. Atherosclerosis 2014;234(2):279; with permission.)

was greater in those plaques that subsequently demonstrated thrombus formation, and therefore deemed vulnerable, than those that remained quiescent.[14]

Clinical 18F-Fluorodeoxyglucose

The first clinical cardiovascular investigation of ^{18}F-FDG occurred in the setting of stroke where uptake in symptomatic carotid plaques was 27% greater than in the contralateral, asymptomatic vessel.[15] Carotid ^{18}F-FDG activity has subsequently been shown to correlate with high-risk plaque features on CT imaging and endarterectomy specimens and to be predictive of recurrent ipsilateral events.[16,17] Similar uptake can be seen in a variety of vascular territories where it is associated with biochemical evidence of increased inflammation and higher prevalence of the metabolic syndrome.[12,18–21] Within the coronary circulation, tracer uptake may be able to identify culprit coronary plaques in patients with acute coronary syndrome,[22] although evidence is conflicting.[23]

Recognition that ^{18}F-FDG provides important information on plaque inflammation has led to investigations of its use as a surrogate endpoint in clinical trials of pharmacologic agents. Two statin studies using ^{18}F-FDG PET imaging of vascular inflammation have shown significant reductions independent of their effect on LDL.[24,25] This lends support to the much discussed pleiotropic effects of this drug class and provides a potential explanation for the clinical benefit of rosuvastatin in patients with normal cholesterol concentrations but elevated C-reactive protein.[26] In contrast, inhibitors of proinflammatory lipoprotein-associated phospholipase A_2 failed to modify vascular inflammation in an early study using PET imaging, which may account for the failure to improve hard clinical endpoints in a subsequent larger clinical trial.[27–29] A similar relationship was seen in a multimodal imaging study of dalcetrapib—a cholesteryl ester transfer protein (CETP) inhibitor—where no impact on vascular inflammation was detected, preempting the negative findings of the later trial assessing clinical endpoints.[30,31] This association between treatment response as determined by ^{18}F-FDG uptake and clinical events raises the possibility of more economically efficient drug development by enabling exploratory research using PET imaging to confirm a therapeutic response before initiating costly long-term large-scale phase III trials.

The key limitation to using ^{18}F-FDG for the identification of coronary plaque inflammation arises as a consequence of its nonspecific uptake by metabolically active tissues, which sees ^{18}F-FDG transported into any cell with significant glucose requirements, including cardiomyocytes. This feature enables myocardial ^{18}F-FDG imaging to assess tissue viability and predict potential benefit from revascularization but unfortunately tends to obscure the signal arising from inflamed coronary plaques. Attempts have been made to suppress this, with patients encouraged to consume low-carbohydrate diets prior to tracer administration, with variable results. In one recent study, more than 50% of coronary segments were not interpretable despite optimal patient preparation.[23] Unless this challenge can be overcome, it may preclude more widespread coronary (but not carotid) research with this agent.

18F-SODIUM FLUORIDE AND ACTIVE MICROCALCIFICATION

Calcium plays a complex and conflicting role in plaque vulnerability. Population-based coronary CT studies have demonstrated an association between calcium scores and cardiovascular risk but this macroscopic calcification merely reflects overall plaque burden and does not allow accurate prediction of individual plaque vulnerability.[32,33] Biomechanical studies have suggested that macrocalcification may increase plaque stability[34] and, for carotid plaques, implies resolution of inflammation and lower stroke risk.[35,36] Instead, newer evidence supports a more nuanced role for calcium in plaque rupture with risk inversely related to mineral density.[37] It is now recognized that the process of calcium formation begins in the earliest stages of plaque evolution, with matrix vesicles acting as a nidus for the deposition of nanocrystalline hydroxyapatite.[38,39] Ex vivo micro-CT imaging has confirmed the presence of microcalcifications (5–50 μm in diameter) within the fibrous caps of a third of fibroatheromas whereas finite element analysis has demonstrated the dramatic amplification of tensile stress within the cap that these deposits produce.[40] Further studies have confirmed a critical window of microcalcification size between 5 and 65 μm to generate the sufficient stress concentration to overcome the structural integrity of the fibrous cap.[41–44] Over time, these smaller particles coalesce into larger nodules resulting in a degree of plaque stabilization before the particles are large enough to be detected with either clinical CT or IVUS, which has limits of resolution of approximately 200 μm.

One promising development in the in vivo detection of calcification on this microscopic scale is PET imaging with ^{18}F-NaF. This tracer demonstrates avid binding to hydroxyapatite and as a consequence has been used for detecting bony metastases for several decades. It was subsequently found to accumulate in a variety of vascular wall locations with its uptake associated with cardiovascular risk factors.[45–47] Intriguingly, this localization is not always concordant with CT-determined calcification as evidenced by one study where 41% of patients with coronary artery calcium scores greater than 1000 demonstrated no ^{18}F-NaF uptake.[47,48] Instead, by revealing early active microcalcification, it predicts the development of CT-determined, advanced calcification within the cardiovascular system.[49] This ability arises as a consequence of the reduction in the total exposed surface area available for ^{18}F-NaF binding that occurs as the large number of small microcalcifications gradually amalgamate to form macroscopic deposits (**Fig. 2**). Similar to early vascular studies of ^{18}F-FDG, carotid endarterectomy specimens from a cohort of patients with acute stroke have provided histologic proof of principle. Tracer uptake was consistently localized to regions of increased calcification activity and macroscopically determined plaque rupture. These sites also exhibited additional high-risk plaque features, including macrophage infiltration and cell apoptosis. A parallel study, where the tracer was administered to a cohort with clinically stable ischemic heart disease, identified 45% that had at least one coronary plaque with focal tracer uptake. Virtual histology of these plaques using IVUS showed a clear relationship between tracer uptake and high-risk features, such as spotty calcification and large necrotic cores. Finally, within a cohort of 40 patients with recent acute myocardial infarction imaged with ^{18}F-NaF, 93% of culprit plaques demonstrated increased uptake.[23]

In contrast to ^{18}F-FDG, ^{18}F-NaF uptake is not typically seen in the myocardium (**Fig. 3**). However, other fibrous structures in the heart, such as the mitral annulus and aortic valvular cusps, are recognized to develop calcification in pathologic states, and the ability to detect early stages in this process is being investigated as a technique for predicting aortic stenosis progression (NCT02132026).

ONGOING LIMITATIONS OF CORONARY PET IMAGING

The early results of clinical studies using ^{18}F-FDG and ^{18}F-NaF CT-PET imaging show promise for improving the ability to detect features of plaque vulnerability in vivo and noninvasively. Several technical challenges, however, remain to be overcome.

Accurate Tracer Localization and Coronary Motion Correction

The physics underpinning PET imaging creates fundamental limits in resolution principally related to positron range prior to annihilation and photon noncolinearity. With regards to clinical imaging with ^{18}F, this limit of resolution is 2 to 4 mm.[50] Unfortunately, imaging of the coronary circulation creates an additional obstacle to tracer localization in the form of cardiac and respiratory motion. The PET signal is obtained continuously over a prolonged period, often in excess of 15 minutes, which is then coregistered with an ECG-gated CT image captured in less than 15 seconds during a period of cardiac diastole when coronary motion is minimal. An approximation of CT gating can be achieved by only using PET data obtained during the third quarter of the ECG-determined cardiac cycle but this results in a 75% reduction in PET signal, which degrades the signal-to-noise ratio and still does not allow for the effects of respiratory motion.

Alternative approaches are, therefore, required. Cardiac motion can be modeled from list-mode PET data and used to correct for both cardiac and respiratory motion, potentially without losing

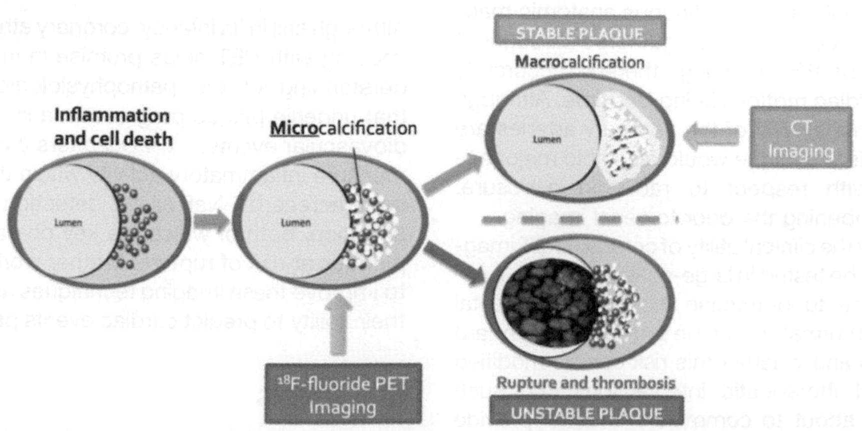

Fig. 2. 18F-fluoride binds to regions of microcalcification prior to the presence of CT-determined macrocalcification.

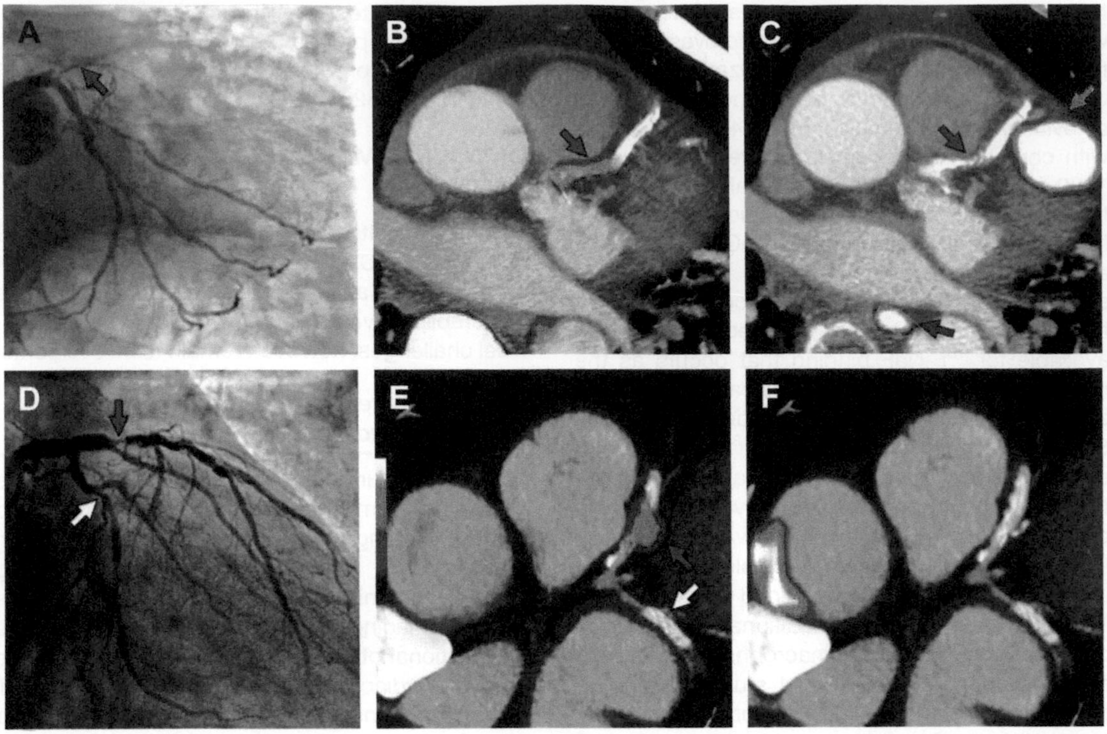

Fig. 3. Focal 18F-fluoride ^{18}F-NaF and ^{18}F-FDG uptake in patients with myocardial infarction. Patient with acute ST-segment elevation myocardial infarction with (*A*) proximal occlusion (*red arrow*) of the left anterior descending artery on invasive coronary angiography and (*B*) intense focal 18F-fluoride. Corresponding ^{18}F-FDG PET-CT image (*C*) showing no uptake at the site of the culprit plaque. Note the significant myocardial uptake overlapping with the coronary artery (*yellow arrow*) and uptake within the esophagus (*blue arrow*). Patient with anterior non–ST-segment elevation myocardial infarction with (*D*) culprit (left anterior descending artery [*red arrow*]) and bystander nonculprit (circumflex artery [*white arrow*]) lesions on invasive coronary angiography that were both stented during the index admission. Only the culprit lesion had increased 18F-fluoride uptake on PET-CT (*E*) after percutaneous coronary intervention. Corresponding ^{18}F-FDG PET-CT showing no uptake either at the culprit or the bystander stented lesion (*F*). Note intense uptake within the ascending aorta. (*From* Joshi NV, Vesey AT, Williams MC, et al. 18F-fluoride positron emission tomography for identification of ruptured and high-risk coronary atherosclerotic plaques: a prospective clinical trial. Lancet 2014;383(9918):709; with permission.)

any data.[51] Alternatively, the recent introduction of PET-MRI should allow continuous anatomic magnetic resonance data to be gathered throughout the period of PET imaging, thereby accurately tracking cardiac motion during this time. Although improvements in MRI of the coronary arteries are required, this technique would also hold major advantages with respect to radiation exposure, potentially opening the door to serial imaging.

Ultimately the clinical utility of coronary PET imaging needs to be tested in large-scale prospective imaging studies to determine whether incremental prognostic information can be provided to standard approaches and whether this risk can be modified by targeted therapeutic intervention. Two such studies are about to commence and will provide an indication as to the future role of this approach (NCT02278211 and NCT02110303).

SUMMARY

Although still in its infancy, coronary atherosclerosis imaging with PET holds promise in improving understanding of the pathophysiologic processes that underlie plaque progression and adverse cardiovascular events. ^{18}F-FDG offers the potential to measure inflammatory activity within the plaque itself whereas ^{18}F-NaF allows detection of microcalcification, both of which are key characteristics of plaques at risk of rupture. Further work is required to improve these imaging techniques and to assess their ability to predict cardiac events prospectively.

REFERENCES

1. Arbab-Zadeh A, Nakano M, Virmani R, et al. Acute coronary events. Circulation 2012;125(9):1147–56.

2. Virmani R, Burke AP, Farb A, et al. Pathology of the vulnerable plaque. J Am Coll Cardiol 2006;47(8 Suppl):C13–8.
3. Kubo T, Maehara A, Mintz GS, et al. The dynamic nature of coronary artery lesion morphology assessed by serial virtual histology intravascular ultrasound tissue characterization. J Am Coll Cardiol 2010;55(15):1590–7.
4. Stone GW, Maehara A, Lansky AJ, et al. A prospective natural-history study of coronary atherosclerosis. N Engl J Med 2011;364(3):226–35.
5. Yonetsu T, Kakuta T, Lee T, et al. In vivo critical fibrous cap thickness for rupture-prone coronary plaques assessed by optical coherence tomography. Eur Heart J 2011;32(10):1251–9.
6. Narula J, Nakano M, Virmani R, et al. Histopathologic characteristics of atherosclerotic coronary disease and implications of the findings for the invasive and noninvasive detection of vulnerable plaques. J Am Coll Cardiol 2013;61(10):1041–51.
7. Musunuru K, Kral BG, Blumenthal RS, et al. The use of high-sensitivity assays for C-reactive protein in clinical practice. Nat Clin Pract Cardiovasc Med 2008;5(10):621–35.
8. Blaha MJ, Rivera JJ, Budoff MJ, et al. Association between obesity, high-sensitivity C-reactive protein >/=2 mg/L, and subclinical atherosclerosis: implications of JUPITER from the Multi-Ethnic Study of Atherosclerosis. Arterioscler Thromb Vasc Biol 2011; 31(6):1430–8.
9. Sherer Y, Shoenfeld Y. Mechanisms of disease: atherosclerosis in autoimmune diseases. Nat Clin Pract Rheumatol 2006;2(2):99–106.
10. Tarkin JM, Joshi FR, Rudd JH. PET imaging of inflammation in atherosclerosis. Nat Rev Cardiol 2014;11(8):443–57.
11. Newsholme P, Curi R, Gordon S, et al. Metabolism of glucose, glutamine, long-chain fatty acids and ketone bodies by murine macrophages. Biochem J 1986;239(1):121–5.
12. Alie N, Eldib M, Fayad ZA, et al. Inflammation, atherosclerosis, and coronary artery disease: PET/CT for the evaluation of atherosclerosis and inflammation. Clin Med Insights Cardiol 2014;8(Suppl 3): 13–21.
13. Wenning C, Kloth C, Kuhlmann MT, et al. Serial F-18-FDG PET/CT distinguishes inflamed from stable plaque phenotypes in shear-stress induced murine atherosclerosis. Atherosclerosis 2014;234(2):276–82.
14. Zhao QM, Zhao X, Feng TT, et al. Detection of vulnerable atherosclerotic plaque and prediction of thrombosis events in a rabbit model using 18F-FDG -PET/CT. PLoS One 2013;8(4):e61140.
15. Rudd JH, Warburton EA, Fryer TD, et al. Imaging atherosclerotic plaque inflammation with [18F]-fluorodeoxyglucose positron emission tomography. Circulation 2002;105(23):2708–11.
16. Figueroa AL, Subramanian SS, Cury RC, et al. Distribution of inflammation within carotid atherosclerotic plaques with high-risk morphological features: a comparison between positron emission tomography activity, plaque morphology, and histopathology. Circ Cardiovasc Imaging 2012;5(1):69–77.
17. Marnane M, Merwick A, Sheehan OC, et al. Carotid plaque inflammation on 18F-fluorodeoxyglucose positron emission tomography predicts early stroke recurrence. Ann Neurol 2012;71(5):709–18.
18. Tahara N, Kai H, Yamagishi S, et al. Vascular inflammation evaluated by [18F]-fluorodeoxyglucose positron emission tomography is associated with the metabolic syndrome. J Am Coll Cardiol 2007; 49(14):1533–9.
19. Rudd JH, Myers KS, Bansilal S, et al. (18)Fluorodeoxyglucose positron emission tomography imaging of atherosclerotic plaque inflammation is highly reproducible: implications for atherosclerosis therapy trials. J Am Coll Cardiol 2007;50(9):892–6.
20. Rudd JH, Myers KS, Bansilal S, et al. Atherosclerosis inflammation imaging with 18F-FDG PET: carotid, iliac, and femoral uptake reproducibility, quantification methods, and recommendations. J Nucl Med 2008;49(6):871–8.
21. Tahara N, Kai H, Nakaura H, et al. The prevalence of inflammation in carotid atherosclerosis: analysis with fluorodeoxyglucose-positron emission tomography. Eur Heart J 2007;28(18):2243–8.
22. Rogers IS, Nasir K, Figueroa AL, et al. Feasibility of FDG imaging of the coronary arteries: comparison between acute coronary syndrome and stable angina. JACC Cardiovasc Imaging 2010;3(4): 388–97.
23. Joshi NV, Vesey AT, Williams MC, et al. 18F-fluoride positron emission tomography for identification of ruptured and high-risk coronary atherosclerotic plaques: a prospective clinical trial. Lancet 2014; 383(9918):705–13.
24. Ishii H, Nishio M, Takahashi H, et al. Comparison of atorvastatin 5 and 20 mg/d for reducing F-18 fluorodeoxyglucose uptake in atherosclerotic plaques on positron emission tomography/computed tomography: a randomized, investigator-blinded, open-label, 6-month study in Japanese adults scheduled for percutaneous coronary intervention. Clin Ther 2010;32(14):2337–47.
25. Tahara N, Kai H, Ishibashi M, et al. Simvastatin attenuates plaque inflammation: evaluation by fluorodeoxyglucose positron emission tomography. J Am Coll Cardiol 2006;48(9):1825–31.
26. Ridker PM, Danielson E, Fonseca FA, et al. Rosuvastatin to prevent vascular events in men and women with elevated C-reactive protein. N Engl J Med 2008;359(21):2195–207.
27. Tawakol A, Singh P, Rudd JH, et al. Effect of treatment for 12 weeks with rilapladib, a lipoprotein-associated

phospholipase A2 inhibitor, on arterial inflammation as assessed with 18F-fluorodeoxyglucose-positron emission tomography imaging. J Am Coll Cardiol 2014;63(1):86–8.
28. White HD, Held C, Stewart R, et al. Darapladib for preventing ischemic events in stable coronary heart disease. N Engl J Med 2014;370(18):1702–11.
29. O'Donoghue ML, Braunwald E, White HD, et al. Effect of darapladib on major coronary events after an acute coronary syndrome: the SOLID-TIMI 52 randomized clinical trial. JAMA 2014;312(10): 1006–15.
30. Fayad ZA, Mani V, Woodward M, et al. Safety and efficacy of dalcetrapib on atherosclerotic disease using novel non-invasive multimodality imaging (dal-PLAQUE): a randomised clinical trial. Lancet 2011;378(9802):1547–59.
31. Schwartz GG, Olsson AG, Abt M, et al. Effects of dalcetrapib in patients with a recent acute coronary syndrome. N Engl J Med 2012;367(22):2089–99.
32. Thilo C, Gebregziabher M, Mayer FB, et al. Correlation of regional distribution and morphological pattern of calcification at CT coronary artery calcium scoring with non-calcified plaque formation and stenosis. Eur Radiol 2010;20(4):855–61.
33. Detrano R, Guerci AD, Carr JJ, et al. Coronary calcium as a predictor of coronary events in four racial or ethnic groups. N Engl J Med 2008;358(13):1336–45.
34. Lin TC, Tintut Y, Lyman A, et al. Mechanical response of a calcified plaque model to fluid shear force. Ann Biomed Eng 2006;34(10):1535–41.
35. Wahlgren CM, Zheng W, Shaalan W, et al. Human carotid plaque calcification and vulnerability. Relationship between degree of plaque calcification, fibrous cap inflammatory gene expression and symptomatology. Cerebrovasc Dis 2009;27(2):193–200.
36. Shaalan WE, Cheng H, Gewertz B, et al. Degree of carotid plaque calcification in relation to symptomatic outcome and plaque inflammation. J Vasc Surg 2004;40(2):262–9.
37. Hutcheson JD, Maldonado N, Aikawa E. Small entities with large impact: microcalcifications and atherosclerotic plaque vulnerability. Curr Opin Lipidol 2014;25(5):327–32.
38. Roijers RB, Debernardi N, Cleutjens JP, et al. Microcalcifications in early intimal lesions of atherosclerotic human coronary arteries. Am J Pathol 2011; 178(6):2879–87.
39. New SE, Aikawa E. Cardiovascular calcification. Circ J 2011;75(6):1305–13.
40. Kelly-Arnold A, Maldonado N, Laudier D, et al. Revised microcalcification hypothesis for fibrous cap rupture in human coronary arteries. Proc Natl Acad Sci U S A 2013;110(26):10741–6.
41. Maldonado N, Kelly-Arnold A, Cardoso L, et al. The explosive growth of small voids in vulnerable cap rupture; cavitation and interfacial debonding. J Biomech 2013;46(2):396–401.
42. Vengrenyuk Y, Cardoso L, Weinbaum S. Micro-CT based analysis of a new paradigm for vulnerable plaque rupture: cellular microcalcifications in fibrous caps. Mol Cell Biomech 2008;5(1):37–47.
43. Bluestein D, Alemu Y, Avrahami I, et al. Influence of microcalcifications on vulnerable plaque mechanics using FSI modeling. J Biomech 2008;41(5):1111–8.
44. Rambhia SH, Liang X, Xenos M, et al. Microcalcifications increase coronary vulnerable plaque rupture potential: a patient-based micro-CT fluid-structure interaction study. Ann Biomed Eng 2012;40(7): 1443–54.
45. Derlin T, Richter U, Bannas P, et al. Feasibility of 18F-sodium fluoride PET/CT for imaging of atherosclerotic plaque. J Nucl Med 2010;51(6):862–5.
46. Derlin T, Wisotzki C, Richter U, et al. In vivo imaging of mineral deposition in carotid plaque using 18F-sodium fluoride PET/CT: correlation with atherogenic risk factors. J Nucl Med 2011;52(3):362–8.
47. Dweck MR, Chow MW, Joshi NV, et al. Coronary arterial 18F-sodium fluoride uptake: a novel marker of plaque biology. J Am Coll Cardiol 2012;59(17): 1539–48.
48. Li Y, Berenji GR, Shaba WF, et al. Association of vascular fluoride uptake with vascular calcification and coronary artery disease. Nucl Med Commun 2012;33(1):14–20.
49. Dweck MR, Jenkins WS, Vesey AT, et al. 18F-sodium fluoride uptake is a marker of active calcification and disease progression in patients with aortic stenosis. Circ Cardiovasc Imaging 2014;7(2):371–8.
50. Moses WW. Fundamental limits of spatial resolution in PET. Nucl Instrum Methods Phys Res A 2011; 648(Suppl 1):S236–40.
51. Slomka PJ, Diaz-Zamudio M, Dey D, et al. Automatic registration of misaligned CT attenuation correction maps in Rb-82 PET/CT improves detection of angiographically significant coronary artery disease. J Nucl Cardiol 2015. [Epub ahead of print].

Translational Molecular Nuclear Cardiology

James T. Thackeray, PhD*, Frank M. Bengel, MD

KEYWORDS

• PET • SPECT • Cardiovascular disease • Translational imaging

KEY POINTS

- Established translational nuclear imaging agents target critical and common molecular pathways of cardiac pathologies.
- Translational strategies are essential for effective identification and characterization of high-potential candidate tracers.
- The characterization of translational imaging compounds should strive to achieve reliable quantification, demonstrate diagnostic and/or prognostic benefit, and allow for monitoring therapeutic efficacy.

INTRODUCTION

The widespread expansion of dedicated small animal imaging systems has provided a research framework for the accelerated development of novel molecular nuclear imaging agents. Current tracers target a number of critical axes in the development and progression of cardiovascular disease, including myocardial metabolism, sympathetic neuronal activation, local and systemic inflammation, molecular biomarkers of ventricular and vascular remodeling, and monitoring of regenerative therapy. Some of these imaging agents have been approved for routine clinical application (**Box 1**). Other novel compounds remain under investigation, at variable stages of translation from lab bench to clinical evaluation (**Box 2**). There remain a number of challenges to wider clinical deployment of novel radiotracers and imaging techniques, particularly (1) absolute, reliable, and reproducible quantification; (2) demonstration of added diagnostic and/or prognostic value for risk stratification; and (3) capacity to measure disease progression and regression to therapy. Here, we discuss the current state of preclinical nuclear molecular imaging research and translation to clinical practice.

MYOCARDIAL METABOLISM

The preeminent test case of molecular imaging is the diagnostic and prognostic application of positron emission tomography (PET) with fludeoxyglucose F 18 (^{18}F-FDG) to assess myocardial glucose metabolism. More thorough metabolic analyses incorporate tracers of fatty acid metabolism, such as ^{99m}Tc-β-methyl-iodophenyl-pentadecanoic acid (^{99m}Tc-BMIPP, fatty acid transport), ^{18}F-fluoro-6-thia-heptadecanoic acid (^{18}F-FTHA, nonesterified fatty acid transport), ^{11}C-palmitate (β-oxidation), and ^{11}C-acetate (oxidative metabolism).

There remain challenges for the absolute quantification of glucose utilization in mice and rats, particularly with regard to accurate calculation of the input function.[1,2] In mice, this complication is accentuated and can contribute to suboptimal image reproducibility and high population variability. A number of hybrid analysis approaches have been proposed,[3–5] but true quantification of

Conflict of Interest: The authors declare that they have no conflict of interest.
Department of Nuclear Medicine, Hannover Medical School, Carl Neuberg-Street 1, Hannover D-30625, Germany
* Corresponding author.
E-mail address: Thackeray.James@mh-hannover.de

Cardiol Clin 34 (2016) 187–198
http://dx.doi.org/10.1016/j.ccl.2015.08.004
0733-8651/16/$ – see front matter

Box 1
Established translational radiotracers in routine clinical practice

Tracer	Target/Measurement
Myocardial metabolism	
^{18}F-FDG (fludeoxyglucose F 18)	Glucose uptake, metabolism Activated inflammatory cells, macrophages
^{99m}Tc-BMIPP (^{99m}Tc-β-methyl-iodophenylpentadecanoic acid)	Fatty acid uptake, metabolism
^{11}C-Acetate	Oxidative metabolism
Myocardial innervation	
^{123}I-MIBG (metaiodobenzylguanidine)	Norepinephrine reuptake and release
^{11}C-Hydroxyephedrine	Norepinephrine reuptake and release
^{11}C-Epinephrine	Norepinephrine reuptake, release, and metabolism
Other molecular targets	
^{18}F-Fluoride	Calcification, mineralization
^{11}C-Methionine	De novo protein synthesis
^{99m}Tc-Annexin	Apoptosis

glucose utilization in the rodent heart remains somewhat elusive.

Due in part to limited accuracy of ^{18}F-FDG kinetic quantification and complications due to continuous anesthesia, there has been a relative dearth of quantitative preclinical studies. More recent molecular metabolism imaging studies have focused on genetically modified animals,

Box 2
Novel translational radiotracers in preclinical and clinical testing

Tracer	Target/Measurement
Myocardial metabolism	
^{18}F-FTHA (^{18}F-fluoro-6-thia-heptadecanoic acid)	Fatty acid uptake
^{11}C-Palmitate	Fatty acid uptake and oxidation
Myocardial innervation	
^{11}C-Phenylephrine	Norepinephrine reuptake, release, and metabolism
^{18}F-LMI1195	Norepinephrine reuptake and release
^{11}C-MQNB	Muscarinic receptors
^{18}F-A85380	Nicotinic receptors
^{11}C-CGP12177	Beta-adrenergic receptors
^{11}C-CGP12388	Beta-adrenergic receptors
^{11}C-GB67	Alpha-adrenergic receptors
Other molecular targets	
^{68}Ga-Dotatate	Somatostatin receptor type 2, macrophages
^{18}F-Mannose	Mannose receptor, glucose uptake
^{99m}Tc-Anti-RAGE	Receptor for advanced glycation endproducts, glycation
Elastin glycoprotein	Activated elastin, matrix remodeling
99mTc-Anti-LOX-1	Oxidized lipid, atherosclerotic plaques
^{18}F-Fluorbetabir	Amyloid plaques
^{99m}Tc-RP782	Matrix metalloproteinases
^{99m}Tc-RP805	Matrix metalloproteinases
^{11}C-KR31173	Angiotensin receptor type 1 (AT_1R)
^{99m}Tc-CRIP	Arginine-glycine-aspartate (RGD) protein sequence, angiogenesis, inflammation
^{18}F-Galacto-RGD	RGD protein sequence, angiogenesis, inflammation
^{64}Cu-DOTA-vMIP-II	Chemokine receptors (nonspecific)
^{68}Ga-Pentixafor	Chemokine receptor CXCR4
^{68}Ga-SDF1	Chemokine receptor CXCR4
^{18}F-FBzBMS	Endothelin receptors
^{18}F-Fucoidan	P-selectin, thrombosis
^{18}F-FXIII	Plasma transglutaminase factor XIII

including cardiac restricted knockout of metabolic genes[6,7] or transgenic mice expressing a specific metabolic mutation[8] derived from a clinical population (**Fig. 1**).[9] Moreover, multitracer metabolic imaging has provided insight on the temporal progression of cardiovascular disease in polygenic animal models, such as spontaneously hypertensive rats,[10] Zucker diabetic fatty rats,[11,12] or multifactorial diabetes.[13] Molecular imaging in animal models provides mechanistic insight on the development of metabolic perturbations and cardiovascular disease.

An in vivo, noninvasive, and serial measurement of myocardial metabolism is desirable and easily translatable to clinical application. Cardiac ^{18}F-FDG PET has been demonstrated to contribute to improved patient care and assist in clinical decision making.[14] Preclinical studies provide additional impetus for wider application of quantitative imaging measurements in the management of cardiovascular disease.

SYMPATHETIC NEURONAL ACTIVATION

Neuronal Imaging

Recent clinical trials with norepinephrine analogues ^{123}I-metaiodobenzylguanidine (^{123}I-MIBG) for single-photon emission computed tomography (SPECT)[15,16] or ^{11}C-meta-hydroxyephedrine (^{11}C-HED) for PET[17] have established the added value of sympathetic neuronal imaging in risk stratification among cardiac patients. Coupled with imaging characterization studies in rodents,[18,19] this stronger clinical foothold has led to wider neuronal imaging in animal models of cardiovascular disease (**Fig. 2**). The development of an ^{18}F-labeled analogue of ^{123}I-MIBG, i.e. ^{18}F-LMI1195, has shown some promise and may provide for wider application of sympathetic neuronal PET imaging.[20]

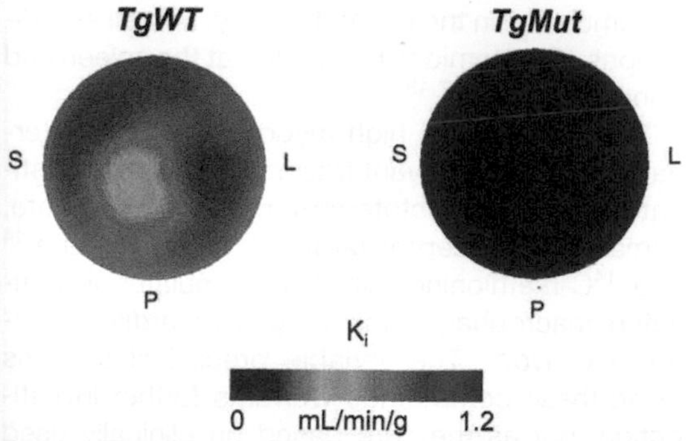

Fig. 1. ^{18}F-FDG imaging of glucose uptake in mice with a genetic mutation contributing to impaired myocardial glycogen storage. Representative left ventricle polar maps demonstrate reduced Patlak ki in transgenic mutant mice (TgMut) compared with wild type (TgWT). L, lateral left ventricle wall; P, posterior; S, septal. (*From* Thorn SL, Gollob MH, Harper ME, et al. Chronic AMPK activity dysregulation produces myocardial insulin resistance in the human Arg302Gln-PRKAG2 glycogen storage disease mouse model. EJNMMI Res 2013;3:48; with permission.)

Image quantification remains a hindrance for neuronal imaging, considering the dynamic uptake and release of sympathetic tracers, which can lead to inconsistency between scans, subjects, and centers. There can be discrepancies between different tracers in small animal imaging, particularly with agents that exhibit high extraneuronal uptake-2 transport, such as ^{123}I-MIBG or ^{18}F-LMI1195.[21–23] Combining measurements of tracer uptake (standardized uptake values, retention index) with washout (k_{mono}) may improve reproducibility.[24,25]

In rodents, innervation imaging studies have focused on diabetic autonomic neuropathy, establishing the progressive decline of myocardial norepinephrine reuptake during the progression of diabetes,[26–28] and association with physiologic measurements of sympathetic neuronal activity.[29] With improvements in ^{11}C-HED quantification, serial imaging studies have emerged to assess the impact of therapy on myocardial sympathetic neuronal integrity, including reperfusion in a pig model of hibernating myocardium[30] and antiglycemic therapy in diabetic rat models.[31,32]

Arrhythmia

Sympathetic neuronal imaging has emerged as a valuable approach in assessing risk of sudden cardiac death and ventricular arrhythmia. The extent of the innervation defect in patients with perfusion-viability mismatch has been associated with sudden cardiac death and implantable cardioverter defibrillator discharge in patients.[17] Large animal models have recapitulated clinical data on lethal arrhythmia. Studies in pigs have identified the interrelationship between reduced sympathetic neuronal tracer accumulation and the onset of ventricular fibrillation,[33–35] and provide valuable insight into the initiation of ventricular tachycardia and fibrillation.

Postsynaptic Imaging

In addition to presynaptic imaging, a limited number of preclinical studies have evaluated postsynaptic targets using radiolabeled CGP12177 and its analogues in rats[36,37] or the α-adrenergic antagonist ^{11}C-GB67.[38] The clinical relevance of postsynaptic measurements may precipitate more extensive evaluation of downstream targets, including β-adrenoceptors and second messengers.[39,40]

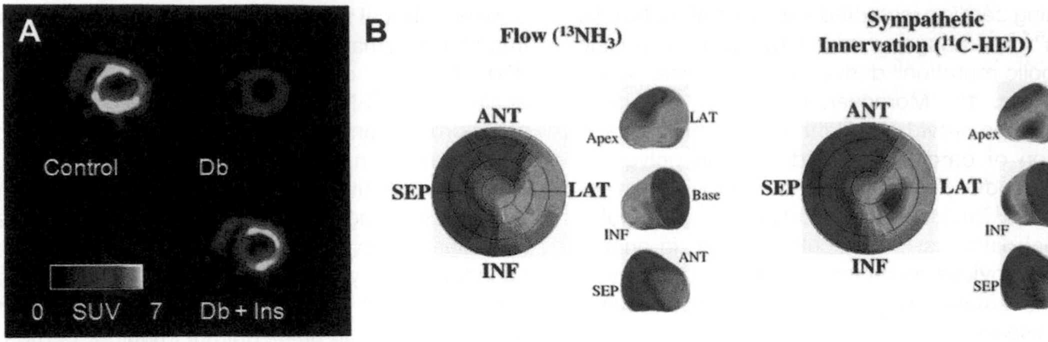

Fig. 2. Translational imaging of myocardial innervation using ^{11}C-hydroxyphedrine in rats and humans. (*A*) Diabetic rats (Db) exhibit progressive impairment of sympathetic neuronal innervation and ^{11}C-HED standardized uptake value (SUV) which is improved by insulin (Ins) treatment. (*B*) Defect in ^{11}C-hydroxyephedrine uptake exceeds the defect in perfusion measured by ^{13}N-ammonia PET in ischemic cardiomyopathy patients. ANT, anterior; INF, inferior; LAT, lateral left ventricle wall; SEP, septal. ([*A*] *Modified from* Thackeray JT, deKemp RA, Beanlands RS, et al. Early diabetes treatment does not prevent sympathetic dysinnervation in the streptozotocin diabetic rat heart. J Nucl Cardiol 2014;21:834, with kind permission from Springer Science and Business media; and [*B*] *Adapted from* Fallavollita JA, Heavey BM, Luisi AJ Jr, et al. Regional myocardial sympathetic denervation predicts the risk of sudden cardiac arrest in ischemic cardiomyopathy. J Am Coll Cardiol 2014;63:144, with permission.)

Parasympathetic Nervous System

Moreover, recent years have seen renewed interest in tracers of the parasympathetic nervous system, particularly muscarinic receptor antagonists ^{11}C-methyl-quinuclidinyl benzilate (^{11}C-MQNB), quinolone analogues,[41] and nicotinic receptor antagonists.[42] Preclinical evaluation in disease models and response to therapy is not well established.

LOCAL AND SYSTEMIC INFLAMMATION

Due to its critical involvement in the healing process following myocardial infarction and relation to plaque rupture in atherosclerosis, inflammation has emerged as an important imaging target. Although ^{18}F-FDG has been the primary workhorse, alternative tracers and approaches are under investigation in search of a more specific and reliable inflammation signal, without the complication of high cardiomyocyte uptake.

Myocardial Infarction

^{18}F-FDG uptake has been identified within the infarct territory and peri-infarct border zone in the acute stages after myocardial infarction (**Fig. 3**).[43,44] Tracer uptake could be suppressed by leukocyte depletion, and magnetic cell sorting for CD11b identified high tracer uptake by inflammatory leukocytes.[43] Despite this selective accumulation of ^{18}F-FDG, uptake by endogenous healthy cardiomyocytes persists, necessitating methods to suppress myocardial glucose transport. Ketamine-xylazine anesthesia inhibits pancreatic glucose sensing, resulting in elevated blood glucose levels and markedly lower myocardial ^{18}F-FDG transport, at the expense of severely reduced heart rate and a nonphysiologic metabolic state. More clinically relevant strategies, such as rigid fasting,[2,45] heparin administration,[46] or limiting anesthesia, have been evaluated with some success. The ease of translating ^{18}F-FDG imaging to clinical practice is appealing, and heparin-based and fasting-based cardiomyocyte suppression strategies have been successful in the clinical setting. Indeed, preliminary PET/MR studies in patients show demarcated ^{18}F-FDG accumulation in the infarct territory, as well as indications of systemic inflammation at the spleen and bone marrow.[43,47,48]

To overcome the high myocardial signal, alternative clinically relevant tracers have been investigated, including lactoferrin-targeted ^{68}Ga-citrate, somatostatin-receptor-targeted ^{68}Ga-dotatate,[44] and ^{14}C-methionine, which accumulates in activated macrophages following myocardial infarction ex vivo.[49] The variable preclinical success using these compounds warrants further investigation, but as they are based on clinically used agents, the translation to patient application may be simplified.

Atherosclerosis

Inflammation is a hallmark characteristic of unstable or vulnerable plaque, which has precipitated a myriad of studies targeting inflammatory markers in atherosclerosis models. As with postinfarct inflammation, ^{18}F-FDG remains a common tracer

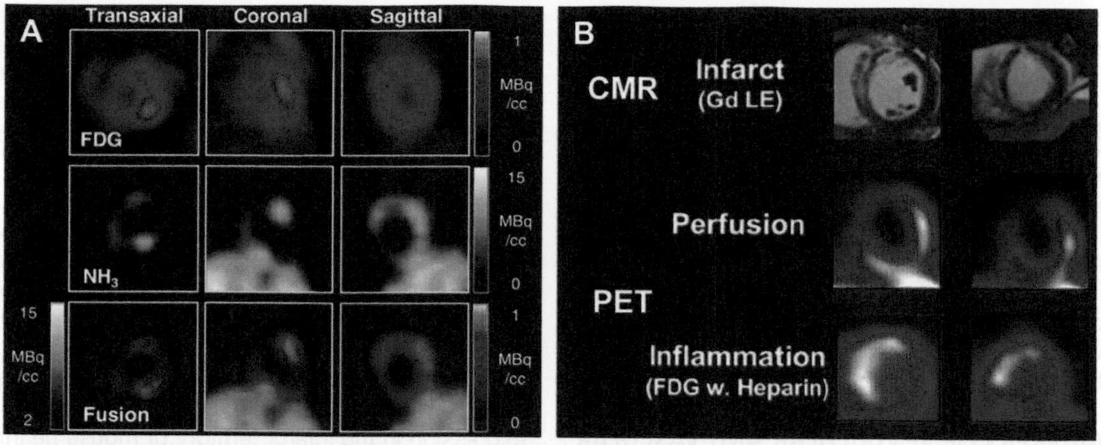

Fig. 3. Translational imaging of acute myocardial inflammation following myocardial infarction using ^{18}F-FDG with suppression of cardiomyocyte uptake in mice and humans. (*A*) Focal uptake of ^{18}F-FDG in the infarct and border zone regions defined by ^{13}N-ammonia fusion images in mice after coronary artery occlusion represents localized inflammation. (*B*) Acute ^{18}F-FDG PET imaging in patients after myocardial infarction defines regional uptake colocalized to cardiac magnetic resonance (CMR) and gadolinium late enhancement (Gd LE), reflecting acute inflammation. (*From* [*A*] Thackeray JT, Bankstahl JP, Wang Y, et al. Targeting post-infarct inflammation by PET imaging: comparison of (68) Ga-citrate and (68)Ga-DOTATATE with (18)F-FDG in a mouse model. Eur J Nucl Med Mol Imaging 2015;42:323; with permission.)

in the identification of atherosclerotic plaque inflammation, particularly for translation to clinical practice. Some variability in ^{18}F-FDG uptake by atherosclerotic plaques is thought to relate to age and high fat feeding duration,[50] suggesting a requirement for standardized methods. Nevertheless, ^{18}F-FDG imaging in atherosclerosis has become entrenched in clinical research,[51] and shows good correlation with molecular markers of plaque inflammation, including macrophage content and neovascularization,[52] as well as C-reactive protein levels and, interestingly, elevated splenic ^{18}F-FDG activity,[53] supporting systemic inflammation in atherosclerosis.

More recent studies have focused on improved resolution of coronary artery inflammation in patients using ^{18}F-FDG, employing suppression techniques to reduced cardiomyocyte uptake[54,55] and focal analysis methods.[56] Increased ^{18}F-FDG accumulation has been identified at the site of culprit lesions in acute coronary syndrome patients, suggesting feasibility for imaging of coronary plaques.[57]

The sequential homing and infiltration of first proinflammatory M1 and second anti-inflammatory phagocytic M2 macrophages has perpetuated an interest in imaging specific leukocyte subpopulations. Cell culture studies have demonstrated preferential uptake of ^{18}F-FDG in M1 compared with M2 polarized macrophages, with the reciprocal true of iron oxide, reflecting the phagocytic activity of M2 macrophages.[58] Evaluation of 2-deoxy-2-^{18}F-fluoro-D-mannose to selectively identify mannose-receptor-expressing M2 macrophages in comparison with ^{18}F-FDG revealed comparable uptake of mannose and ^{18}F-FDG within atherosclerotic plaques in a rabbit model,[59] suggesting an incapacity to distinguish the subpopulation of macrophages.

Alternatively, uptake of ^{18}F-sodium fluoride (NaF) denoting active microcalcification has been suggested as a marker of plaque vulnerability. In a retrospective clinical analysis, accumulation of ^{18}F-NaF in major arteries and coronary vessels was significantly correlated with cardiovascular events, with higher focal uptake incidence in those patients with worse outcome.[60] More recently, a prospective study identified increased ^{18}F-NaF uptake in the culprit coronary lesion among patients with acute myocardial infarction.[61] This concept has been extended to valvular disease, with comparable increase in ^{18}F-NaF binding patterns with respect to valve calcification.[62] In each case, the low ^{18}F-NaF signal from cardiomyocytes allowed for more reliable localization of signal as compared to ^{18}F-FDG imaging.

Other molecular targets for vulnerable plaque include somatostatin type 2 receptors on macrophages using ^{68}Ga-DOTATATE,[63,64] ^{64}Cu-labeled glycoprotein binding to elastin,[65] RAGE-targeting with a ^{99m}Tc-labeled antibody,[66] and liposomes targeted to oxidized low-density lipoprotein receptor (LOX-1) and labeled with indium-111.[67] Although these approaches have shown some success in imaging plaque biology, extended prospective and therapy regression studies are necessary to define the ultimate utility of these compounds in identifying vulnerable plaque inflammation.

Systemic Inflammation

An expanded role of ^{18}F-FDG PET imaging has been in systemic inflammatory diseases such as in sarcoidosis, wherein the presence of patchy or focal ^{18}F-FDG uptake is indicative of cardiac involvement.[68] Moreover, imaging approaches to characterize cardiac amyloidosis have emerged, with preliminary studies using amyloid-targeted tracers, such as ^{18}F-florbetabir.[69,70]

MARKERS OF VENTRICULAR AND VASCULAR REMODELING

The progression of heart failure is directly related to maladaptive ventricular remodeling, encompassing several physiologic pathways at various stages of disease. Importantly, many of the pathways implicated in ventricular remodeling are also postulated to contribute to vascular remodeling and atherosclerotic plaque vulnerability. Several putative targets have been identified and imaging agents developed.

Apoptosis

^{99m}Tc-Annexin targets exposed phosphatidylserine on the cell membrane of apoptotic cells.[71] More recently, annexin has been applied to assess therapeutic efficacy in preclinical studies,[72] with some evidence that binding can provide an early predictive index for infarct size.[73] Alternative apoptotic markers are concurrently being explored, including the caspase-3-targeted ^{18}F-CP18, which displayed increased cardiac binding in a mouse model of anthracycline-induced cardiotoxcity.[74]

Matrix Remodeling

Changes in the extracellular matrix and the multiphasic patterns of expression and activation of matrix metalloproteinases provides a prognostic biomarker of left ventricular adaptive remodeling progression. Extensive preclinical characterization of matrix metalloproteinase (MMP)-targeted tracers has been undertaken, particularly with the analogous SPECT tracers ^{111}In-RP782 and ^{99m}Tc-RP805.[75] MMP tracers exhibit increased focal accumulation in vasculature of mice with atherosclerosis,[76] wire-injury,[77] and abdominal aortic aneurysm,[78] as well as in hearts of pigs after myocardial infarction.[75] Importantly, several studies have demonstrated a regression of RP782 binding in response to therapy, supporting a clinical application. Although translation to clinical studies has not yet been published, the wider versatility of MMP imaging as a myocardial and vascular remodeling biomarker, may be invaluable to navigation through the regulatory process.

Renin-Angiotensin System

Activation of the renin-angiotensin system during the progression of heart failure and the myriad of therapeutic agents that modulate angiotensin signaling precipitated the development of molecular imaging agents targeted to this axis. Temporal increases in angiotensin type 1 (AT_1) receptor expression in the infarct territory of mouse hearts within 1 week of coronary artery occlusion has been demonstrated using a ^{99m}Tc-losartan analogue with SPECT[79] and in the ischemic territory in rats using ^{11}C-KR31173 with PET.[80] The increase in ^{11}C-KR31173 binding was attenuated by angiotensin-converting enzyme (ACE) inhibitor therapy, suggesting that the PET tracer may play a role in directing therapeutic efforts to modify ventricular remodeling. These findings have led to further translational evaluation in a pig model and first-in-man studies.[81]

Integrins

Since the initial characterization of the arginine-glycine-aspartate (RGD) peptide sequence as a target for α-integrins, a wide array of radiolabeled tracers continue to be evaluated for imaging of $\alpha_v\beta_3$ integrins in pathobiology. The multimodal ^{99m}Tc-labeled Cy5.5-RGD imaging peptide (CRIP) displayed increased uptake in the infarct territory of mouse hearts[82] associated with an increase in myocardial collagen deposition, and refractory to therapeutic combinations of aldosterone receptor antagonist, angiotensin receptor blocker, or ACE inhibitor.[83] The degree of CRIP uptake was correlated to the decline of left ventricular ejection fraction and rotation, as well as increased myocardial strain.

Taking advantage of higher spatial resolution afforded by PET, ^{18}F-galacto-RGD displayed enhanced binding in aortic plaques of atherosclerotic mice,[84] correlated to markers of cell infiltration and neovascularization. High-fat diet withdrawal partially reduced this increase in uptake.[85] Preliminary clinical imaging trials identified patients with high integrin expression in high-grade stenosis, with high levels of β_3 integrin expression, macrophage infiltration, and neovascularization.[86]

Analogous RGD-targeted tracers have been applied for vascular remodeling in abdominal aortic aneurysm[87] and hindlimb ischemia.[88] The versatility of the target supports a wider rollout of specific agents for preclinical and clinical evaluation.

Emerging Targets

In addition to these more established compounds, a number of novel targets are emerging as molecular prognostic biomarkers of cardiovascular disease.

Chemokine receptors

Chemokines are involved in the mobilization and recruitment of immune cells participating in the endogenous healing process. Tracers targeting various chemokine receptors are under development for myocardial and vascular injury, including ^{64}Cu-DOTA-vMIP-II,[89] ^{68}Ga-SDF-1,[90] and ^{68}Ga-pentixafor.[91]

Endothelin receptors

Endothelin receptor signaling has been linked to positive remodeling in experimental heart failure. In autoradiography studies, the endothelin subtype A receptor ligand ^{18}F-FBzBMS displays persistent uptake in the infarct wall (defined by ^{201}Tl) over 6 months after coronary artery ligation in rats.[92]

Thrombosis

^{99m}Tc-Fucoldan, a polysaccharide ligand of P-selectin, exhibits hot-spot uptake at the site of wire-induced vascular injury, associated with intraluminal thrombi in abdominal aortic aneurysm, valve vegetation in endocarditis, and the area at risk in myocardial ischemia.[93]

Plasma transglutinase FXIII

Uptake of radiofluorinated affinity peptide (^{18}F-FXIII), a substrate for plasma transglutaminase factor XIII, an enzyme involved in infarct healing,[94] was increased in the infarct territory of mice 4 days after coronary ligation.[95]

REGENERATION

In addition to pharmacologic treatment, molecular imaging offers the opportunity to noninvasively monitor cell-based therapy, either by direct labeling of stem cells or the expression of a reporter gene.

Cell Tracking

Direct cell labeling allows for a short-term visualization of stem cell distribution following administration. ^{18}F-FDG labeling of therapeutic cells can be tracked over the short term.[96] Membrane labeling with ^{111}In-oxine, used clinically for leukocyte scans, allows for longer term SPECT/CT tracking of therapeutic cells in mice.[97]

Reporter gene labeling of transplanted cells has been more widely deployed in preclinical imaging studies, using a variety of multimodal labeling techniques, therapeutic cell types, and animal models. Transduction of the sodium iodide symporter (NIS) allows effective tracking for up to 6 days after transplantation in a rat coronary occlusion model using either ^{99m}Tc-pertechnetate or radioiodine.[98] NIS reporter gene tracking has been used in pig models with human-induced pluripotent stem cells for up to 15 weeks after intramyocardial injection.[99] Postmortem analysis suggested NIS-positive stem cells had differentiated to endothelial cells.

Alternatively, the herpes simplex virus thymidine kinase gene (HSV-TK) combined with other modality reporters has been used for multimodal monitoring of cell therapy. Transplant of stably transduced human cardiac progenitor cells could be effectively imaged over 4 weeks by the HSV-TK

Table 1
Current trends in translational nuclear cardiology

Trend/Challenge	Direction
Absolute quantification	Metabolic rate Kinetics of innervation measurements Quantitative inflammation Standardization of protocols, reproducibility studies
Novel tracers	Prognostic markers of remodeling Identification of novel biomarkers
Streamlined tracer development	Evaluation in genetically modified animals Evaluation in cardiovascular disease models Versatile application, widest potential use
Prognostic benefit	Study design to predict outcome Added value over traditional markers/diagnostics

ligand ^{18}F-9(4-fluoro-3-hydroxy-methyl-butyl)guanine (^{18}F-FHBG) with PET. Higher cell engraftment represented by elevated ^{18}F-FHBG signal at 1 day was proportional to improved left ventricular contractility at 2 weeks.[100] Reporter gene constructs lend themselves to theranostic approaches, incorporating therapeutic genes into the engineered cells, although at present, such studies remain exploratory.

FUTURE PROSPECTS AND CHALLENGES

The wider array of potential targets and tracers present a number of challenges and opportunities for continued research and development (**Table 1**).

Quantification

As the number of available targeted molecular radiotracers has increased, there is a requirement for more extensive evaluation of tracer kinetics and accurate quantification of tracer uptake. For innervation and inflammation, true quantification is particularly crucial, to define an accurate threshold of disease that can be reliably compared between studies and institutions. This challenge is best illustrated by preclinical studies with ^{18}F-FDG, for which the calculation of glucose utilization kinetics, routinely applied in clinical imaging, is frequently disparate between reports, speaking to a lack of standardization in preclinical image acquisition and analysis. Strategies to improve the accuracy and reproducibility of preclinical measurements will lend credence and credibility to these techniques.

Novel Markers of Remodeling

The expanding catalog of molecular imaging targets and tracers provides a wealth of information on the pathophysiology of cardiovascular disease. The development of tracers requires a definitive connection to both clinical need and biological relevance, necessitating clear communication among physicians, biologists, and radiochemists, as well as modeling physicists.

Streamlined Development

Preclinical imaging in animal models provides a foundational step in the accelerated development of novel radiotracers. Standardized characterization studies identify high potential candidate tracers, which are then tested in an array of relevant disease models. Highly specific binding, low background, and versatility (ie, definitive differences in binding in multiple disease models) provides greater impetus for clinical translation of novel compounds.

Prognostic Imaging

Recent years have seen a more intensive focus on imaging markers that can monitor disease regression as well as progression, providing evidence for molecular imaging to effectively monitor therapy. Thorough investigation of the physiologic relevance of altered tracer binding is invaluable to the translation of preclinical findings to clinical application. Moreover, demonstration of modified tracer accumulation in response to clinically relevant therapy is a crucial step in the effective preclinical development of novel radiotracers.

SUMMARY

The changing paradigms in cardiology bear significant influence over the development of novel imaging probes and techniques. As cardiology shifts focus from diagnosis to prognosis, from disease management to risk stratification, translational molecular imaging is uniquely positioned to service the change in medical philosophy. Building on well-established and concurrent clinical translation of myocardial metabolism, as well as more recent experience with sympathetic neuronal imaging, novel imaging biomarkers, identified and targeted in preclinical imaging studies, can provide added value in studying mechanisms of disease, development of novel therapies, and evolution to personalized medicine.

REFERENCES

1. Cusso L, Vaquero JJ, Bacharach S, et al. Comparison of methods to reduce myocardial 18F-FDG uptake in mice: calcium channel blockers versus high-fat diets. PLoS One 2014;9:e107999.
2. Kreissl MC, Stout DB, Wong KP, et al. Influence of dietary state and insulin on myocardial, skeletal muscle and brain [F]-fluorodeoxyglucose kinetics in mice. EJNMMI Res 2011;1:8.
3. Thorn SL, deKemp RA, Dumouchel T, et al. Repeatable noninvasive measurement of mouse myocardial glucose uptake with 18F-FDG: evaluation of tracer kinetics in a type 1 diabetes model. J Nucl Med 2013;54:1637–44.
4. Zhong M, Kundu BK. Optimization of a model corrected blood input function from dynamic FDG-PET images of small animal heart. IEEE Trans Nucl Sci 2013;60:3417–22.
5. Lanz B, Poitry-Yamate C, Gruetter R. Image-derived input function from the vena cava for 18F-FDG PET studies in rats and mice. J Nucl Med 2014;55:1380–8.
6. Cheng C, Nakamura A, Minamimoto R, et al. Evaluation of organ-specific glucose metabolism by (1)(8)F-FDG in insulin receptor substrate-1 (IRS-1)

knockout mice as a model of insulin resistance. Ann Nucl Med 2011;25:755–61.
7. Ciccarelli M, Chuprun JK, Rengo G, et al. G protein-coupled receptor kinase 2 activity impairs cardiac glucose uptake and promotes insulin resistance after myocardial ischemia. Circulation 2011;123:1953–62.
8. Thorn SL, Gollob MH, Harper ME, et al. Chronic AMPK activity dysregulation produces myocardial insulin resistance in the human Arg302Gln-PRKAG2 glycogen storage disease mouse model. EJNMMI Res 2013;3:48.
9. Ha AC, Renaud JM, Dekemp RA, et al. In vivo assessment of myocardial glucose uptake by positron emission tomography in adults with the PRKAG2 cardiac syndrome. Circ Cardiovasc Imaging 2009;2:485–91.
10. Hernandez AM, Huber JS, Murphy ST, et al. Longitudinal evaluation of left ventricular substrate metabolism, perfusion, and dysfunction in the spontaneously hypertensive rat model of hypertrophy using small-animal PET/CT imaging. J Nucl Med 2013;54:1938–45.
11. Shoghi KI, Gropler RJ, Sharp T, et al. Time course of alterations in myocardial glucose utilization in the Zucker diabetic fatty rat with correlation to gene expression of glucose transporters: a small-animal PET investigation. J Nucl Med 2008;49:1320–7.
12. Nemanich S, Rani S, Shoghi K. In vivo multi-tissue efficacy of peroxisome proliferator-activated receptor-gamma therapy on glucose and fatty acid metabolism in obese type 2 diabetic rats. Obesity (Silver Spring) 2013;21:2522–9.
13. Menard SL, Croteau E, Sarrhini O, et al. Abnormal in vivo myocardial energy substrate uptake in diet-induced type 2 diabetic cardiomyopathy in rats. Am J Physiol Endocrinol Metab 2010;298:E1049–57.
14. Beanlands RS, Nichol G, Huszti E, et al. F-18-fluorodeoxyglucose positron emission tomography imaging-assisted management of patients with severe left ventricular dysfunction and suspected coronary disease: a randomized, controlled trial (PARR-2). J Am Coll Cardiol 2007;50:2002–12.
15. Jacobson AF, Senior R, Cerqueira MD, et al. Myocardial iodine-123 meta-iodobenzylguanidine imaging and cardiac events in heart failure. Results of the prospective ADMIRE-HF (AdreView Myocardial Imaging for Risk Evaluation in Heart Failure) study. J Am Coll Cardiol 2010;55:2212–21.
16. Boogers MJ, Borleffs CJ, Henneman MM, et al. Cardiac sympathetic denervation assessed with 123-iodine metaiodobenzylguanidine imaging predicts ventricular arrhythmias in implantable cardioverter-defibrillator patients. J Am Coll Cardiol 2010;55:2769–77.
17. Fallavollita JA, Heavey BM, Luisi AJ Jr, et al. Regional myocardial sympathetic denervation predicts the risk of sudden cardiac arrest in ischemic cardiomyopathy. J Am Coll Cardiol 2014;63:141–9.
18. Law MP, Schafers K, Kopka K, et al. Molecular imaging of cardiac sympathetic innervation by 11C-mHED and PET: from man to mouse? J Nucl Med 2010;51:1269–76.
19. Tipre DN, Fox JJ, Holt DP, et al. In vivo PET imaging of cardiac presynaptic sympathoneuronal mechanisms in the rat. J Nucl Med 2008;49:1189–95.
20. Yu M, Bozek J, Lamoy M, et al. Evaluation of LMI1195, a novel 18F-labeled cardiac neuronal PET imaging agent, in cells and animal models. Circ Cardiovasc Imaging 2011;4:435–43.
21. Rischpler C, Fukushima K, Isoda T, et al. Discrepant uptake of the radiolabeled norepinephrine analogues hydroxyephedrine (HED) and metaiodobenzylguanidine (MIBG) in rat hearts. Eur J Nucl Med Mol Imaging 2013;40:1077–83.
22. Higuchi T, Yousefi BH, Kaiser F, et al. Assessment of the 18F-labeled PET tracer LMI1195 for imaging norepinephrine handling in rat hearts. J Nucl Med 2013;54:1142–6.
23. Yu M, Bozek J, Kagan M, et al. Cardiac retention of PET neuronal imaging agent LMI1195 in different species: impact of norepinephrine uptake-1 and -2 transporters. Nucl Med Biol 2013;40:682–8.
24. Thackeray JT, Renaud JM, Kordos M, et al. Test-retest repeatability of quantitative cardiac 11C-meta-hydroxyephedrine measurements in rats by small animal positron emission tomography. Nucl Med Biol 2013;40:676–81.
25. Matsunari I, Aoki H, Nomura Y, et al. Iodine-123 metaiodobenzylguanidine imaging and carbon-11 hydroxyephedrine positron emission tomography compared in patients with left ventricular dysfunction. Circ Cardiovasc Imaging 2010;3:595–603.
26. Kiyono Y, Iida Y, Kawashima H, et al. Norepinephrine transporter density as a causative factor in alterations in MIBG myocardial uptake in NIDDM model rats. Eur J Nucl Med Mol Imaging 2002;29:999–1005.
27. Schmid H, Forman LA, Cao X, et al. Heterogeneous cardiac sympathetic denervation and decreased myocardial nerve growth factor in streptozotocin-induced diabetic rats: implications for cardiac sympathetic dysinnervation complicating diabetes. Diabetes 1999;48:603–8.
28. Kusmic C, L'Abbate A, Sambuceti G, et al. Improved myocardial perfusion in chronic diabetic mice by the up-regulation of pLKB1 and AMPK signaling. J Cell Biochem 2010;109:1033–44.
29. Thackeray JT, Radziuk J, Harper ME, et al. Sympathetic nervous dysregulation in the absence of systolic left ventricular dysfunction in a rat model of

insulin resistance with hyperglycemia. Cardiovasc Diabetol 2011;10:75.
30. Fallavollita JA, Banas MD, Suzuki G, et al. 11C-meta-hydroxyephedrine defects persist despite functional improvement in hibernating myocardium. J Nucl Cardiol 2010;17:85–96.
31. Thackeray JT, deKemp RA, Beanlands RS, et al. Insulin restores myocardial presynaptic sympathetic neuronal integrity in insulin-resistant diabetic rats. J Nucl Cardiol 2013;20:845–56.
32. Thackeray JT, deKemp RA, Beanlands RS, et al. Early diabetes treatment does not prevent sympathetic dysinnervation in the streptozotocin diabetic rat heart. J Nucl Cardiol 2014;21:829–41.
33. Sasano T, Abraham MR, Chang KC, et al. Abnormal sympathetic innervation of viable myocardium and the substrate of ventricular tachycardia after myocardial infarction. J Am Coll Cardiol 2008;51:2266–75.
34. Luisi AJ Jr, Suzuki G, Dekemp R, et al. Regional 11C-hydroxyephedrine retention in hibernating myocardium: chronic inhomogeneity of sympathetic innervation in the absence of infarction. J Nucl Med 2005;46:1368–74.
35. Lautamaki R, Sasano T, Higuchi T, et al. Multiparametric molecular imaging provides mechanistic insights into sympathetic innervation impairment in the viable infarct border zone. J Nucl Med 2015; 56:457–63.
36. Thackeray JT, Parsa-Nezhad M, Kenk M, et al. Reduced CGP12177 binding to cardiac beta-adrenoceptors in hyperglycemic high-fat-diet-fed, streptozotocin-induced diabetic rats. Nucl Med Biol 2011;38:1059–66.
37. de Jong RM, Willemsen AT, Slart RH, et al. Myocardial beta-adrenoceptor downregulation in idiopathic dilated cardiomyopathy measured in vivo with PET using the new radioligand (S)-[11C] CGP12388. Eur J Nucl Med Mol Imaging 2005; 32:443–7.
38. Park-Holohan SJ, Asselin MC, Turton DR, et al. Quantification of [11C]GB67 binding to cardiac alpha1-adrenoceptors with positron emission tomography: validation in pigs. Eur J Nucl Med Mol Imaging 2008;35:1624–35.
39. Caldwell JH, Link JM, Levy WC, et al. Evidence for pre- to postsynaptic mismatch of the cardiac sympathetic nervous system in ischemic congestive heart failure. J Nucl Med 2008;49:234–41.
40. Kenk M, Thackeray JT, Thorn SL, et al. Alterations of pre- and postsynaptic noradrenergic signaling in a rat model of adriamycin-induced cardiotoxicity. J Nucl Cardiol 2010;17:254–63.
41. Mazzadi AN, Pineau J, Costes N, et al. Ventricular muscarinic receptor remodeling in patients with and without primary ventricular fibrillation. An imaging study. J Nucl Cardiol 2012;19:1017–25.
42. Bucerius J, Manka C, Schmaljohann J, et al. Feasibility of [18F]-2-Fluoro-A85380-PET imaging of human vascular nicotinic acetylcholine receptors in vivo. JACC Cardiovasc Imaging 2012;5:528–36.
43. Lee WW, Marinelli B, van der Laan AM, et al. PET/MRI of inflammation in myocardial infarction. J Am Coll Cardiol 2012;59:153–63.
44. Thackeray JT, Bankstahl JP, Wang Y, et al. Targeting post-infarct inflammation by PET imaging: comparison of (68)Ga-citrate and (68)Ga-DOTATATE with (18)F-FDG in a mouse model. Eur J Nucl Med Mol Imaging 2015;42:317–27.
45. Toyama H, Ichise M, Liow JS, et al. Evaluation of anesthesia effects on [18F]FDG uptake in mouse brain and heart using small animal PET. Nucl Med Biol 2004;31:251–6.
46. Thackeray JT, Bankstahl JP, Wang Y, et al. Clinically relevant strategies for lowering cardiomyocyte glucose uptake for 18F-FDG imaging of myocardial inflammation in mice. Eur J Nucl Med Mol Imaging 2015;42:771–80.
47. Wollenweber T, Roentgen P, Schafer A, et al. Characterizing the inflammatory tissue response to acute myocardial infarction by clinical multimodality noninvasive imaging. Circ Cardiovasc Imaging 2014;7:811–8.
48. Kim EJ, Kim S, Kang DO, et al. Metabolic activity of the spleen and bone marrow in patients with acute myocardial infarction evaluated by 18f-fluorodeoxyglucose positron emission tomographic imaging. Circ Cardiovasc Imaging 2014;7:454–60.
49. Taki J, Wakabayashi H, Inaki A, et al. 14C-Methionine uptake as a potential marker of inflammatory processes after myocardial ischemia and reperfusion. J Nucl Med 2013;54:431–6.
50. Silvola JM, Saraste A, Laitinen I, et al. Effects of age, diet, and type 2 diabetes on the development and FDG uptake of atherosclerotic plaques. JACC Cardiovasc Imaging 2011;4:1294–301.
51. Rudd JH, Warburton EA, Fryer TD, et al. Imaging atherosclerotic plaque inflammation with [18F]-fluorodeoxyglucose positron emission tomography. Circulation 2002;105:2708–11.
52. Taqueti VR, Di Carli MF, Jerosch-Herold M, et al. Increased microvascularization and vessel permeability associate with active inflammation in human atheromata. Circ Cardiovasc Imaging 2014;7:920–9.
53. Emami H, Singh P, MacNabb M, et al. Splenic metabolic activity predicts risk of future cardiovascular events: demonstration of a cardiosplenic axis in humans. JACC Cardiovasc Imaging 2015; 8:121–30.
54. Wykrzykowska J, Lehman S, Williams G, et al. Imaging of inflamed and vulnerable plaque in coronary arteries with 18F-FDG PET/CT in patients with suppression of myocardial uptake using a

low-carbohydrate, high-fat preparation. J Nucl Med 2009;50(4):563–8.
55. Bucerius J, Duivenvoorden R, Mani V, et al. Prevalence and risk factors of carotid vessel wall inflammation in coronary artery disease patients: FDG-PET and CT imaging study. JACC Cardiovasc Imaging 2011;4(11):1195–205.
56. Emami H, Vucic E, Subramanian S, et al. The effect of BMS-582949, a P38 mitogen-activated protein kinase (P38 MAPK) inhibitor on arterial inflammation: A multicenter FDG-PET trial. Atherosclerosis 2015;240(2):490–6.
57. Rogers IS, Nasir K, Figueroa AL, et al. Feasibility of FDG imaging of the coronary arteries: comparison between acute coronary syndrome and stable angina. JACC Cardiovasc Imaging 2010;3(4):388–97.
58. Satomi T, Ogawa M, Mori I, et al. Comparison of contrast agents for atherosclerosis imaging using cultured macrophages: FDG versus ultrasmall superparamagnetic iron oxide. J Nucl Med 2013;54:999–1004.
59. Tahara N, Mukherjee J, de Haas HJ, et al. 2-deoxy-2-[18F]fluoro-D-mannose positron emission tomography imaging in atherosclerosis. Nat Med 2014;20:215–9.
60. Li Y, Berenji GR, Shaba WF, et al. Association of vascular fluoride uptake with vascular calcification and coronary artery disease. Nucl Med Commun 2012;33(1):14–20.
61. Joshi NV, Vesey AT, Williams MC, et al. 18F-fluoride positron emission tomography for identification of ruptured and high-risk coronary atherosclerotic plaques: a prospective clinical trial. Lancet 2014;383(9918):705–13.
62. Dweck MR, Jones C, Joshi NV, et al. Assessment of valvular calcification and inflammation by positron emission tomography in patients with aortic stenosis. Circulation 2012;125(1):76–86.
63. Li X, Bauer W, Kreissl MC, et al. Specific somatostatin receptor II expression in arterial plaque: (68)Ga-DOTATATE autoradiographic, immunohistochemical and flow cytometric studies in apoE-deficient mice. Atherosclerosis 2013;230:33–9.
64. Schatka I, Wollenweber T, Haense C, et al. Peptide receptor targeted radionuclide therapy alters inflammation in atherosclerotic plaques. J Am Coll Cardiol 2013;62:2344–5.
65. Bigalke B, Phinikaridou A, Andia ME, et al. Positron emission tomography/computed tomographic and magnetic resonance imaging in a murine model of progressive atherosclerosis using (64)Cu-labeled glycoprotein VI-Fc. Circ Cardiovasc Imaging 2013;6:957–64.
66. Tekabe Y, Li Q, Rosario R, et al. Development of receptor for advanced glycation end products—directed imaging of atherosclerotic plaque in a murine model of spontaneous atherosclerosis. Circ Cardiovasc Imaging 2008;1:212–9.
67. Li D, Patel AR, Klibanov AL, et al. Molecular imaging of atherosclerotic plaques targeted to oxidized LDL receptor LOX-1 by SPECT/CT and magnetic resonance. Circ Cardiovasc Imaging 2010;3:464–72.
68. Schatka I, Bengel FM. Advanced imaging of cardiac sarcoidosis. J Nucl Med 2014;55:99–106.
69. Dorbala S, Vangala D, Semer J, et al. Imaging cardiac amyloidosis: a pilot study using (1)(8)F-florbetapir positron emission tomography. Eur J Nucl Med Mol Imaging 2014;41:1652–62.
70. Antoni G, Lubberink M, Estrada S, et al. In vivo visualization of amyloid deposits in the heart with 11C-PIB and PET. J Nucl Med 2013;54:213–20.
71. Bennink RJ, van den Hoff MJ, van Hemert FJ, et al. Annexin V imaging of acute doxorubicin cardiotoxicity (apoptosis) in rats. J Nucl Med 2004;45:842–8.
72. Godier-Furnemont AF, Tekabe Y, Kollaros M, et al. Noninvasive imaging of myocyte apoptosis following application of a stem cell-engineered delivery platform to acutely infarcted myocardium. J Nucl Med 2013;54:977–83.
73. Todica A, Zacherl MJ, Wang H, et al. In-vivo monitoring of erythropoietin treatment after myocardial infarction in mice with [(6)(8)Ga]Annexin A5 and [(1)(8)F]FDG PET. J Nucl Cardiol 2014;21:1191–9.
74. Su H, Gorodny N, Gomez LF, et al. Noninvasive molecular imaging of apoptosis in a mouse model of anthracycline-induced cardiotoxicity. Circ Cardiovasc Imaging 2015;8:e001952.
75. Sahul ZH, Mukherjee R, Song J, et al. Targeted imaging of the spatial and temporal variation of matrix metalloproteinase activity in a porcine model of postinfarct remodeling: relationship to myocardial dysfunction. Circ Cardiovasc Imaging 2011;4:381–91.
76. Razavian M, Tavakoli S, Zhang J, et al. Atherosclerosis plaque heterogeneity and response to therapy detected by in vivo molecular imaging of matrix metalloproteinase activation. J Nucl Med 2011;52:1795–802.
77. Tavakoli S, Razavian M, Zhang J, et al. Matrix metalloproteinase activation predicts amelioration of remodeling after dietary modification in injured arteries. Arterioscler Thromb Vasc Biol 2011;31:102–9.
78. Golestani R, Razavian M, Nie L, et al. Imaging vessel wall biology to predict outcome in abdominal aortic aneurysm. Circ Cardiovasc Imaging 2014;8. pii:e002471.
79. Verjans JW, Lovhaug D, Narula N, et al. Noninvasive imaging of angiotensin receptors after myocardial infarction. JACC Cardiovasc Imaging 2008;1:354–62.

80. Higuchi T, Fukushima K, Xia J, et al. Radionuclide imaging of angiotensin II type 1 receptor upregulation after myocardial ischemia-reperfusion injury. J Nucl Med 2010;51:1956–61.
81. Fukushima K, Bravo PE, Higuchi T, et al. Molecular hybrid positron emission tomography/computed tomography imaging of cardiac angiotensin II type 1 receptors. J Am Coll Cardiol 2012;60: 2527–34.
82. van den Borne SW, Isobe S, Verjans JW, et al. Molecular imaging of interstitial alterations in remodeling myocardium after myocardial infarction. J Am Coll Cardiol 2008;52:2017–28.
83. van den Borne SW, Isobe S, Zandbergen HR, et al. Molecular imaging for efficacy of pharmacologic intervention in myocardial remodeling. JACC Cardiovasc Imaging 2009;2:187–98.
84. Laitinen I, Saraste A, Weidl E, et al. Evaluation of alphavbeta3 integrin-targeted positron emission tomography tracer 18F-galacto-RGD for imaging of vascular inflammation in atherosclerotic mice. Circ Cardiovasc Imaging 2009;2:331–8.
85. Saraste A, Laitinen I, Weidl E, et al. Diet intervention reduces uptake of alphavbeta3 integrin-targeted PET tracer 18F-galacto-RGD in mouse atherosclerotic plaques. J Nucl Cardiol 2012;19: 775–84.
86. Beer AJ, Pelisek J, Heider P, et al. PET/CT imaging of integrin alphavbeta3 expression in human carotid atherosclerosis. JACC Cardiovasc Imaging 2014;7:178–87.
87. Kitagawa T, Kosuge H, Chang E, et al. Integrin-targeted molecular imaging of experimental abdominal aortic aneurysms by (18)F-labeled Arg-Gly-Asp positron-emission tomography. Circ Cardiovasc Imaging 2013;6:950–6.
88. Liu Y, Pressly ED, Abendschein DR, et al. Targeting angiogenesis using a C-type atrial natriuretic factor-conjugated nanoprobe and PET. J Nucl Med 2011;52:1956–63.
89. Liu Y, Pierce R, Luehmann HP, et al. PET imaging of chemokine receptors in vascular injury-accelerated atherosclerosis. J Nucl Med 2013;54:1135–41.
90. Zacherl M, Lehner S, Todica A, et al. Quantification of CXCR4-expression by 68Ga-SDF-1(alpha) PET for serial in-vivo therapy monitoring and for risk stratification in the murine model of myocardial infarction. J Nucl Med 2014;55:80.
91. Herrmann K, Lapa C, Wester HJ, et al. Biodistribution and radiation dosimetry for the chemokine receptor CXCR4-targeting probe 68Ga-pentixafor. J Nucl Med 2015;56:410–6.
92. Higuchi T, Rischpler C, Fukushima K, et al. Targeting of endothelin receptors in the healthy and infarcted rat heart using the PET tracer 18F-FBzBMS. J Nucl Med 2013;54:277–82.
93. Rouzet F, Bachelet-Violette L, Alsac JM, et al. Radiolabeled fucoidan as a p-selectin targeting agent for in vivo imaging of platelet-rich thrombus and endothelial activation. J Nucl Med 2011;52: 1433–40.
94. Nahrendorf M, Hu K, Frantz S, et al. Factor XIII deficiency causes cardiac rupture, impairs wound healing, and aggravates cardiac remodeling in mice with myocardial infarction. Circulation 2006; 113:1196–202.
95. Majmudar MD, Keliher EJ, Heidt T, et al. Monocyte-directed RNAi targeting CCR2 improves infarct healing in atherosclerosis-prone mice. Circulation 2013;127:2038–46.
96. Terrovitis J, Lautamaki R, Bonios M, et al. Noninvasive quantification and optimization of acute cell retention by in vivo positron emission tomography after intramyocardial cardiac-derived stem cell delivery. J Am Coll Cardiol 2009;54: 1619–26.
97. Kircher MF, Grimm J, Swirski FK, et al. Noninvasive in vivo imaging of monocyte trafficking to atherosclerotic lesions. Circulation 2008;117:388–95.
98. Terrovitis J, Kwok KF, Lautamaki R, et al. Ectopic expression of the sodium-iodide symporter enables imaging of transplanted cardiac stem cells in vivo by single-photon emission computed tomography or positron emission tomography. J Am Coll Cardiol 2008;52:1652–60.
99. Templin C, Zweigerdt R, Schwanke K, et al. Transplantation and tracking of human-induced pluripotent stem cells in a pig model of myocardial infarction: assessment of cell survival, engraftment, and distribution by hybrid single photon emission computed tomography/computed tomography of sodium iodide symporter transgene expression. Circulation 2012;126:430–9.
100. Liu J, Narsinh KH, Lan F, et al. Early stem cell engraftment predicts late cardiac functional recovery: preclinical insights from molecular imaging. Circ Cardiovasc Imaging 2012;5:481–90.

Index

Note: Page numbers of article titles are in **boldface** type.

Cardiol Clin 34 (2016) 199–205
http://dx.doi.org/10.1016/S0733-8651(15)00119-8
0733-8651/16/$ – see front matter

Q

R

Printed and bound by CPI Group (UK) Ltd, Croydon, CR0 4YY
03/10/2024
01040377-0002